MOWRY'S

BASIC NUTRITION AND DIET THERAPY

Times Mirror/Mosby
Series In Nutrition

MOWRY'S

BASIC NUTRITION AND DIET THERAPY

SUE RODWELL WILLIAMS, Ph.D., M.P.H., M.R.Ed., R.D.

President and Director, The Berkeley Nutrition Group,
SRW Productions, Inc.; Field Faculty, M.P.H.–
Dietetic Internship Program, and Coordinated Undergraduate
Program in Dietetics, University of California, Berkeley, California;
formerly Chief, Nutrition Program, Kaiser-Permanente Medical Center,
Oakland, California

SEVENTH EDITION

Illustrated

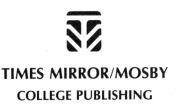

TIMES MIRROR/MOSBY
COLLEGE PUBLISHING

ST. LOUIS • TORONTO • SANTA CLARA 1984

Editor: Nancy K. Roberson
Assistant editor: Catherine H. Converse
Manuscript editor: Linda L. Duncan
Book design: Gail Morey Hudson
Cover design: Diane Beasley
Production: Barbara Merritt, Judy England

SEVENTH EDITION

Library of Congress Cataloging in Publication Data

Mowry, Lillian.
    Mowry's Basic nutrition and diet therapy.

    Includes bibliographies and index.
    1. Diet therapy. 2. Nutrition. I. Williams, Sue Rodwell, 1922-   . II. Title. III. Title: Basic nutrition and diet therapy. [DNLM: 1. Diet therapy. 2. Nutrition. WB 400 M936n]
RM216.M64   1984   615.8'54   83-13239
ISBN 0-8016-5580-3

GW/VH/VH 9 8 7 6 5 4 3   03/C/328

To
all those whose efforts in the past
have made possible our present knowledge of nutrition
and its role in preserving human health
and in advancing diet therapy

Preface

From its beginning, this text has provided a sound basic learning resource for support level personnel in health care. It has filled a practical need among various allied health workers and students for a realistic and easily comprehended reference.

However, the field of nutrition has been expanding and changing since publication of earlier editions. Two main factors have contributed to this expansion. First, the science of nutrition has grown with basic research, which has challenged some traditional ideas and developed new ones. This is especially true in the application of nutritional science to preventive health care in younger populations and to the management of chronic disease in older persons. Second, increasing attention of the media to nutrition and health matters has awakened popular awareness and concern. Interest in nutrition has grown, and patients are raising more questions and seeking answers. They want sound information to deal intelligently with common misinformation and fads, as well as with legitimate controversy. They want to be more personally involved in their health care. As a result of these expanding developments in nutrition and health, and my commitment along with that of my publisher to maintain a useful basic resource for students and health workers, I have rewritten and reorganized much of the material in the previous edition to help meet these current needs.

Objectives of the book

This text is designed primarily for students and health workers in beginning assistant level programs for practical or licensed vocational nurses (LVNs), as well as for diet technicians or diet aides. It assumes limited background in nutrition-related basic sciences. Thus its general purpose is to introduce basic nutrition principles and present some of their applications in the care of persons in health and disease. In addition, I have three personal concerns: (1) that this introduction will lead students and readers to enjoy learning about nutrition and stimulate further reading in personal interest areas, (2) that these caretakers will be alert to nutrition news and to questions raised by their patients, and

(3) that contact and communication will be made with professional nutrition resource persons to build a team approach to clinical nutrition problems in patient care.

Features of the book

Balance of content. The range of topics in each section has been revised and expanded to provide more breadth, still maintaining the style of discussion at a level of clarity appropriate for beginning students. In each section the material has been extensively reorganized and rewritten to reflect current knowledge and trends. In Part One, "Principles of Nutrition," the major nutrients are introduced, along with their basic functions in the body, their sources in a variety of foods, and their relations to health. The newer U.S. Dietary Goals, in addition to the current Recommended Dietary Allowances, are used as a basis for planning a balanced diet. Discussion of minerals in relation to fluid and electrolyte balance, trace elements, vitamins, dietary fiber, and energy balance, for example, has been expanded. New summary tables are provided in the sections on vitamins, minerals, digestion, and absorption.

In Part Two, "Community Nutrition and the Life Cycle," a greater emphasis is placed on nutritional needs of various age groups, food safety, and food habits among various ethnic groups. The chapters on menu planning and cooking have been deleted to reflect changes in function of support level personnel.

In Part Three, "Diet Therapy," several changes indicate newer trends in clinical nutrition and provide better organization of material. For example, the chapter on diet modifications has been deleted as such and the representative diets have been moved to their related disease discussions. In the discussion of gastrointestinal problems the traditional "bland" diet therapy in peptic ulcer disease has been deleted in favor of the liberal individual approach now in general use. Each of the remaining chapters on various clinical problems has been reorganized and updated, and two new chapters on surgical nutrition and nutrition and cancer have been added.

Chapter learning aids and organizers. A number of new learning aids have been used in the revision of this text. An outline of each chapter is clearly indicated by the division headings and subheadings throughout each discussion. This should help the student to organize the material and relate the main ideas in each section. In addition, a number of new visual materials have been added to clarify concepts, including illustrations, graphs, tables, and photographs. Terms used for basic concepts are defined clearly in the text. At the end of each chapter a number of different types of review questions are given for the student to use in responding to the material presented. Also, in the section on clinical nutrition case studies and clinical problems provide opportunity for further application of the diet therapy material discussed.

Acknowledgments

A realistic and useful textbook always depends on the valuable contributions of a number of people for its development and production. I am grateful to many individuals who have helped to bring this book to its present form. First, I am particularly indebted to the reviewers of the text: Karen Thrasher, Somerset State Vocational-Technical School; Jane Venen, Willoughby-Eastlake School of Practical Nursing; and Dolores Zopf, Atlantic Vocational-Technical School Center. These experienced teachers contributed many valuable suggestions from their own teaching experience for developing the material. Second, I owe much to my guiding editors at Mosby, Catherine H. Converse, Nancy K. Roberson, and Kathy Spengel, for their tremendous help in putting this entire project together and to Linda L. Duncan, manuscript editor, who guided the manuscript through to its finished book form. These skillful and competent editors and all of their assistants provided immense support to me all the way and are largely responsible for bringing the final product into being. To all of these friends and to the publisher, I am grateful.

Finally, but certainly not least, to my faithful research assistant and typist (word-processor), Ruth Williams, I am indebted for helping to produce the finished manuscript through many revisions. Her efforts through tedious hours made the final version possible.

I hope that those who use this text will continue to give me feedback and suggestions for future editions. It is my continuing purpose to provide students with a beginning text that will help bring about a clear understanding of some of the elemental principles of nutritional science and a realistic concern for applying them in personalized patient care.

Sue Rodwell Williams

Contents

MOWRY'S
BASIC NUTRITION AND DIET THERAPY

PART ONE

PRINCIPLES OF NUTRITION

1

The importance of a balanced diet

FOOD, NUTRITION, AND HEALTH

Nutrition concerns the food people eat and how their bodies use it. Nutritional science is the study of the scientific laws governing the food requirements of human beings for maintenance, growth, activity, reproduction, and lactation. Dietetics is the practical application of these laws to persons and groups of persons in various conditions of health and disease. Good nutrition is essential to good health throughout life, beginning with prenatal life and extending through old age.

Food has always been one of the prime necessities of life. Too many people, however, are concerned only with food that relieves their hunger or satisfies their appetites but are not concerned with whether it supplies their bodies with all the components of good nutrition.

The physician, nurse, and nutritionist or dietitian are all aware of the important part that food plays in maintaining good health in normal people and in the recovery of ill people. Chronic ill health in patients cannot be accepted without checking on food habits as possible contributing factors. Thus, a primary activity in planning care in any situation is assessing the patients' nutritional status and identifying nutritional needs.

Evidence of good nutrition is a well-developed body, ideal weight for body size, and good muscles. The skin is smooth and clear, the hair is glossy, and the eyes are clear and bright. Posture is good, and the facial expression is alert. Appetite, digestion, and elimination are good. More detailed characteristics of good and poor states of nutrition are presented in Table 1-1.

Well-nourished people are much more likely to be alert, both mentally and physically, and to have a happy outlook on life. They are also more able to resist infectious diseases than are undernourished people. Proper diet not only makes them healthier persons but also extends the period of their normal activity for more years.

Table 1-1. Clinical signs of nutritional status

Features	Good	Poor
General appearance	Alert, responsive	Listless, apathetic; cachexia
Hair	Shiny, lustrous; healthy scalp	Stringy, dull, brittle, dry, depigmented
Neck glands	No enlargement	Thyroid enlarged
Skin, face and neck	Smooth, slightly moist; good color, reddish pink mucous membranes	Greasy, discolored, scaly
Eyes	Bright, clear; no fatigue circles	Dryness, signs of infection, increased vascularity, glassiness, thickened conjunctivae
Lips	Good color, moist	Dry, scaly, swollen, angular lesions (stomatitis)
Tongue	Good pink color; surface papillae present; no lesions	Papillary atrophy, smooth appearance; swollen, red, beefy (glossitis)
Gums	Good pink color; no swelling or bleeding; firm	Marginal redness or swelling; receding, spongy
Teeth	Straight, no crowding; well-shaped jaw; clean, no discoloration	Unfilled cavities, absent teeth, worn surfaces; mottled, malpositioned
Skin, general	Smooth, slightly moist; good color	Rough, dry, scaly, pale, pigmented, irritated; petechiae, bruises
Abdomen	Flat	Swollen
Legs, feet	No tenderness, weakness, swelling; good color	Edema, tender calf; tingling, weakness
Skeleton	No malformations	Bowlegs, knock-knees, chest deformity at diaphragm, beaded ribs, prominent scapulae
Weight	Normal for height, age, body build	Overweight or underweight
Posture	Erect, arms and legs straight, abdomen in, chest out	Sagging shoulders, sunken chest, humped back
Muscles	Well developed, firm	Flaccid, poor tone; undeveloped, tender
Nervous control	Good attention span for age; does not cry easily; not irritable or restless	Inattentive, irritable
Gastrointestinal function	Good appetite and digestion; normal, regular elimination	Anorexia, indigestion, constipation or diarrhea
General vitality	Endurance; energetic; sleeps well at night; vigorous	Easily fatigued, no energy, falls asleep in school, looks tired, apathetic

FUNCTIONS OF FOOD AND NUTRIENTS

The nutrients in food must perform three basic functions within the body: provide energy sources, build tissue, and regulate metabolic processes. Metabolism refers to the sum of all body processes that sustain life.

ENERGY. Fuel for heat and energy is provided primarily by carbohydrate and fat and secondarily by part of the protein consumed in the diet.

TISSUE BUILDING. Protein provides building units, or amino acids, for necessary construction materials to build and repair body tissues. This is a constant process that provides for growth and maintenance of a strong body structure.

REGULATION AND CONTROL. All of the multiple chemical processes in the body required for providing energy and building tissue must be carefully regulated and controlled to maintain a smooth, balanced operation. Otherwise, there would be chaos within the body systems, and death would result. Life and health result from a dynamic balance among all the body parts and processes. Among the control agents that help to maintain this state of balance within the body are vitamins and minerals. These nutrients, along with water and fiber, that perform these marvelous basic body functions have sometimes been called "the seven wonders of the world."

Nutrients that build or repair {
Carbohydrates
Fats
Proteins
Minerals
Water
Vitamins
Cellulose

} Nutrients that produce energy

Nutrients that regulate body processes

Good nutrition, then, means that a person receives and uses substances that are obtained from a diet containing carbohydrates, fats, proteins, certain minerals, vitamins, water, and cellulose in optimum amounts. The optimum amounts of these nutrients should be greater than the minimum requirements to make provision for variations in health and disease and for the accumulation of some reserves. Dietary surveys have shown that approximately one third of the U.S. population are living on diets below the optimum level. This does not necessarily mean that one third of Americans are undernourished. Some persons can maintain good health on somewhat less than the optimum amounts of the various nutrients. On the average, however, a person receiving less than the optimum amounts will have a greater risk of physical illness than a person receiving the proper amounts.

NUTRIENT STANDARDS

Most of the developed countries of the world have set up nutrition standards for the major nutrients to serve as guidelines for maintaining healthy populations. These standards, however, are not intended to indicate individual requirements or therapeutic needs; rather, they are intended to serve as a reference for levels of intake of the essential nutrients considered, on the basis of available scientific knowledge, to be adequate to meet the known nutritional needs of most healthy population groups. Although these standards are similar in different countries, they may vary somewhat according to the philosophy of scientists and practitioners in a particular country. For example, the U.S. standard allows for a "margin of safety" to meet the variable needs of a broad population base. In the United States these standards are called the *Recommended Dietary Allowances* (RDAs).

U.S. standard (RDA)

The U.S. nutrient standard is developed and maintained by a group of leading scientists and practitioners in the field of nutrition, working through the National Academy of Sciences in Washington, D.C. The Academy has numerous divisions of councils and is supported by the National Institutes of Health. The working group of nutrition scientists responsible for the RDAs make up the Food and Nutrition Board of the National Research Council. Each 5 or 6 years the Research Council publishes a revision of the standard based on current research. The current standard for major nutrients is presented in Table 1-2 (see also Table 5-3, p. 39, and Table B, pp. 292-293 of the Appendix).

Other standards

Canadian and British standards are similar to the U.S. standard. Workers in less developed countries look to standards such as those set by the Food and Agriculture Organization of the World Health Organization, in which such factors as quality of protein foods available must be considered. Nonetheless, in all of these standards a guideline is provided to help health workers in a variety of population groups promote good health through sound nutrition.

FOOD GUIDES

To interpret and apply sound nutrient standards, practical food guides have been developed to assist health workers in nutrition education and food planning with individuals and families. Such tools include the Basic Four Food Groups, the U.S. Dietary Goals, and the Food Exchange System.

Basic four food groups

This basic tool was developed by the U.S. Department of Agriculture as a food guide for planning a well-balanced diet. Although it has limitations, it provides a practical general basis for planning meals and evaluating a person's overall food intake pattern. Additional calories as needed may come from increased servings of the foods listed or from adding other food items. An outline of this food guide is presented in Table 1-3. A daily plan consists of three or more meals, each supplying a portion of the total day's food needs. Following is a sample plan for daily meals:

Breakfast

    Fruit rich in vitamin C
    Cereal and/or
    Toast, roll or hot bread
    Butter or fortified margarine
    Milk for cereal and beverage
    Egg served frequently (When eggs are not served, include extra milk for necessary animal protein.)
    Coffee for adults

Lunch

    Main dish—should contain eggs, cheese, meat, fish, or poultry (could be soup, salad, sandwich, or a casserole dish)
    Vegetable, preferably raw
    Bread and *butter* or fortified margarine
    Simple dessert, such as custard, gelatin, ice cream, or fruit
    Milk for children

Dinner

    Meat, poultry, or *fish,* at least 2 oz per person
    Vegetables (2) (1 may be potatoes and the other a green leafy or yellow vegetable)
    Salad, vegetable or fruit
    Dessert—a fruit if a vegetable salad has been used unless fruit was used for dessert at noon
    Milk for children

U.S. Dietary Goals

A recent general food guide, the U.S. Dietary Goals, or Dietary Guidelines for Americans, has developed as a result of concern about chronic health problems in an aging population and a changing food environment. Although no guidelines can guarantee health or well-being, and although people differ widely in their food needs, these general statements can lead people to evaluate their food habits and move toward general improvements. Good food habits based on moderation and variety can help to build sound healthy bodies. Seven statements that comprise the U.S. Dietary Goals follow:

1. *Eat a variety of foods.* About 40 different nutrients are needed to stay healthy. No single food can supply all the essential nutrients in the amounts needed. Thus the greater the variety of foods used, the less likely a person is to develop either a deficiency or an excess of any single nutrient. One way to ensure a variety, and with it a well-balanced diet, is to select foods each day from all of the major food groups.

2. *Maintain ideal weight.* Excessive fatness is associated with some chronic disorders such as hypertension and diabetes, which in turn relate to

Table 1-2. Recommended daily dietary allowances, revised 1980[a]

	Age (yr)	Weight		Height		Protein (gm)	Fat-soluble vitamins			Vita-min C (mg)
		kg	lb	cm	in		Vita-min A (µg RE)[b]	Vita-min D (µg)[c]	Vita-min E (mg α-TE)[d]	
Infants	0.0-0.5	6	13	60	24	kg × 2.2	420	10	3	35
	0.5-1.0	9	20	71	28	kg × 2.0	400	10	4	35
Children	1-3	13	29	90	35	23	400	10	5	45
	4-6	20	44	112	44	30	500	10	6	45
	7-10	28	62	132	52	34	700	10	7	45
Males	11-14	45	99	157	62	45	1000	10	8	50
	15-18	66	145	176	69	56	1000	10	10	60
	19-22	70	154	177	70	56	1000	7.5	10	60
	23-50	70	154	178	70	56	1000	5	10	60
	51+	70	154	178	70	56	1000	5	10	60
Females	11-14	46	101	157	62	46	800	10	8	50
	15-18	55	120	163	64	46	800	10	8	60
	19-22	55	120	163	64	44	800	7.5	8	60
	23-50	55	120	163	64	44	800	5	8	60
	51+	55	120	163	64	44	800	5	8	60
Pregnant						+30	+200	+5	+2	+20
Lactating						+20	+400	+5	+3	+40

From Food and Nutrition Board, National Academy of Sciences–National Research Council: Recom-
[a]The allowances are intended to provide for individual variations among most normal persons as they live foods to provide other nutrients for which human requirements have been less well defined. See text for and heights by individual year of age. See Table 5-3 for suggested average energy intakes.
[b]Retinol equivalents. 1 retinol equivalent = 1 µg retinol or 6 µg β-carotene. See text for calculation of
[c]As cholecalciferol. 10 µg cholecalciferol = 400 IU vitamin D.
[d]α-Tocopherol equivalents. 1 mg d-α-tocopherol = 1 α-TE. See text for variation in allowances and
[e]1 XY (alacin equivalent) is equal to 1 mg of niacin or 60 mg of dietary tryptophan.
[f]The folacin allowances refer to dietary sources as determined by *Lactobacillus casei* assay after treatment
[g]The FDA for vitamin B_{12} in infants is based on average concentration of the vitamin in human milk. The Pediatrics) and consideration of other factors such as intestinal absorption (see text).
[h]The increased requirement during pregnancy cannot be met by the iron content of habitual American is recommended. Iron needs during lactation are not substantially different from those of nonpregnant replenish stores depleted by pregnancy.

heart disease. What is "ideal" weight, however, must be determined individually, for many factors are involved, such as body composition, body metabolism, genetics, and physical activity.

3. *Avoid too much fat, saturated fat, and cholesterol.* Some persons apparently cannot tolerate fat, and extra fat intake leads to high levels of blood fats or lipids. Elevated levels of blood fats are associated with a higher risk of heart disease. Also, the American population as a whole

Water-soluble vitamins						Minerals					
Thiamin (mg)	Riboflavin (mg)	Niacin (mg ME)[e]	Vitamin B6 (mg)	Folacin[f] (μg)	Vitamin B12 (μg)	Calcium (mg)	Phosphorus (mg)	Magnesium (mg)	Iron (mg)	Zinc (mg)	Iodine (μg)
0.3	0.4	6	0.3	30	0.5[g]	360	240	50	10	3	40
0.5	0.6	8	0.6	45	1.5	540	360	70	15	5	50
0.7	0.8	9	0.9	100	2.0	800	800	150	15	10	70
0.9	1.0	11	1.3	200	2.5	800	800	200	10	10	90
1.2	1.4	16	1.6	300	3.0	800	800	250	10	10	120
1.4	1.6	18	1.8	400	3.0	1200	1200	350	18	15	150
1.4	1.7	18	2.0	400	3.0	1200	1200	400	18	15	150
1.5	1.7	19	2.2	400	3.0	800	800	350	10	15	150
1.4	1.6	18	2.2	400	3.0	800	800	350	10	15	150
1.2	1.4	16	2.2	400	3.0	800	800	350	10	15	150
1.1	1.3	15	1.8	400	3.0	1200	1200	300	18	15	150
1.1	1.3	14	2.0	400	3.0	1200	1200	300	18	15	150
1.1	1.3	14	2.0	400	3.0	800	800	300	18	15	150
1.0	1.2	13	2.0	400	3.0	800	800	300	18	15	150
1.0	1.2	13	2.0	400	3.0	800	800	300	10	15	150
+0.4	+0.3	+2	+0.6	+400	+1.0	+400	+400	+150	[h]	+5	+25
+0.5	+0.5	+5	+0.5	+100	+1.0	+400	+400	+150	[h]	+10	+50

mended dietary allowances, ed. 9, Washington, D.C., 1980, The Academy.
in the United States under usual environmental stresses. Diets should be based on a variety of common
detailed discussion of allowances and of nutrients not tabulated. [See Table B in the Appendix for weights

vitamin A activity of diets as retinol equivalents.

calculation of vitamin E activity of the diet as α-tocopherol equivalents.

with enzymes ("conjugases") to make polyglutamyl forms of the vitamin available to the test organism.
allowances after weaning are based on energy intake (as recommended by the American Academy of

diets or by the existing iron stores of many women; therefore the use of 30-60 mg of supplemental iron
women, but continued supplementation of the mother for 2-3 months after parturition is advisable to

consumes a high-fat diet. Thus it seems wise to consider cutting down on fats, using them in moderation.

4. *Eat foods with adequate starch and fiber.* Complex carbohydrate foods (starches) are better fuel sources for energy than are fats and simple carbohydrates (sugars). Starches also contain many essential nutrients in addition to needed calories for energy. Furthermore, the American diet is relatively low in fiber, with the increased use of processed and refined

Table 1-3. Daily food guide—the Basic Four Food Groups

Food group	Main nutrients	Daily amounts*
Milk		
Milk, cheese, ice cream, or other products made with whole or skimmed milk	Calcium Protein Riboflavin	Children under 9: 2-3 cups Children 9 to 12: 3 or more cups Teenagers: 4 or more cups Adults: 2 or more cups Pregnant women: 3 or more cups Nursing mothers: 4 or more cups (1 cup = 8 oz fluid milk or designated milk equivalent†)
Meats		
Beef, veal, lamb, pork, poultry, fish, eggs	Protein Iron Thiamin	2 or more servings Count as one serving: 2-3 oz lean, boneless, cooked meat, poultry, or fish
Alternates: dry beans and peas, nuts, peanut butter	Niacin Riboflavin	2 eggs 1 cup cooked dry beans or peas 4 tbs peanut butter
Vegetables and fruits		4 or more servings Count as 1 serving: ½ cup vegetable or fruit or a portion such as 1 medium apple, banana, orange, potato, or half a medium grapefruit or melon
	Vitamin A	Include: 1 dark green or deep yellow vegetable or fruit rich in vitamin A, at least every other day
	Vitamin C (ascorbic acid)	1 citrus or other fruit or vegetable rich in vitamin C daily
	Smaller amounts of other vitamins and minerals	Other vegetables and fruits, including potatoes
Bread and cereals		4 or more servings of whole-grain, enriched, or restored Count as 1 serving:
	Thiamin Niacin Riboflavin Iron Protein	1 slice bread 1 oz (1 cup) ready-to-eat cereal, flake or puff varieties ½-¾ cup cooked cereal ½-¾ cup cooked pasta (macaroni, spaghetti, noodles) Crackers: 5 saltines, 2 squares graham crackers, and so forth

*Use additional amounts of these foods or added butter, margarine, oils, sugars, and so forth as desired or needed.
†Milk equivalents: 1 oz cheddar cheese, 3 servings cottage cheese, 1 cup fluid skimmed milk, 1 cup buttermilk, ¼ cup dry skimmed milk powder, 1 cup ice milk, 1⅔ cup ice cream, ½ cup evaporated milk.

foods. Increasing the use of complex carbohydrates will also help to increase dietary fiber. In turn there is some indication that this increase will help control certain chronic bowel diseases, as well as contribute to better blood sugar control for diabetics. Starches, then, may be substituted for fats and sugars.

5. *Avoid too much sugar*. The major health hazard from eating too much sugar is tooth decay (dental caries). Contrary to common opinion, too much sugar does not in itself cause diabetes. It can only contribute to poorer control of diabetes in persons who have inherited the disease. However, most Americans consume a relatively large amount of sugar: about 130 pounds per person per year. Much of this intake comes through many processed foods in which sugar is a regular ingredient. Again, moderation is the key.

6. *Avoid too much sodium*. Excessive sodium or salt is contraindicated for persons who have high blood pressure. In general, however, since many processed foods contain extra sodium and most Americans eat more sodium than is needed, it seems wise to moderate the use of added salt and "salty" foods.

7. *If you drink alcohol, do so in moderation*. Alcoholic beverages tend to be high in calories and low in other nutrients. Limited food intake may accompany large alcohol intake. Also, heavy drinking contributes to chronic liver disease and some neurological disorders, as well as to some throat and neck cancers. Thus moderation is the key if alcohol is used at all.

Food exchange system

Another food guide in general use, especially for modified diets such as those for diabetes or weight control, is the Food Exchange System. There are six food groups in this system: milk, vegetables, fruits, breads and other starches, meats and other protein foods, and fats. These foods are grouped according to their similarity in calories and food values. Thus measured amounts of these foods within the group may be traded off, or "exchanged," in meals. This provides an easy way for anyone to learn to balance a meal, not only for special needs but also for general needs. These food exchange groups are found in Table 19-1 on p. 209.

Whatever type of food guide that may be used, health workers must remember that meal patterns will vary with individual living situations and energy demands. However, usually the person who eats nutritionally well-balanced meals at the beginning of the day and continuing fairly evenly throughout the remainder of the day can work more efficiently and sustain a more even energy supply.

With the food environment rapidly changing in recent years to include more processed food items of variable or unknown nutrient quality, in some ways American dietary habits have deteriorated. Despite a plentiful food supply surveys give evidence of malnutrition, even among hospitalized patients. All nurses and other health workers have an important responsibility here. In general, however, it is encouraging to note that Americans are gradually learning that what they eat does influence their health. More than ever, people are being more selective about what they eat.

FOOD MISINFORMATION

Some persons seem more ready than others to believe false information given out by quacks and health food faddists. These persons may be seeking to preserve youthful vigor, relieve the pain of a chronic illness, or enhance beauty or athletic ability. More effort is now being made by health workers to teach the public the importance of a balanced diet.

The communication of sound nutritional information in a manner that meets individual needs provides the basis for building sound food habits. A real danger in nutritional misinformation, especially for persons with health problems, is that they often postpone obtaining the proper medical attention until it is too late. The American Medical Association has estimated that nutritional quackery costs 10 million Americans several million dollars a year. Sound knowledge of foods and nutrition can help counteract the influence of food faddists.

Questions on the importance of a balanced diet

1. Define nutrition.
2. What is dietetics?
3. What functions must food perform within the body?
4. What nutrients are necessary to provide good nutrition?
5. Why should the optimum required amounts of nutrients be taken?
6. How has the American diet changed in the last few years?
7. Plan a day's menu in accordance with a suggested food guide.
8. What are some evidences of good nutrition?
9. Make a list of ways in which you could help to combat food misinformation.

True-false

Circle *T* if the statement is true. Circle *F* if it is false, and then write the correct statement.

T   F   1. The U.S. Dietary Goals stress the two basic concepts of variety and moderation in food habits.

T   F   2. Food processing has little influence on food taste, appearance, safety, or nutrient values.

T   F   3. Some specific foods are called *complete foods* because they contain all the nutrients essential for full growth and health and are therefore essential in everyone's diet.

Multiple choice

Circle the letter in front of the correct answer.

1. Nutrients are:
   a. chemical elements or compounds in foods that have specific metabolic functions
   b. foods that are necessary for good health
   c. metabolic control substances such as enzymes
   d. nourishing materials used to cure certain illnesses
2. All nutrients needed by the body:
   a. must be obtained by specific food combinations
   b. must be obtained by vitamin and mineral supplements in pills
   c. have a variety of functions and uses in the body
   d. are supplied by a variety of foods in many different combinations
3. All persons throughout life, as indicated by the RDA, need:
   a. the same nutrients but in varying amounts
   b. the same amount of nutrients in any state of health
   c. the same nutrients at any age in the same amounts
   d. different nutrients in varying amounts
4. Signs of good nutritional status and health include:
   a. smooth, clear skin that is slightly moist, with good color
   b. firm muscle development
   c. appropriate weight for body size and body composition
   d. all of the above

Suggestions for additional study

1. Keep a notebook throughout the course. Cut out any articles on nutrition. Bring them to class for discussion and evaluation and then paste them in your notebook.
2. Make a list of your food intake for 3 days and analyze each day in accordance with the Basic Four Food Groups.
3. At some time during the first half of the course, each student gives a special report on some phase of nutrition. Students may choose a subject from the phase of nutrition that interests them most. This report is given before the class and then placed in the notebook.

Suggested readings

Food and Nutrition Board, National Academy of Sciences–National Reserach Council: Recommended dietary allowances, ed. 9, Washington, D.C., 1980, The Academy.

Guthrie, H.A.: Introductory nutrition, ed. 5, St. Louis, 1983, The C.V. Mosby Co.

U.S. Department of Agriculture and U.S. Department of Health and Human Services: *Nutrition and your health: Dietary Guidelines for Americans*, Home and Garden Bulletin, no. 232, Washington, D.C., 1980, U.S. Government Printing Office.

Williams, S.R.: Nutrition and diet therapy, ed. 4, St. Louis, 1981, The C.V. Mosby Co.

Williams, S.R.: Essentials of nutrition and diet therapy, ed. 3, St. Louis, 1982, The C.V. Mosby Co.

2

Carbohydrates

FUNCTIONS OF CARBOHYDRATE
Primary energy function

The main function of carbohydrate in nutrition is to provide the primary fuel for the body's energy needs. To meet this primary energy need, carbohydrate burns in the body at a rate of 4 kilocalories (kcal) per gram. This rate is called the *fuel factor*. Thus the fuel factor for carbohydrate is 4. This readily available energy is needed by the body not only for physical activities but also for all the work of all the body cells.

Under normal circumstances, carbohydrate supplies this primary fuel to meet about two thirds of an individual's total energy needs. When sufficient carbohydrate is not available in the food consumed, the body first turns to its stored glycogen reserve. When this reserve is depleted, tissue fat and protein are broken down to meet energy demands.

The ease with which carbohydrate can be converted to glycogen adds greatly to its usefulness as a primary energy source. Glycogen is found in several tissues of the body, mainly in the liver and muscles. Although this body reserve of liver and muscle glycogen is not large, it is readily available for quick energy and is constantly being replaced.

Functions related to other nutrients

Another important function of carbohydrate relates to protein metabolism. When the diet contains sufficient carbohydrate to meet major energy needs, less protein has to be diverted to help supply energy and thus can be used to build tissue. This is called the *protein-sparing* function of carbohydrate.

Also, carbohydrate has a significant function in relation to fat metabolism. When the diet does not contain sufficient carbohydrate to meet primary energy demands, fat is burned more rapidly to fill these needs. This rapid burning of fats produces excess materials called *ketones,* which result from incomplete fat oxidation in the cells. These ketones are strong acids, so this condition is called acidosis, or *ketosis*. This condition upsets the normal acid-base balance of the body and can become serious, as is the case in uncontrolled diabetes mellitus (see Chapter 21). This ability of carbohydrate to prevent the excess formation of ketones from fats is called the *antiketogenic* function of carbohydrate.

Functions related to vital organs

Carbohydrate also performs important functions for two vital organ systems, the heart and the central nervous system. The heart must always have sufficient energy supply, for heart action is life-sustaining muscle exercise. The stored glycogen in cardiac muscle is a vital emergency source of energy for contractions of the muscle to sustain the heartbeat. In a damaged heart a low carbohydrate intake, or poor glycogen stores, can threaten proper heart action and cause heart problems and chest pains.

The central nervous system also depends on carbohydrate for proper functioning. This is true for all nerve tissue but is especially true for the brain. Since the brain contains no stored supply of glucose, it depends on a minute-to-minute supply of glucose from the blood at all times. If this supply is not present, profound hypoglycemic (low blood sugar) shock may cause irreversible brain damage. Thus a constant supply of sufficient carbohydrate in the diet is necessary for the proper functioning of the entire central nervous system.

FOOD SOURCES OF CARBOHYDRATE

STARCHES. A major source of dietary carbohydrate is starch, or the *complex* carbohydrate foods. These are important foods in the diet and should supply the major energy source. The myth that starches are so-called fattening foods needs to be dispelled, for they help to supply many essential nutrients and maintain a steady source of blood sugar for fuel to the cells. Complex carbohydrate foods include starches such as breads and cereal grains, beans and peas and other legumes, and potatoes and other vegetables.

SUGARS. Food sugars, or *simple* carbohydrates, are found in foods such as fruits and milk, as well as in sweets. The United States is one of the world's biggest consumers of sugar and products made from sugar. Sweets in general are expensive and nutritionally poor sources of energy calories. Also, too much sugar in the diet dulls the appetite for foods that are needed to supply necessary vitamins and minerals, is irritating to the inner lining of the stomach, and ferments readily, causing gas. When sugars are absorbed in amounts that exceed the body's ability to use the accumulated glycogen, they are converted into fat and stored as such.

RECOMMENDED AMOUNTS OF DIETARY CARBOHYDRATE

RECOMMENDED DIETARY ALLOWANCES (RDA). There is no recommended dietary allowance for carbohydrate as such in the RDAs. In this standard nutrient guide energy needs are listed as total calories, which would include energy intake from fat and protein, as well as from carbohydrate.

U.S. DIETARY GOALS. The recommendation for the relative amount of carbohydrate in the diet outlined in the U.S. Dietary Goals is given in terms of percent of total calories. To achieve a better balance, it is recommended that 55% to 60% of the total calories in the diet come from carbohydrate foods, with the majority of these foods being *complex* carbohydrates, or starches. Generally, in practical application, it is wise to plan for 50% to 60% of the diet's calories to come from carbohydrate foods, mainly in the form of starches.

CLASSES OF CARBOHYDRATE

Carbohydrates are classified into three main groups, monosaccharides, disaccharides, and polysaccharides, with three subgroups in each main class.

Monosaccharides

These are the simple single sugars:
1. *Glucose*. The basic single sugar in body metabolism is glucose. This is the sugar form circulating in the blood and serving as the primary fuel source for the cells. It is not usually found as such in the diet but is derived mainly from the digestion of starch.
2. *Fructose*. This single sugar is found mainly in fruits, from which it gets its name. The amount of this sugar in fruits depends somewhat on the degree of ripeness. As the fruit ripens, some of the stored starch turns to sugar.
3. *Galactose*. This single sugar also is not usually found as such in the diet but is derived mainly from the digestion of milk sugar, or lactose.

All of the monosaccharides, or simple single sugars, require no digestion. They are therefore quickly absorbed from the intestine into the bloodstream and carried to the liver, where they are converted by liver enzymes into glycogen. This glycogen form of carbohydrate is similar in structure to starch.

Disaccharides

These are the simple double sugars:
1. *Sucrose*. One of the most common dietary sugars is sucrose. It is the common sugar—granulated, powdered, or brown, produced from sugarcane or sugar beets. Molasses, a by-product of sugar production, is also a form of sucrose.
2. *Lactose*. The sugar in milk is lactose. It is the only common sugar not found in plants. It is less soluble and less sweet than sucrose. It remains in the intestines longer than other sugars and encourages the growth of certain useful bacteria. Lactose is formed in the mammary glands and comprises about 40% of the milk solids. There is 4.8% lactose in cow's milk and 7% in human milk. Since lactose aids calcium and phosphorus absorption, the presence of all three of these nutrients in one natural

"package" food is a fortunate circumstance. Also, since lactose is less sweet than any other one of the sugars, it can be added to fruit juices to increase caloric intake without detracting from the palatability of the beverage.

3. *Maltose*. This simple double sugar is not found usually as such in the diet but is derived in the intermediate digestive breakdown of starch. Its dietary uses would be as a sweetener in various commercial products.

Polysaccharides

These are the complex carbohydrates composed of many sugar units:

1. *Starches*. These larger structures of carbohydrate, the starches, are found in grains, legumes and other vegetables, and in minute amounts in fruits. Starches are more complex than sugars and therefore take a longer time to digest. For starch to be used more promptly by the body, the outer membrane can be broken down by grinding or cooking. Heat, especially if moisture is present, causes the outer membrane to break apart, and the starch granules then absorb water and swell. Long application of dry heat will also cause starch to break down.

2. *Glycogen*. This polysaccharide is similar in structure to starch and is therefore sometimes called *animal starch*. It is found in the liver and muscles. Glycogen is constantly being "recycled" in the body—broken down to form glucose for immediate energy needs and resynthesized for liver and muscle storage.

3. *Fiber*. Several of the types of dietary fiber are polysaccharides. These include cellulose and hemicellulose, which form the framework of dietary plant foods such as fruits, vegetables, and whole grains. Pectin is a similar dietary fiber also found in fruits. Since humans lack the necessary enzymes to digest dietary fiber, these substances have no direct nutrient value as do other carbohydrates. However, it is this very indigestibility that makes these materials important dietary assets. They furnish bulk in the intestinal food mass, which is essential for normal peristaltic muscle action and elimination of waste products in the feces. Usually a person requires about 6 g of fiber in the diet each day. This amount, for example, could be supplied by two vegetables, two fruits, and four servings of whole-grain bread or cereal. Other forms of fiber, not usually in the diet, have special uses. For example, agar, which is obtained from seaweed, can absorb many times its weight in water and so is used in the treatment of constipation. Alginate, also found in seaweed, is used in making commercial ice cream to give it a smooth texture. Pectins, obtained from fruits, are useful for their gelling properties. Pectin is also used in the treatment of diarrhea because it absorbs the toxins and bacteria in the intestines and adds bulk to the intestinal contents.

Questions on carbohydrates

1. What are the chief sources of carbohydrate?
2. What are the chief functions of carbohydrate?
3. Why is it not good to have too much sugar in the diet?
4. What are the three principal groups of carbohydrates?
5. Where are the single sugars found?
6. What is sucrose?
7. Which sugar is not found in plants?
8. How does lactose differ from other carbohydrates?
9. What is necessary to make starch more readily available to the body?
10. What is glycogen, and where is it found?
11. What is cellulose, and why is it advantageous in the normal diet?
12. How may a person be assured of receiving enough dietary fiber?
13. Where is dietary fiber found?
14. What use is made of agar, alginate, and pectin?
15. Why do humans need an adequate amount of carbohydrate in the diet?

True-false

Circle *T* if the statement is true. Circle *F* if it is false, and then write the correct statement.

T   F   1. The main carbohydrate in the diet is starch, a complex carbohydrate.

T   F   2. Modern processing and refinement of foods have reduced the amount of fiber in the American diet.

T   F   3. Lactose is a very sweet simple sugar found in a number of carbohydrate foods.

T   F   4. Glucose is the form in which sugar circulates in the blood and supplies energy to cells.

T   F   5. Glycogen is an important long-term storage form of energy deposited in relatively large amounts in the liver and muscles.

Multiple choice

Circle the letter in front of the correct answer.

1. Carbohydrates provide the primary fuel source for body energy. Which of the following carbohydrate foods provides the *quickest* source of energy?
   a. glass of milk
   b. slice of bread
   c. glass of orange juice
   d. bowl of cooked cereal
   e. chocolate candy bar
2. A quickly available form of energy, although limited in amount, is stored in the liver by conversion of glucose to:
   a. tissue fat
   b. amino acids
   c. glycerol
   d. glycogen

Suggestions for additional study

1. Cut pictures from magazines illustrating carbohydrate foods and put them in a notebook.

2. Add 2 tbs lactose to $\frac{1}{2}$ cup orange juice and compare the taste with that of plain orange juice.
3. Compare the taste of a ripe banana with that of one only partially ripe and describe the difference.
4. Make a list of foods high in carbohydrate that are usually consumed between meals.
5. Read the labels on five different products in a grocery market and list the carbohydrate value of each.

Suggested readings

Guthrie, H.A.: Introductory nutrition, ed. 5, St. Louis, 1983, The C.V. Mosby Co.

Williams, S.R.: Nutrition and diet therapy, ed. 4, St. Louis, 1981, The C.V. Mosby Co.

Williams, S.R.: Essentials of nutrition and diet therapy, ed. 3, St. Louis, 1982, The C.V. Mosby Co.

3

Proteins

FUNCTIONS OF PROTEIN
Primary tissue-binding function

The primary function of protein is to repair worn-out, wasted, or damaged tissue and to build new tissue. Thus protein provides for growth needs and maintains tissue health during adult years. Protein is the fundamental structural material of every cell in the body. In fact the largest percentage of the body, excluding the water content, is made up of protein that must be constantly repaired and replaced. Protein not only makes up the bulk of the muscles, internal organs, brain, nerves, skin, hair, and nails but also is a vital part of regulatory substances such as hormones, enzymes, and blood plasma.

Additional body functions

In addition to its basic tissue-building function, protein has other body functions. These functions relate to energy, water balance, metabolism, and the body defense system:
1. *Energy*. If needed, protein may furnish heat and energy to the body. This is a secondary backup source to carbohydrate and fat, however, and will be called on to provide an additional energy source only when there is an insufficient amount of primary fuel sources. The available fuel factor of protein is 4 calories per gram.
2. *Water balance*. Plasma protein, especially albumin, helps to control water balance throughout the body by exerting osmotic pressure to maintain normal circulation of tissue and blood vessel fluids.
3. *Metabolism*. Protein aids metabolic functions in two main ways. First, protein combines with iron to form hemoglobin, which carries oxygen to the cells for cell oxidation processes. The protein compound hemoglobin also gives the red coloring to the corpuscles. About 10,000 atoms make up a hemoblogin molecule, and about 100 million molecules make up a corpuscle. Second, protein is used to manufacture agents that control metabolic processes, such as digestive and cell enzymes, as well as hormones.

4. *Body defense system*. Protein is used to build special white blood cells (lymphocytes) and antibodies as part of the body's immune system to help defend against disease and infection.

STRUCTURAL NATURE OF PROTEIN
Amino acids

Protein is made up of small building units or compounds known as amino acids. These amino acids are joined in specific chain combinations to form specific proteins. When protein foods are eaten, the food protein is broken down into its amino acids in the digestive process. Amino acids are then reassembled in the body in the proper order to form needed body tissue protein. There are 22 known amino acids, some of which are essential amino acids and others that are termed nonessential:

1. *Essential amino acids*. Eight of the amino acids are called essential amino acids because the body cannot manufacture them. Thus *essential* means that they are needed in the diet. These eight essential amino acids are tryptophan, threonine, isoleucine, leucine, lysine, methionine, phenylalanine, and valine. During the growth years, histidine and arginine are also essential to meet normal childhood growth demands.
2. *Nonessential amino acids*. Nonessential is rather a misleading term, for all amino acids have essential tissue building and metabolic functions in the body. However, as used in this way, the term refers to the remaining amino acids that the body can synthesize, so they are nonessential in the diet.

METABOLIC FUNCTIONS OF AMINO ACIDS. In addition to their role in basic tissue building, certain amino acids also have specific metabolic functions. For example, methionine serves as a source of *labile methyl groups* (CH_3) for the synthesis of choline or creatine. Arginine is also involved in the synthesis of creatine. Phenylalanine furnishes the nucleus for the synthesis of thyroxine.

NITROGEN

Protein is unique among the primary nutrients in that it contains the element nitrogen. Unlike carbohydrate and fat, which contain no nitrogen, protein contains approximately 16% nitrogen. In addition, some proteins contain small but valuable amounts of sulfur, phosphorus, iron, and iodine.

Nitrogen balance

The balance of nitrogen in the body is an indication of how well the body tissues are being maintained. The amount of protein consumed in the diet and used by the body is measured by the amount of nitrogen consumed in the dietary protein and the amount of nitrogen excreted in the urine. For example, 1 g of urinary nitrogen results from the digestion and metabolism of 6.25 g of protein. Therefore, if for every 6.25 g of protein consumed, 1 g of nitrogen is excreted in the urine, the body is said to be in nitrogen balance. This is the normal pattern in health.

POSITIVE NITROGEN BALANCE. A positive nitrogen balance means that the body has excreted less nitrogen than it has taken in and is therefore retaining nitrogen. This situation occurs during rapid growth in infancy, childhood, or adolescence or during pregnancy and lactation. It also occurs in persons who have been malnourished and are subsequently being "built back up" with increased nourishment. In such cases protein is being retained within the body to supply its increased needs for tissue building and various associated metabolic functions.

NEGATIVE NITROGEN BALANCE. A negative nitrogen balance means that the body is breaking down some of the body protein. Failure to keep the body in nitrogen balance may not become apparent for some time, but it will eventually cause loss of muscle tissue, impairment of body organs and body functions, and increased susceptibility to infection. In children negative nitrogen balance will cause growth retardation.

FOOD SOURCES OF PROTEIN

Food proteins are classified as complete proteins or incomplete proteins, depending on their amino acid composition.

Complete proteins

A food protein that contains all of the eight essential amino acids in sufficient amounts to meet human requirements is called a complete protein. Complete proteins are sometimes spoken of as proteins of high biological value, which means that they supply all the amino acids needed for building body tissues. In general the complete protein foods of high biological value are from animal sources. These foods are meats (including poultry and fish), eggs, milk, and cheese. Gelatin, although an animal product, is a rather worthless protein, for it lacks three essential amino acids—tryptophan, valine, and isoleucine—and has only small amounts of another essential amino acid, leucine.

Incomplete proteins

Protein foods that contain many amino acids but not all of the essential ones in sufficient amounts are called incomplete proteins. These proteins are found in plant foods: cereal grains, legumes, and certain nuts and seeds. However, these foods make valuable contributions to the total dietary protein.

Complementary proteins

Fortunately, most foods contain a mixture of proteins that complement one another. People combine several foods in one meal, and the protein in one food supplements the protein in other foods. Bread and milk, cereal and milk, and meat, cheese, or egg sandwiches are very logical and useful combinations.

Amino acids that are insufficient in vegetable protein are present in adequate amounts in meat, milk, eggs, and cheese. Thus the overall protein value is improved when foods of animal origin are eaten with foods of vegetable origin. In general this supplementing of amino acids is more efficiently done if the various foods are eaten at the same time. For example, bread protein and milk protein supplement each other better if they are consumed at the same time. One of the important facts of protein nutrition is that although there is no storage of amino acids in the body as such, a metabolic "pool" of amino acids is maintained in the liver to meet constant cell needs. This general metabolic resource helps to ensure a supply of needed amino acids for any specific tissue protein synthesis required.

Vegetarian diets that are nourishing and complete can be built on the complementary protein principle. When meat is eliminated, the remaining animal proteins—milk, cheese, and egg—can still supply the needed complete protein foods. When these animal foods are also omitted, it becomes all the more imperative that plant food proteins are carefully combined so that amino acids that are low in one particular food will be offset by higher amounts in another food. It is important that either some form of complete animal protein or complementary combinations of incomplete plant proteins be included in each meal to ensure that the necessary amino acids for maintaining the cells and tissues are present when needed.

PROTEIN REQUIREMENTS

When protein requirements are established, both quality of the protein in terms of its essential amino acids and quantity of total protein must be considered. The food in a person's diet should contain sufficient protein to provide an intake well above basic needs to ensure an adequate supply of the essential amino acids contained in the complete proteins. Thus a margin of safety is usually built into most of the standards for recommended protein allowances. After all of the tissue protein needs of the body are met, any amino acids not needed for protein synthesis are carried back to the liver, where they are divided into two parts: the part carrying the nitrogen and the remainder. The nitrogen part is used in other products or converted into urea for excretion through the kidneys. The remaining part, the "carbon skeleton," is then routed through the same channels as carbohydrate and is used to provide added energy for general body needs.

Specific dynamic action of protein

Allowances for the amount of protein needed by an individual in relation to energy or calories required for protein metabolism were based on former assumptions that the so-called specific dynamic action of protein—the work of handling protein in the body—required additional energy. However, current research indicates that this "specific dynamic action" or work of metabolizing protein is far less significant than was formerly assumed. In other words a high-protein diet does not make the body "burn up" more calories than a normal diet does. Thus this theoretical protein-calorie link does not have to be considered in setting protein requirements.

Recommended dietary allowances (RDAs)

The RDA established by the Food and Nutrition Board of the National Research Council has set the current standard for adult protein needs at 0.8 g/kg of body weight. The standard reference man used in the determination weighed 154 pounds (70 kg), and the reference woman weighed 120 pounds (55 kg). The standard set for the daily amount of protein was designed for the maintenance of good nutrition in a healthy person who is engaged in moderate physical activity. Strenuous physical activity does not actually increase the protein need but does greatly increase the energy or calorie need.

The protein needs of children and adults, as set in the U.S. RDA standard, are presented in Table 3-1. The "margin of safety" philosophy of the U.S. standard helps to prevent any incidence of protein deficiency. Actually, nutrition surveys in the United States have not shown particular protein deficiency except in certain poverty situations.

Table 3-1. Required amounts of protein per day

Men (154 lb [70 kg])	56 g
Women (120 lb [55 kg])	44 g
Women (pregnant)	+30 g
Women (lactating)	+20 g
Infants	
0-6 mo	2.2 g/kg of body weight
6-12 mo	2.0 g/kg of body weight
Children	
1-3 yr	23 g
4-6 yr	30 g
7-10 yr	34 g
Boys	
11-14 yr	45 g
15-18 yr	56 g
Girls	
11-14 yr	46 g
15-18 yr	46 g

From Food and Nutrition Board, National Academy of Sciences–National Research Council: Recommended dietary allowances, ed. 9, Washington, D.C., 1980, The Academy.

Of this protein intake, to ensure adequate protein quality, the percentage of complete proteins should be 33% for adults and 50% to 60% for children. Because boys and girls are growing, their protein needs up to the age of 20 years are greater per pound of body weight than are the relative protein needs of adults. There is little difference between the protein needs of boys and those of girls for the first 12 years. However, when they reach adolescence, the protein requirement is higher for boys than for girls because of the increasing muscle mass in boys. A variety of foods high in protein are shown in Table 3-2. These foods may be used in many ways in planning menus for children and adults.

U.S. Dietary Goals

The recently developed U.S. Dietary Goals provide additional guidance for meeting protein requirements. These guidelines for a balanced diet for healthy Americans indicate that about 15% of the total calories in the diet should come from protein. For most Americans this amount is less than is usually consumed. This does not mean that protein requirements are lowered but rather that most

Table 3-2. Foods high in protein

Food	Approximate amount	Protein (g)
Beef, chuck roast	3 oz cooked	23.4
Beef, hamburger	3 oz cooked	20.5
Beef, round	3 oz cooked	24.7
Beef, club steak	4 oz cooked	27.6
Lamb leg	3 oz cooked	21.6
Liver (beef, calf, and pork)	3 oz cooked	20.4
Pork loin	3 oz cooked	20.7
Ham	3 oz cooked	20.7
Veal, leg or shoulder	3 oz cooked	25.2
Chicken	$\frac{1}{4}$ broiler	22.4
Chicken, fryer	$\frac{1}{2}$ breast (4 oz raw)	26.9
Chicken, hen, stewed	1 thigh or $\frac{1}{2}$ breast	26.5
Duck, roasted	3 slices ($3\frac{1}{2} \times 2\frac{3}{4} \times \frac{1}{4}$)	20.6
Goose, roasted	3 slices ($3\frac{1}{2} \times 2\frac{3}{4} \times \frac{1}{4}$)	25.3
Turkey	3 slices ($3\frac{1}{2} \times 2\frac{3}{4} \times \frac{1}{4}$)	27.8
Haddock	3 oz cooked	20.2
Halibut	3 oz cooked	21.0
Oysters	6 medium	15.1
Salmon	$\frac{2}{3}$ cup	20.5
Scallops	5-6 medium	23.8
Tuna	$\frac{1}{2}$ cup	15.9
Peanut butter	4 tbs	15.9
Milk	1 cup	8.5
Cottage cheese	5-6 tbs	19.5
American cheddar cheese	1 oz	7.0
Egg	1 medium	7.0

Americans would be wise to cut down their *overconsumption* of protein foods, especially in the form of meat, which carries considerable animal fat.

Questions on proteins

1. What are the functions of protein in the body?
2. What is the protein that carries oxygen in the blood and gives the red color to blood?
3. Name the eight essential amino acids.
4. What minerals are found in the different proteins?
5. Define nitrogen balance, positive nitrogen balance, and negative nitrogen balance.
6. What are complete proteins, and where are they found?
7. What is meant by high biological value?
8. What are incomplete proteins, and where are they found?
9. Why is it advisable to provide a protein intake above actual needs?
10. What happens to excess protein?
11. What percentage of the protein intake should be from complete proteins for adults and what percentage for children? Why are the percentages different?
12. Underline the complete proteins in the following list: Cream of Wheat, eggs, applesauce, roast beef, coffee, milk.
13. List your protein intake for 1 day, indicating which are complete and which are incomplete.

True-false

Circle *T* if a statement is true. Circle *F* if it is false, and then write the correct statement.

T F 1. Complete proteins of high biological value are found in dried beans and peas (legumes), seeds and nuts, and whole grains.
T F 2. Protein provides the main source of body heat.
T F 3. Protein plays a large role in the body's resistance to disease.
T F 4. The general U.S. standard of protein allowance for adults is about 0.8 g of protein per kilogram of body weight.
T F 5. Because they are smaller, children need less protein per unit of body weight than adults require.
T F 6. The healthy adult is usually in a state of nitrogen balance.
T F 7. Positive nitrogen balance exists during periods of rapid growth, such as in early childhood and during adolescence.

Multiple choice

Circle the letter in front of the correct answer.

1. Twenty-two amino acids are involved in total body metabolism, building and rebuilding various tissues. Of these, eight are called *essential* amino acids. This means that:
   a. the body cannot synthesize these eight amino acids and hence must obtain them in the diet
   b. these eight amino acids can be made by the body because they are essential to life
   c. after synthesizing these eight amino acids, the body then uses them in processes essential for growth
   d. these eight amino acids are essential in various body processes, and the remaining fourteen are not

2. A complete protein food of high biological value would be one that contains:
   a. all twenty-two of the amino acids in sufficient quantity to meet human requirements
   b. most of the twenty-two amino acids from which the body will then make additional amounts of the eight essential amino acids as needed
   c. the eight essential amino acids in any proportion, since the body can always fill in the difference needed
   d. all eight of the essential amino acids in correct proportion to meet human needs
3. A state of negative nitrogen balance exists in the body when tissue breakdown and nitrogen loss exceed nitrogen intake and tissue building. In which of the following situations would such a state of negative nitrogen balance occur?
   a. during pregnancy
   b. during adolescence
   c. after an injury or surgery
   d. during infancy

Suggestions for additional study

1. Place pictures cut from magazines illustrating complete proteins on one page of your notebook and those showing incomplete proteins on another page.
2. List the foods rich in protein that you would normally consume at each of the three daily meals.
3. Prepare for the class a display of actual foods, showing those containing complete proteins and those containing incomplete proteins. Use these foods to demonstrate how you would plan a vegetarian diet to ensure adequate complete protein.
4. Plan a high-protein diet and a low-protein diet for 3 days.

Suggested readings

Food and Nutrition Board, National Academy of Sciences–National Research Council: Recommended dietary allowances, ed. 9, Washington, D.C., 1980, The Academy.

Guthrie, H.A.: Introductory nutrition, ed. 5, St. Louis, 1983, The C.V. Mosby Co.

Lappé, F.M.: Diet for a small planet, ed. 2, New York, 1975, Ballantine Books, Inc.

Pennington, J., and Church, H.N.: Bowes and Church's food values of portions commonly used, ed. 13, Philadelphia, 1980, J.B. Lippincott Co.

Robertson, L., Flinders, C., and Godfrey, B.: Laurel's kitchen, Petalunia, Calif., 1976, Nilgiri Press.

Williams, S.R.: Nutrition and diet therapy, ed. 4, St. Louis, 1981, The C.V. Mosby Co.

Williams, S.R.: Essentials of nutrition and diet therapy, ed. 3, St. Louis, 1982, The C.V. Mosby Co.

4

Fats

FUNCTIONS OF FAT
Primary energy function

Along with carbohydrate, fat serves as one of the body's primary fuels for energy production. Because carbohydrate can be so easily converted to fat, fat serves as an important storage form of body fuel for energy. Fat is a more concentrated source of energy than carbohydrate, yielding 2¼ times as many calories per unit of weight. Each gram of fat burned in the body yields 9 calories. Therefore the fuel factor for fat is 9. However, fat in the diet is still a more expensive source of calories than carbohydrate food.

Additional body functions

The fat not needed for immediate use is stored as fatty tissue. It can be used in an emergency as fuel and also for additional body functions such as regulating body temperature and aiding in developing body structures:
1. *Body temperature.* The layer of fat directly beneath the skin acts as an important tissue in regulating body temperature. This layer of fat acts as a nonconductor and prevents excessive radiation or loss of body heat. It also protects the body from mechanical injury.
2. *Body structures.* Additional fatty tissue is distributed inside the body as a support to the vital organs. It also is an important part of cell wall structure.

Dietary functions

Fat also serves several important functions in the diet in relation to nutrients and to the satisfaction people get from food:
1. *Fat-soluble nutrients.* Fats act as carriers of fat-soluble vitamins A, D, E, and K. Fat also favors absorption of other fat-soluble factors.
2. *Satiety and flavor.* Fat also gives a person a feeling of satisfaction, or *satiety,* after eating. This is caused partly by the slower rate of digestion of fats and partly by the flavor they give to foods.

TYPES OF FAT

Food fat comes from both animal and plant sources. A number of fats and fat compounds are important in health. Five of the most commonly encountered fat-related terms in health care are defined here.

Lipids

The chemical class name for all fats and fat-related compounds is *lipids*. This word comes from the Greek word for fat, *lipos*. The class name *lipids* is found in a number of combination words used for health problems. For example, the condition of an elevated level of blood fats circulating in the body is called *hyperlipidemia*.

Triglycerides

This is the chemical name for fat. The word comes from the chemical structure of fat, which is a base of glycerol with three fatty acids attached to it. Thus any fat, whether it is a food fat from plants or animals or a tissue fat in the body, is called a *triglyceride*.

Fatty acids

Fatty acids that make up various fats have two significant characteristics. These characteristics relate to the concept of saturation and to essential fatty acids.

SATURATED AND UNSATURATED FAT. When any substance is said to be *saturated*, it simply means that it contains all of the material that it is capable of holding. For example, a sponge may be saturated with water when it holds all the water that it is capable of holding. In the same manner fats are called saturated or unsaturated according to whether or not they are filled with the substance they are capable of holding. The substance that fills the structure of fat is hydrogen. Thus a saturated fat is one whose structure is completely filled with all the hydrogen it can hold and as a result is heavier and denser. On the other hand, an unsaturated fat is one that is not completely filled with hydrogen and thus is less heavy and less dense.

For example, a saturated fat usually comes from animal food sources and is solid in nature. An unsaturated fat usually comes from plant sources and is liquid or soft in nature or less solid. Related terms such as *polyunsaturated* are frequently found on labels of food products. This means that the product is one that has many unfilled spaces in the structure of the fat involved. Margarine and shortenings are examples of saturated fats that are made from relatively inexpensive vegetable oils, which are unsaturated fats, by the introduction of hydrogen into the fat molecule of the oil under carefully controlled conditions. These terms, saturated and unsaturated fat, are significant for health workers because current research relates them to elevated or abnormal levels of circulating blood fat and hence to disease conditions associated with blood vessels and the heart.

ESSENTIAL FATTY ACID. A particular fatty acid, linoleic acid, is recognized as the main essential fatty acid because the body cannot synthesize it and it is vital to body processes. Two other fatty acids, linolenic acid and arachidonic acid, have been called essential fatty acids. However, they are not actually dietary essentials because the body can synthesize them. The essential one, linoleic acid, is found primarily in vegetable oils.

Cholesterol

Cholesterol is a member of a chemical group of substances called *sterols*. It is a substance that comes from animal sources, since it is synthesized in animal tissue. Cholesterol is not actually a fat, but it is classified with fat as a fat-related compound because it has the capacity of combining with fatty acids and transporting them in the bloodstream.

Cholesterol is a complex fat-related compound found in practically all body tissues, especially in the brain and nerve tissue, bile, blood, and liver, where most of the cholesterol is synthesized. Cholesterol is synthesized within the body mainly in the intestinal walls and the liver according to need, metabolic balances, and dietary intake. It has been estimated that the human body normally synthesizes about 2 g of cholesterol daily.

Lipoproteins

A significant type of compound in which fat travels in the blood is the group of materials called *lipoproteins*. Since fat is insoluble in water, it cannot travel freely in the bloodstream, which is largely water. This problem is solved by the body by wrapping the small particles of fat with a layer of protein, since protein is soluble in water. Thus, as the name implies, lipoproteins are compounds of fat and protein used for transporting fat by way of the bloodstream to all body tissues. Several of these compounds carry loads of triglycerides, or fat, to and from the cells. Others carry cholesterol to and from cells. These substances are significant in current research relating fats and various fat-related compounds to the blood vessel disease *atherosclerosis*. This underlying problem of fatty deposits on the inside wall of blood vessels is the condition leading to heart disease.

DIETARY FAT AND HEALTH
American diet

Traditionally the American diet has been high in fat. The average American eats approximately 100 pounds of fat a year, which provides about 40% of the total calories. This amount of fat exceeds that needed by the average person.

Not more than 20% to 30% of an average diet need be in the form of fat. If 20% of the total calories come from fat, an adequate amount of the essential fatty acids to meet the physiological needs of the body will be present. With a 2000-calorie diet a person would still be getting 45 to 50 g of fat. It has been demonstrated in Asia and eastern Europe that even 20% to 25% of fat in the diet is not necessary to the health of all persons.

Heart disease risk factor

The current movement in American health care toward prevention of disease through reduction of various risk factors related to chronic disease is a healthy sign. Heart disease is the leading chronic disease in developed countries such as the United States, and much attention has been given to reducing the various risk factors leading to the development of this disease process. The underlying tissue disease within the blood vessels is atherosclerosis, as indicated. This condition, characterized by fatty deposits in the blood vessel walls, leads to a thickening of the wall and potential closure of the vessel, thus cutting off the blood supply to tissues served by that vessel. If this event occurs in a major coronary blood vessel supplying vital oxygen and nutrients to the heart muscle, a heart attack, or *myocardial infarction*, results.

Current research indicates that this heart disease process is a multifactor event. The fat and cholesterol portion of the diet has been identified by only one of these factors. Other related health factors include obesity, diabetes, elevated blood fats, and hypertension. Additional life-style factors include smoking, reduced amount of exercise, and stress. Various studies seem to indicate that a high consumption of dietary cholesterol and animal fats may lead to abnormal levels of cholesterol bodies in the blood in susceptible individuals and that an increased intake of plant fats, especially those containing linoleic acid, lowers the blood cholesterol level. A high blood cholesterol level does not necessarily mean that large cholesterol bodies are deposited in the walls of the blood vessels and vice versa. However, a blood cholesterol level that is higher than 240 mg/100 ml should be a warning sign.

As indicated, approximately 40% of the calories consumed in the American diet are derived from fat. The countries that have a lower fat intake show a much lower incidence of coronary disease. The American public would do well to cut its fat intake from 40% to 20% or 30%, thereby reducing the caloric intake and perhaps lowering the blood cholesterol level. There is less atherosclerosis in countries where the use of saturated or animal fat is low and unsaturated or plant fat is used instead. This is the case, for example, in Japan. Surveys made in Italy, Spain, Africa, and other countries where people's intake of fat is approximatley 20% show that there are lower cholesterol levels and less atherosclerosis in the general population. Thus a middle-aged or older

Table 4-1. Cholesterol content of foods

Food item	Size of serving	Cholesterol per serving (mg)
Muscle meats		
Beef, round		
Medium fat	3⅓ oz	125
Lean	3⅓ oz	95
Lamb	3⅓ oz	70
Veal	3⅓ oz	65-140
Organ meats		
Liver		
Beef	3⅓ oz	320
Calf	3⅓ oz	360
Lamb	3⅓ oz	610
Pork	3⅓ oz	420
Sweetbreads	3⅓ oz	280
Fish		
Cod	3⅓ oz	50
Salmon	3⅓ oz	60
Sardines	1¾ oz	35
Shellfish		
Crab	3⅓ oz	145
Oysters	3⅓ oz	230-470
Shrimp	3⅓ oz	150
Poultry		
Chicken, light	3⅓ oz	90
Chicken, dark	3⅓ oz	60
Duck	3⅓ oz	70
Turkey	3⅓ oz	75
Cheese		
American	2 oz	96
American, processed	2 oz	93
Swiss, processed	2 oz	87
Velveeta	2 oz	96
Miscellaneous		
Butter	1 tbs	40
Egg yolk, fresh	1	333
Milk, whole	1 cup	26
Milk, skim	1 cup	1

Data compiled from Okey, R.: J. Am. Diet. Assoc. **21**:341, 1945; Pennington, J., and Church, H.N.: Bowes and Church's food values of portions commonly used, ed. 13, Philadelphia, 1980, J.B. Lippincott Co.

person who is overweight and who also has a high blood cholesterol level will find it advisable to reduce both weight and consumption of fat, especially animal fat. The cholesterol content of some foods is given in Table 4-1.

FOOD SOURCES OF FATS
Visible and invisible fats

For practical purposes, food fats are generally classified as *visible* fats or *invisible* fats. Visible fats are the more obvious ones in the diet. These include butter, margarine, salad oils and dressings, lard, shortening, fat meat such as bacon and salt pork, and the visible fat of any meat. Invisible fats include those foods in which the fat component is less obvious, including the cream portion of milk, cheese, egg yolk, nuts, seeds, avocado, and lean meat. Even when all of the visible fat has been removed from meat, such as the skin on poultry and the obvious fat on the lean portions, an average of 6% of fat surrounding the muscle fibers will remain.

Margarine and shortenings are made from vegetable oils, such as cottonseed oil, soybean oil, and corn oil, by the introduction of hydrogen into the fat molecule, as described. This process is called *hydrogenation,* a word that appears frequently on the labels of such commercial fat products. To make margarine a substitute for butter, the hydrogenated product is then further processed by being churned with cultured milk to give it the flavor of butter. It is usually fortified with vitamins A and D. Nutritionally, fortified margarine is then the equivalent of butter and has the same caloric value. Margarine, which is economical, tasteful, and lower in saturated fat, is 80% fat and is fortified with vitamin A to supply a minimum of 15,000 IU (international units) per pound.

Digestibility of fats

The digestibility of fat varies somewhat according to the food source and cooking method. Butter digests more completely than meat fat. Fried foods, especially those that are saturated with fat in the frying process, are digested more slowly than boiled or baked foods. Fried foods cooked at too high a temperature are more difficult to digest, and substances in the fat break down into irritating materials. Fried foods should be used sparingly, and the temperature of the fat used in frying should be carefully controlled. In general, as indicated, the health goal is to reduce the amount of all fat used in the diet.

FAT REQUIREMENTS

RECOMMENDED DIETARY ALLOWANCES (RDA). There is no fat requirement stated in the RDA standard. The fat allowance in the diet is included in the general calorie allowances.

U.S. DIETARY GOALS. In line with the health standard for a lowered amount of fat in the diet the U.S. Dietary Goals indicate a recommendation for less fat in the diet, especially in saturated fat and cholesterol. The amount of dietary fat should be limited to no more than 30% of the total calories in the diet. This recommendation is based on the relationships indicated by research between dietary fat and heart disease, as discussed.

WAYS TO LOWER DIETARY FAT

Several practical ways of lowering fat in the diet follow:
1. *Meat*. Use leaner cuts of all meats and more poultry and seafood than red meats. Remove skin from poultry and trim fat from all meats. Avoid added fat in cooking. Use smaller portions.
2. *Eggs*. Use fewer eggs, a limit of approximately two or three a week. Cook and serve without added fat.
3. *Milk and milk products*. Use low-fat or fat-free milk products and lower fat cheeses.
4. *Food preparation*. Avoid fat in cooking as much as possible. Use alternate seasonings such as herbs, spices, lemon juice, onion, garlic, fat-free broth, or wine.

Questions on fats
1. Name three visible fats.
2. Name three sources of invisible fat.
3. How is margarine made? How does it compare nutritionally with butter?
4. What percentage of the total calories in the average diet should be in the form of fat?
5. What purpose does fat serve in the diet?
6. What is the main essential fatty acid? Where is it found?
7. What precautions should be taken in frying foods and why?
8. List six foods high in cholesterol.

True-false

Circle *T* if the statement is true. Circle *F* if it is false, and then write the correct statement.

T   F   1. Corn oil is a saturated fat.
T   F   2. Polyunsaturated fat usually comes from animal sources.
T   F   3. In cold climates smaller amounts of dietary fat are usually consumed.
T   F   4. Lipoproteins are transport forms of fat in the body, produced mainly in the liver and in the intestinal wall.
T   F   5. Fat has approximately the same caloric value as carbohydrate has.

Multiple choice

Circle the letter in front of the correct answer.

1. The energy fuel fat found in food sources is:
   a. glycerol
   b. lipoprotein

c. fatty acid
d. triglyceride
2. Which of the following statements are correct in reference to the saturation of fat?
   (1) The degree of saturation depends on the relative amount of hydrogen in the structure of the fat.
   (2) The more unsaturated fats come from animal sources.
   (3) The more saturated the fat, the harder it tends to be.
   (4) Fats with many empty spaces in their structure, unfilled with hydrogen, are called *polyunsaturated*.
   a. (1) and (2)
   b. (3) and (4) only
   c. (1), (3), and (4)
   d. (2) and (4)

Suggestions for additional study

1. Place pictures of foods containing visible fat on one page of your notebook and pictures of foods containing invisible fat on another page.
2. An average person will consume approximately 90 g of fat, whereas a person with a low-to-moderate fat intake will use approximately 45 g. Illustrate this point by placing 6 tbs (90 g) of a concentrated fat in one jar and 3 tbs (45 g) in another. Discuss the difference from a health and a caloric standpoint (90 g of fat will contain 810 calories, whereas 45 g will contain only 405 calories).
3. Plan your family's meals for 1 day using as little fat as possible. Describe how you would prepare and serve the food to avoid fat.

Suggested readings

Guthrie, H.A.: Introductory nutrition, ed. 5, St. Louis, 1983, The C.V. Mosby Co.
Williams, S.R.: Nutrition and diet therapy, ed. 4, St. Louis, 1981, The C.V. Mosby Co.
Williams, S.R.: Essentials of nutrition and diet therapy, ed. 3, St. Louis, 1982, The C.V. Mosby Co.

5

Energy requirements

BODY ENERGY NEEDS

Energy is needed whenever any work is performed by the body. These actions can be either voluntary or involuntary.

VOLUNTARY WORK AND EXERCISE. Voluntary work by the body includes all those physical activities related to an individual's usual activities, as well as any additional exercise that is done.

INVOLUNTARY BODY WORK. Involuntary body work includes all those activities that go on in the body and that are not consciously performed. These activities include circulation, respiration, digestion, absorption, and other internal activities related to maintaining life.

SOURCES OF FUEL. The energy needed for voluntary and involuntary body work requires fuel. The only nutrients that are burned as body fuel to supply energy are carbohydrate and fat, with protein available as additional fuel as needed. None of the other nutrients has this capability. The body must be supplied with these fuels in the form of food in sufficient amounts to provide energy for work and to keep the body warm. If sufficient food to supply the energy requirements and to furnish heat for the body is not consumed, the body will then borrow from its reserve fat. The average daily food intake should equal the daily energy requirements, except in obesity, in which the intake should be less than the daily energy needs to burn up the surplus fatty tissue.

MEASUREMENT OF ENERGY

CALORIE. In common usage the calorie is the measure of body heat energy that is produced by the burning or oxidation of food. To be more specific, the term *kilocalorie* is sometimes used to designate the large calorie used in nutritional science. In the metric system the unit measure for energy is called the *joule*.

FUEL FACTORS OF ENERGY NUTRIENTS. The three energy nutrients, carbohydrate, fat, and protein as a backup source, have basic fuel factors:

Carbohydrate	4 calories per gram
Fat	9 calories per gram
Protein	4 calories per gram

ENERGY BALANCE

The total overall energy balance in the body is determined by a measure of the energy intake against a measure of the energy output. The body weight then reflects the condition of this balance.

Energy intake

The source of energy for all body work, as indicated, is food. In the foods consumed the three energy nutrients provide the fuel for the body to burn to meet its energy requirements.

Energy output

Humans spend the energy from their food in all the necessary activities of the various organs of the body, mechanical work, regulation of body temperature, and the processes of growth and repair of the body. The total chemical changes that occur during all of these activities are called *metabolism*. This exchange of energy in overall energy balance is usually expressed in calories or, more correctly, in kilocalories (kcal). The energy output of the body is determined by three demands for energy: physical activity, basal metabolism, and effect of food.

PHYSICAL ACTIVITY. For the voluntary work of the body the number of calories required depends largely on the degree of physical activity. The body weight of the person is also a determining factor. Mental work, however, does not require calories. The fatigue a person doing mental work may feel is caused not by the brain work itself but by muscle tensions and movements associated with the process. The varying amounts of calories needed for different activities for an average woman weighing 130 pounds (58.5 kg), for example, are shown in Table 5-1. Every movement, even a slight one, calls for calories to be used. Two individuals may do the same job, yet one will burn more calories than the other because of wasted motions or variances in metabolic need.

BASAL METABOLISM. Energy is needed constantly for the work of the body, even when the body is at rest. A test previously used to determine the basal metabolic rate (BMR) was taken when a person was at complete rest, although awake, in a room where the temperature was comfortable, 12 hours after any food had been consumed, and several hours after strenuous exercise. In this test the normal BMR would vary somewhat according to the size and shape of the body, the age of the person, and the degree of activity of the thyroid gland. Currently, however, the test used for determining thyroid gland activity and consequently BMRs is the measure of the thyroid hormones in the blood. Two

Table 5-1. Calories needed for an average woman during different activities

Form of activity	Calories per hour, including basal needs
Sleeping	56
Sitting quietly	85
Standing relaxed	90
Standing at attention	96
Light exercise	143
Active exercise	244
Walking moderately fast	254
Walking downstairs	307
Walking upstairs	935

compounds are measured: T_4 (total serum thyroxine) and T_3 (the prethyroxine compound in the serum). A measure then called the *free thyroxine index* is the product of these two hormone measures ($T_3 \times T_4$). Since the thyroid hormone, or thyroxine, is the controlling agent of the body's overall metabolic rate, these blood measures provide a much more easily determined test for basal metabolism.

The average basal energy requirement for a man is about 1650 calories daily and for a woman 1350 calories daily. For a particular individual the basal energy requirement may be calculated with the following formula: 1 calorie per kilogram of body weight (weight in pounds divided by 2.2) per hour.

EFFECT OF FOOD. Any time food is consumed, an increase in energy needs results. This energy is required for the digestion, absorption, and transportation of the nutrients in the foods consumed. This effect, requiring additional energy, has been referred to as the *specific dynamic effect* of food, or more recently as *dietary thermogenesis*. Although hard evidence of precise need is undetermined, it is still generally believed that the effect of food on body energy requirements amounts to about 10% of the total energy needed for both basal metabolism and activity.

Weight maintenance

The body weight, as indicated, reflects the energy balance. However, it is difficult to determine what an ideal body weight is for a specific individual because these weights vary widely. Newer concepts of body weight are taking this individual variance into account.

IDEAL BODY WEIGHT. An estimate of the energy needs of a moderately active woman may be made by allowing 18 calories per pound of ideal weight and of a moderately active man by allowing 20.5 calories per pound of ideal weight. For the man who is doing strenuous labor the allowance may need to

Table 5-2. Gradual reduction of calorie needs during adulthood, in added percent decreases for each decade past the age of 25

Age	Calorie reduction for maintenance of ideal weight (%)
30-40	3.0
40-50	3.0
50-60	7.5
60-70	7.5
70-80	10.0

Table 5-3. Approximate caloric allowances for ages 1 month to 19 years

Age	Calories per pound	Age	Calories per pound
Infants		Boys	
1-3 mo	54.5	13-15 yr	30.0
4-9 mo	49.5	16-19 yr	25.5
10-12 mo	45.5	Girls	
Children		13-15 yr	24.3
1-3 yr	45.0	16-19 yr	20.0
4-6 yr	40.0		
7-9 yr	40.0		
10-12 yr	32.0		

be raised to as high as 28 calories for each pound of ideal body weight. The calculation for a woman follows:

$$\begin{array}{r} \text{Ideal weight of woman} = \quad 120 \text{ pounds (54 kg)} \\ \underline{\times\, 18} \\ 2160 \text{ calories} \end{array}$$

Thus 2160 calories are usually needed by a woman weighing 120 pounds (54 kg) to maintain her present weight if she is moderately active. If by necessity or choice she becomes less active, she will need to lower her caloric intake accordingly. Energy needs can be estimated only approximately because of the varying amounts of time spent in activity and resting. Currently the traditional height-weight charts have been modified somewhat to make allowance for these variables.

A person's ideal weight at 25 years of age should be maintained throughout life. As the adult grows older the caloric intake needs to be gradually reduced from 30 years of age onward to maintain this ideal weight. Table 5-2 gives an approximation of this need for gradual calorie reduction as a person grows older. Energy requirements for children are greater per pound than those for adults.

Table 5-4. Mean heights and weights and recommended energy intake*

Category	Age (years)	Weight kg	Weight lb	Height cm	Height in	Energy needs (with range) kcal	Energy needs (with range) MJ
Infants	0.0-0.5	6	13	60	24	kg × 115 (95-145)	kg × .48
	0.5-1.0	9	20	71	28	kg × 105 (80-135)	kg × .44
Children	1-3	13	29	90	35	1300 (900-1800)	5.5
	4-6	20	44	112	44	1700 (1300-2300)	7.1
	7-10	28	62	132	52	2400 (1650-3300)	10.1
Males	11-14	45	99	157	62	2700 (2000-3700)	11.3
	15-18	66	145	176	69	2800 (2100-3900)	11.8
	19-22	70	154	177	70	2900 (2500-3300)	12.2
	23-50	70	154	178	70	2700 (2300-3100)	11.3
	51-75	70	154	178	70	2400 (2000-2800)	10.1
	76+	70	154	178	70	2050 (1650-2450)	8.6
Females	11-14	46	101	157	62	2200 (1500-3000)	9.2
	15-18	55	120	163	64	2100 (1200-3000)	8.8
	19-22	55	120	163	64	2100 (1700-2500)	8.8
	23-50	55	120	163	64	2000 (1600-2400)	8.4
	51-75	55	120	163	64	1800 (1400-2200)	7.6
	76+	55	120	163	64	1600 (1200-2000)	6.7
Pregnancy						+300	
Lactation						+500	

From Food and Nutrition Board, National Academy of Sciences–National Research Council: Recommended dietary allowances, Washington, D.C., 1980, The Academy.

*The data in this table have been assembled from the observed median heights and weights of children shown in Table 1-2, together with desirable weights for adults given in Table B for the mean heights of men (70 inches) and women (64 inches) between the ages of 18 and 34 years as surveyed in the U.S. population (HEW/NCHS data).

The energy allowances for the young adults are for men and women doing light work. The allowances for the two older age groups represent mean energy needs over these age spans, allowing for a 2% decrease in basal (resting) metabolic rate per decade and a reduction in activity of 200 kcal/day for men and women between 51 and 75 years, 500 kcal for men over 75 years, and 400 kcal for women over 75. The customary range of daily energy output is shown for adults in parentheses and is based on a variation in energy needs of ± 400 kcal at any one age (see text and Garrow, 1978), emphasizing the wide range of energy intakes appropriate for any group of people.

Energy allowances for children through age 18 are based on median energy intakes of children these ages observed in longitudinal growth studies. The values in parentheses are 10th and 90th percentiles of energy intake, to indicate the range of energy consumption among children of these ages.

The approximate calorie allowances per pound for the various age groups are presented in Table 5-3. There should be gradual addition of calories from one age group to another as a child grows older.

Newer concepts of body weight

More recently, however, it has been recognized that persons consuming the same amount of food maintain greatly different weights, or even that an overweight person may actually require fewer calories for weight maintenance than a thinner person. This has led researchers to study more carefully the so-called set point theory of body weight. The theory holds that some persons are "programmed" by their genetic makeup to maintain a greater amount of body weight. However, increased exercise can lower this "set point" for an individual, and thus increased physical activity assumes a larger emphasis in any weight management program.

ENERGY REQUIREMENTS

RECOMMENDED DIETARY ALLOWANCES (RDA). The RDAs for energy needs at all ages are given in Table 5-4. As indicated, these allowances are based on estimates of need for population groups. Individual needs within these age groups may vary widely. A recognition of this variance is shown in the RDA table in the wide variance of total calories recommended for each of the age groups.

U.S. DIETARY GOALS. Energy needs are indicated in two ways in the U.S. Dietary Goals. First, there is a recommendation for maintenance of ideal body weight and the avoidance of obesity as a health measure. Second, there is a recommendation for reduced use of fat, the most concentrated source of calories in the diet, as a means of controlling total calories in the diet. The recommendation for limited use of simple carbohydrates or sweets would also help in this management of excess calories. Instead of fats and sweets, complex carbohydrates are recommended as the major fuel source.

Questions on energy requirements

1. What is the difference between voluntary and involuntary actions of the body?
2. When is it advisable to have the daily food intake less than the daily energy requirements?
3. How many calories does 1 g of carbohydrate produce? One g of protein? One g of fat?
4. What is meant by the basal metabolism rate? How is it usually measured?
5. What are some of the causes of normal variations in the basal rate in different persons?
6. What is the average basal energy requirement for a man? For a woman?
7. Does mental work increase caloric needs?
8. Determine the number of calories needed by a woman whose ideal weight is 130 pounds (58.5 kg)
9. Calculate the number of calories needed by a 175-pound (78.7 kg) man at hard labor.

True-false

Circle *T* if a statement is true. Circle *F* if it is false, and then write the correct statement.

T   F   1. Calories are nutrients in foods.
T   F   2. Thyroid hormone controls the rate of overall body metabolism.
T   F   3. Energy requirements for children are less per pound than for adults because they are smaller in size.
T   F   4. Mental work requires extra calories.
T   F   5. Different persons doing the same amount of physical activity will all require the same number of calories.

Multiple choice

Circle the letter in front of the correct answer.

1. In human nutrition the calorie, or the kilocalorie, is used:
   a. to provide nutrients
   b. to measure body heat energy
   c. to control energy reactions
   d. as a measure of electrical energy
2. In this family of four, who has the highest energy needs per unit of body weight?
   a. the 32-year-old mother
   b. the 2-month-old son
   c. the 35-year-old father
   d. the 70-year-old grandmother
3. Which of the following foods has the highest energy value per unit of weight?
   a. potato
   b. bread
   c. meat
   d. butter
4. If a slice of bread contains 2 g of protein and 15 g of carbohydrate in the form of starch, which is its calorie value?
   a. 17 calories
   b. 42 calories
   c. 68 calories
   d. 92 calories
5. Which of the following persons is using the most energy?
   a. a woman walking uphill
   b. a student studying for final examinations
   c. a teenager playing basketball
   d. a man driving a car

Suggestions for additional study

1. Figure the number of calories you would need to maintain your own ideal weight.
2. If the composition of one slice of bread is 2 g of protein, 1 g of fat, and 12 g of carbohydrate, what is the caloric value of that slice of bread?
3. Figure the caloric value of the following:

Food	Grams carbohydrate	Grams protein	Grams fat	Calories
1 cup milk	12	8	10	_____
¼ pint vanilla ice cream	15	3	9	_____
½ cup cooked carrots	7	2	0	_____
½ small grapefruit	10	0	0	_____

Suggested readings

Bennett, W., and Gurin, J.: The dieter's dilemma, New York, 1982, Basic Books, Inc. *A discussion of the "set point" theory of body weight.*

Food and Nutrition Board, National Academy of Sciences–National Research Council: Recommended dietary allowances, Washington, D.C., 1980, The Academy.

Guthrie, H.A.: Introductory nutrition, ed. 5, St. Louis, 1983, The C.V. Mosby Co.

Williams, S.R.: Nutrition and diet therapy, ed. 4, St. Louis, 1981, The C.V. Mosby Co.

Williams, S.R.: Essentials of nutrition and diet therapy, ed. 3, St. Louis, 1982, The C.V. Mosby Co.

6

Vitamins

THE NATURE OF VITAMINS

Vitamins are organic compounds that regulate metabolism and make possible more efficient use of carbohydrate, protein, and fat within the body. Vitamins themselves are totally lacking in caloric value. They are like the ignition spark, which furnishes no fuel but keeps the motor running in an orderly fashion. Two characteristics of these compounds identify them as vitamins: (1) they cannot be synthesized by the body, and (2) they are necessary substances to control specific cell metabolism functions. Thus on the basis of both of these characteristics vitamins are essential to life. The amount of these materials required by the body is usually very small, unless some special state or condition has created a greater need in a particular individual. The total volume of vitamins that a healthy person would normally require would barely fill a teaspoon. However, these materials are essential to existence.

THE DISCOVERY OF VITAMINS

The history of vitamin discoveries is largely related to work on cures for classic disease states believed to be related to deficiencies in the diet. For example, as early as 1753, Dr. James Lind, a surgeon in the British navy, discovered that scurvy, the curse of sailors, was caused by some dietary deficiency. On long voyages the sailors were forced to live on very limited rations, since no fresh foods were available. It was learned that when certain fresh foods, such as lemons and limes, were given to the sailors, no one had scurvy. Thus originated the nickname of "limeys" for British sailors.

Later, in 1906, Dr. Frederich Hopkins, working at Cambridge University in England, performed an experiment in which he fed a group of white rats a diet consisting of a synthetic mixture of protein, fat, carbohydrate, mineral salts, and water. As a result, the animals became sick and died. With the next group, Dr. Hopkins added milk to the purified ration, and the rats all lived and grew normally. Thus an important discovery was made—that there are accessory food factors present in *natural* foods that in some way are essential to life. Much additional research followed this early work to make possible the knowledge about vitamins from which persons benefit today.

GENERAL FUNCTIONS OF VITAMINS

Although each vitamin has specific functions, two general functions may be ascribed to vitamins as a group: control of cell metabolism and structure of body tissue.

CONTROL AGENT: COENZYME PARTNER. For basic chemical reactions to occur in the cells, many of them require the presence of a partner to the main enzyme regulating the reaction. In chemical reactions an enzyme is a necessary material to control the reaction by acting as a catalyst. In many of the cell reactions a vitamin is also required as a specific coenzyme factor. Together these two substances allow the reaction to proceed. For example, several of the B-complex vitamins—thiamin, niacin, and riboflavin—are essential components of the cell enzyme systems that metabolize glucose to produce energy.

STRUCTURAL MATERIALS. Some of the vitamins also function as components related to tissue building. For example, vitamin C (ascorbic acid) helps to deposit a cementlike substance in the intercellular spaces to produce strong tissue. This material is sometimes called a "ground substance" and is similar to collagen. In fact the word *collagen* comes from a Greek word meaning "glue."

VITAMIN DEFICIENCY STATES

The word *deficiency* is usually used to indicate varying degrees of shortages of various nutrients. For example, a deficiency of an essential substance may be mild, moderate, severe, or complete. Deficiency diseases are usually the result of deficiencies in more than one vitamin or other essential food factor. Subclinical deficiency states, which precede frank vitamin deficiency diseases, usually cause such vague symptoms that they are seldom brought to the attention of a physician or clinical nutritionist. If these early warning signs are heeded, more serious illness may often be avoided.

Only vitamins A and D are stored in the body in any quantity, primarily in the liver. Other vitamins are stored in such small amounts, or excreted readily, that it is important for all persons to be certain that they have an adequate intake of each of the vitamins every day. Usually this intake can be ensured by a well-balanced diet. However, in some situations, such as during pregnancy or nutritional rehabilitation in malnourished states, added vitamin supplements are necessary.

CLASSIFICATION OF VITAMINS

Vitamins are usually classified on the basis of their solubility as either fat soluble or water soluble. Although this is a somewhat arbitrary grouping with little real significance, the traditional classification will be used here. The fat-soluble vitamins are A, D, E, and K. The water-soluble vitamins are C (ascorbic acid) and the family of B vitamins.

Fat-soluble vitamins

VITAMIN A

Functions. Vitamin A performs the following functions in the body:

1. It maintains the mucous membranes in the nose, throat, alimentary tract, eyes, and genitourinary tract in a healthy condition. A lack of vitamin A will aggravate an infection that may be present in the bronchial tubes, sinuses, or lungs.
2. It is essential in regenerating visual purple in the eye, a substance necessary for good vision. A mild deficiency in vitamin A will manifest itself by night blindness, slow adaptation to darkness, or glare blindness.
3. It is essential to growth. For example, lack of vitamin A, especially in growing children, retards skeletal growth.
4. It prevents xerosis, which is caused by a deficiency in vitamin A and is characterized by itching and burning of the eyes, with redness of the lids and some inflammation.
5. It prevents xerophthalmia, which is caused by severe deficiency in vitamin A and which often produces permanent blindness before the disease can be controlled.

Human requirements. The recommended daily allowance for the average adult is 800 μg RE (retinol equivalents) for women and 1000 μg for men. The recommended daily allowance for a pregnant woman is 1000 μg RE during pregnancy and 1200 μg RE during lactation.

Recommended daily allowances for children follow:

Birth-6 mo	420 μg RE	7-10 yr	700 μg RE
6 mo-1 yr	400 μg RE	11-22 yr	
1-3 yr	400 μg RE	Males	1000 μg RE
4-6 yr	500 μg RE	Females	800 μg RE

Sources. Among the best sources of preformed vitamin A (retinol) are fish liver oils, liver, egg yolk, butter, and cream. Carotene is a pigment in dark green and yellow vegetables and fruits that is changed into vitamin A within the body. Some good sources of carotene are carrots, leafy green vegetables, yellow corn, sweet potatoes, apricots, and peaches. Both carotene and preformed vitamin A require the presence of bile salts for proper absorption in the intestine. In the absence of bile, carotene and vitamin A are not absorbed from the intestinal tract unless bile salts are administered orally. The bile salts act as an antioxidant to protect and stabilize the easily oxidized vitamin, and they also provide a vehicle of transport through the intestinal wall.

Stability. Vitamin A is unstable in heat in contact with air. Cooking vegetables in an open kettle is more destructive to vitamin A than heating the product in a pan with a lid.

Heating for a shorter time at a higher temperature is less destructive to the vitamin than heating for a longer period at a lower temperature.

If fats are rancid or vegetables are wilted, the majority of vitamin A has been destroyed.

VITAMIN D

Functions. The following body functions are performed by vitamin D:

1. It is essential in the proper absorption and metabolism of calcium and phosphorus to produce normal growth of bone structures. However, vitamin D does not decrease the requirements for calcium and phosphorus.

2. In adequate amounts it prevents rickets in children, provided that there is also enough calcium and phosphorus in the diet. In rickets the bones become pliable, and deformities such as bowlegs and knock-knees occur when children begin to walk. The long bones of arms and legs are usually the ones most affected, and a roentgenogram (x-ray picture) will show incomplete calcification on the ends of these bones. Profuse sweating and restlessness are early symptoms of rickets in infants. However, growth may not be retarded, and infants may outwardly appear to be in perfect health, but when they start to walk, the deficiency will be manifested. The same deficiency usually leads to malformation of teeth that are forming in the gums.

Human requirements. The recommended daily allowance is 10 μg cholecalciferol for all persons up to 18 years of age and 10 to 15 μg for pregnant and lactating women. An adult does not outgrow the need for vitamin D. However, if people eat balanced diets and have general exposure to sunlight, they will surely receive a sufficient amount of vitamin D.

Sources. Small but nutritionally insignificant amounts are present in cream, butter, eggs, and liver. Good sources are fish liver oils, milk enriched with vitamin D, and exposure to sunlight under favorable conditions.

One quart of milk enriched with vitamin D contains 400 IU of vitamin D (10 μg cholecalciferol), which is the recommended daily amount for children of all ages. Milk is a very logical product to which vitamin D can be added because milk is also an excellent source of calcium and phosphorus.

Stability. Vitamin D is very stable in heat, during aging, and in storage.

VITAMIN E

Functions. Although exact mechanisms are unclear, recent studies indicate several significant functions of vitamin E in relation to human metabolism:

1. It is an effective antioxidant and as such is being used in commercial

products to retard spoilage. It is added to therapeutic forms of vitamin A to protect the vitamin from oxidizing before it is absorbed.

2. It seems to preserve the integrity of red blood cells by protecting them from breakdown of their cell walls. Vitamin E therapy has effectively controlled certain anemias in infants.
3. It may also protect the structure and function of muscle tissue. Various stages and forms of muscle degeneration and lesions have been found in patients with low plasma vitamin E levels, for example, patients with cystic fibrosis or kwashiorkor.
4. It protects unsaturated essential fatty acids, such as linoleic acid, from oxidative breakdown. The amount of vitamin E required by people has been directly linked with the amount of polyunsaturated fatty acids in their diets.

Human requirements. Vitamin E is clearly an essential nutrient. In recognition of this fact the National Research Council made a statement in 1968 concerning vitamin E requirements for the first time and continued it in the 1980 revision of the Recommended Dietary Allowances (RDA). The RDA (in α-tocopherol equivalents) for men is 10 mg daily and for women 8 mg., increased to 10 mg during pregnancy and 11 mg during lactation. Children's needs range from 3 to 4 mg for infants, 5 to 7 mg for young children, and 8 to 10 mg for boys and girls 10 to 18 years of age.

Sources. The richest sources of vitamin E are the vegetable oils. It is interesting that they are also the richest sources of polyunsaturated fatty acids, which vitamin E protects. Other food sources include milk, eggs, muscle meats, fish, cereals, and leafy vegetables.

Stability. Vitamin E is stable to heat and also to acids but not to alkalis. It is insoluble in water.

VITAMIN K

Functions. Vitamin K is essential in clotting of the blood, since it is necessary to the formation of prothrombin, the clotting agent in blood. This vitamin is often used in the control and prevention of certain types of hemorrhages.

Vitamin K is absorbed more completely if bile salts are also present. Patients in whom the flow of bile to the intestines is reduced usually have blood with low clotting ability. However, if bile salts are given with vitamin K concentrate, the clotting time becomes normal.

Human requirements. For most people the intestinal bacteria normally synthesize a constant supply. As yet there is no general agreement on the amount of vitamin K needed by the body.

Vitamin K is usually given to a mother before delivery and to an infant immediately after birth as a precautionary measure.

Sources. Small amounts of vitamin K are found in green leafy vegetables, pork liver, and soybean and other vegetable oils. The main source, however,

Table 6-1. A summary of fat-soluble vitamins

Vitamin	Function	Results of deficiency	Food sources
A (retinol); provitamin A (carotene)	Vision cycle—adaptation to light and dark; tissue growth, especially skin and mucous membranes; toxic in large amounts	Night blindness, xerophthalmia, susceptibility to epithelial infection, changes in skin and membranes and in tooth formation	Retinol (animal food): liver, egg yolk, cream, butter or fortified margarine, whole milk; carotene (plant foods): green and yellow vegetables, fruits
D (calciferol)	Absorption of calcium and phosphorus, calcification of bones; toxic in large amounts	Rickets, faulty bone growth, poor tooth development	Fortified or irradiated milk, sunshine, fish oils
E (tocopherol)	Antioxidant—protection of materials that oxidize easily; normal growth; reproduction (in animals)	Protection of Vitamin A and unsaturated fatty acids, breakdown of red blood cells, anemia, sterility (in rats)	Vegetable oils, vegetable greens
K (menadione)	Normal blood clotting; toxic in large amounts	Bleeding tendencies, hemorrhagic disease	Green leafy vegetables, cheese, egg yolk, liver; intestinal bacteria synthesis—main source

is that of intestinal bacteria synthesis. Usually a deficiency in vitamin K is the result of poor absorption.

Stability. Vitamin K is fairly stable, although sensitive to light and irradiation. Thus clinical preparations of vitamin K should be kept in dark bottles.

A summary of the fat-soluble vitamins is given in Table 6-1.

Water-soluble vitamins

VITAMIN C (ASCORBIC ACID)

Functions. Vitamin C performs or assists in the performance of the following body functions:

1. It is essential in the formation and maintenance of the capillary walls.
2. It is essential in the normal healing of wounds and is frequently given following surgical procedures.
3. It prevents the tendency to bleed easily. Pinpoint hemorrhages under the skin, which show up as black-and-blue spots, indicate a lack of vitamin C.
4. It prevents scurvy, which is caused by an extreme deficiency of vitamin C. The symptoms are loss of appetite, skin tender to touch, sore mouth with bleeding gums and loosened teeth, black-and-blue spots on the skin, and tenderness of the knee joints.

5. It aids in cementing body cells together and in strengthening the walls of the blood vessels.
6. It helps to guard against infection by stimulating white blood cells.
7. It is necessary in forming new tissue and regenerating existing tissue.
8. It is implicated in preventing fatigue, since lack of ascorbic acid results in the extreme fatigue that occurs after strenuous exercise.
9. It increases the amount of iron absorbed when food is ingested simultaneously.

Human requirements. Vitamin C recommendations were changed in the National Research Council's 1980 RDA revisions. The optimum requirements are 60 mg for the average man and woman. In women the need is 80 mg during pregnancy and 100 mg during lactation.

For children and adolescents the requirements are as follows:

Birth-1 yr	35 mg
1-10 yr	45 mg
11-14 yr	50 mg
15-18 yr	60 mg

Sources. The best sources are citrus fruits. Additional sources include tomatoes, cabbage and other raw leafy vegetables, strawberries, melons, and potatoes. Potatoes are not so high in vitamin C as some of the other sources, but because of the quantity in which they are consumed, they serve as a valuable source.

Stability. Vitamin C is easily destroyed by heat and exposure to air. Because an alkaline medium is very destructive to vitamin C, soda should never be

Table 6-2. A summary of vitamin C (ascorbic acid)

Functions	Clinical applications	Food sources
Intercellular cement substance; firm capillary walls and collagen formation	Scurvy (deficiency disease)	Citrus fruits, tomatoes, cabbage, potatoes, strawberries, melons, chili peppers, broccoli, chard, turnip greens, green peppers, asparagus
	Sore gums	
Helps prepare iron for absorption and release to tissues for red blood cell formation	Hemorrhages, especially around bones	
	Tendency to bruise easily	
	Stress reactions	
	Growth periods	
	Fevers and infections	
	Wound healing, tissue formation	
	Anemia	

added to food when it is cooked. Acid fruits and vegetables retain their vitamin C content more completely than nonacid fruits and vegetables.

Vitamin C is very soluble in water; therefore only small amounts of water should be used for cooking. Vegetables should not be cut into small pieces until one is ready to cook them, because the more surface exposed to air, the greater is the destruction of vitamin C.

A summary of the functions, clinical applications, and food sources of vitamin C (ascorbic acid) is given in Table 6-2.

THE B-COMPLEX VITAMINS. The large family of B vitamins are all water soluble. Each of them performs specific tasks in the body metabolism and is a unique separate substance. However, for general discussion here, they may be grouped according to function as classic deficiency disease factors, more recently discovered coenzyme factors, and cell growth and blood-forming factors.

Classic deficiency disease factors

THIAMIN

Functions. Thiamin performs or assists in the performance of the following body functions:

1. It is essential in maintaining good muscle tone, good nerves, and good function of the digestive system. Lack of adequate thiamin is usually accompanied by diminished gastric secretion.
2. It is essential in the metabolism of carbohydrate in the body. The amount of thiamin that is needed is in proportion to the amount of calories consumed; 0.5 mg for each 1000 calories is considered adequate. Therefore in the diet of an average man 1.5 mg of thiamin would be adequate for a 3000-calorie diet.
3. It prevents beriberi, which is the manifestation of a severe deficiency of thiamin.
4. It helps maintain a healthy appetite and general well-being. A mild deficiency may cause loss of appetite, certain forms of constipation, poor muscular tone of the intestines, fatigue, and irritability.

Human requirements. The Food and Nutrition Board recommends 1.2 to 1.5 mg for the average man and 1 to 1.1 mg for the average woman, increased during pregnancy and lactation to 1.4 to 1.6 mg.

Men doing hard physical work especially need the optimum amount of thiamin daily, or they will show physical exhaustion.

The recommended amounts for children follow:

Infants	
Birth-6 mo	0.3 mg
6 mo-1 yr	0.5 mg
Children	
1-3 yr	0.7 mg
4-6 yr	0.9 mg
6-10 yr	1.2 mg
Boys 11-14 yr	1.4 mg

Girls 11-14 yr	1.1 mg
Boys 15-18 yr	1.4 mg
Girls 15-18 yr	1.1 mg

Sources. Thiamin is present in wheat germ, pork, liver and other organ meats, enriched or whole-grain bread and cereals, and potatoes.

Stability. Thiamin is destroyed by prolonged heating at a high temperature. An alkaline medium is also destructive to thiamin. Thiamin is very soluble in water; therefore small amounts of water should be used in cooking vegetables. Thiamin in cooked cereals is retained because the water is retained with the cereal.

NIACIN (NICOTINIC ACID)

Functions. Niacin performs or assists in the performance of the following body functions:

1. It forms a part of certain enzymes.
2. It is essential to growth and to the metabolism of carbohydrate.
3. It is necessary to the normal function of the digestive tract and the nervous system.
4. It prevents pellagra, which is manifested by dermatitis, diarrhea, dementia, weakness, vertigo, and anorexia. Before the practice of cereal enrichment began, pellagra occurred most frequently among underprivileged persons in southern states where the diet consisted largely of cornmeal, molasses, and salt pork. When therapeutic doses of niacin and a balanced diet are given, pellagra clears up.

Human requirements. The amount recommended by the Food and Nutrition Board is 16 to 19 mg niacin equivalents for the average man and 13 to 14 mg for the average woman, increased to 15 or 16 mg during pregnancy and to 18 or 19 mg during lactation.

The recommended amounts for infants and children follow:

Infants	
Birth-6 mo	6 mg
6 mo-1 yr	8 mg
Children	
1-3 yr	9 mg
4-6 yr	11 mg
7-10 yr	16 mg
Boys 11-14 yr	18 mg
Girls 11-14 yr	15 mg
Boys 15-18 yr	18 mg
Girls 15-18 yr	14 mg

Sources. Niacin is present largely in meat, poultry, fish, peanut butter, brown rice, and whole-grain breads and cereals. Niacin is also formed from the amino acid tryptophan (60 mg of tryptophan equals 1 mg of niacin). Thus this amount of tryptophan is called a niacin equivalent.

Stability. Niacin is unusually stable and withstands both heat and contact with oxygen. However, it is soluble in water, and large amounts of niacin may be discarded with the water in which vegetables are cooked.

RIBOFLAVIN (VITAMIN B₂)

Functions. Riboflavin is a part of the following body functions:

1. It plays a part in maintaining healthy eyes. A deficiency causes itching and burning of the eyes, sensitivity to light, and headaches.
2. It forms a part of certain enzymes.
3. It is active in maintaining the color and structural tissue of the lips. A deficiency causes the lips to be pale and to split at the corners of the mouth.
4. It is essential to growth.

Human requirements. The Food and Nutrition Board recommends 1.6 mg for the average man and 1.2 mg for the average woman, increased to 1.5 mg during pregnancy and to 1.7 mg during lactation.

The recommended amounts for infants and children follow:

Infants	
Birth-6 mo	0.4 mg
6 mo-1 yr	0.6 mg
Children	
1-3 yr	0.8 mg
4-6 yr	1.0 mg
7-10 yr	1.4 mg
Boys 11-14 yr	1.6 mg
Girls 11-14 yr	1.3 mg
Boys 15-18 yr	1.7 mg
Girls 15-18 yr	1.3 mg

Sources. The most important source of riboflavin is milk. Each quart contains 2 mg. Other sources include organ meats, green leafy vegetables, eggs, enriched bread, and cereals.

Stability. Riboflavin in solution, such as in milk, is rapidly destroyed by light. Milk should not be left outside after delivery unless it is in a dark bottle or paper container. Moreover, for obvious reasons, milk should be refrigerated promptly.

More recently discovered coenzyme factors

PYRIDOXINE (VITAMIN B₆)

Functions. The following body functions are performed by pyridoxine:

1. It is involved in the conversion of tryptophan to niacin.
2. It helps to prevent muscular weakness and certain nervous disorders.

3. It aids in various interconversions of amino acids.

4. It supplies increased metabolic demands during pregnancy.

Human requirements. For the first time, in its 1968 RDAs the National Research Council made a statement concerning pyridoxine requirements and continued it in the 1980 revisions. The recommendation for adults is 2 mg/day for women and 2.2 mg/day for men to assure a margin of safety for variances in individual needs. Children's needs range progressively from 0.3 mg for infants to 1.8 mg for adolescents.

Sources. It occurs freely in many different foods, including pork, glandular meats, lamb, and veal. Lesser amounts are found in fish, beef, legumes, potatoes, oatmeal, bananas, cabbage, and carrots.

Stability. Pyridoxine is stable in heat but it is soluble in water and is sensitive to light and alkalis.

PANTOTHENIC ACID

Functions. Pantothenic acid assists in the performance of the following body functions:

1. It is involved in the metabolism of carbohydrate.

2. It is essential in the synthesis and breakdown of fatty acids, sterols, and steroid hormones.

Human requirements. The amount of pantothenic acid necessary for human beings has not yet been determined.

Sources. Pantothenic acid is present in most ordinary food; therefore there should be no deficiency in the average normal diet. Liver, meat, cereal, and milk are reliable sources. A diet of 2500 calories selected from both animal and plant foods would provide approximately 10 mg a day.

Stability. Pantothenic acid is stable in heat but is water soluble and sensitive to alkalis.

Cell growth and blood-forming factors

Major blood "factories" in the bone marrow produce about 1 million new red blood cells every second to replace an equal number that have completed the life span of approximately 4 months. Every budding red blood cell requires two of the B vitamins at vital stages of its growth. These two vitamins are folic acid and vitamin B_{12}.

FOLACIN (FOLIC ACID)

Functions. Folic acid assists in the performance of the following body functions:

1. It is essential in the formation of all body cells, especially the red blood cells.

2. It contributes to the successful treatment of certain types of anemia when used in combination with vitamin B_{12}.

Table 6-3. A summary of selected B-complex vitamins

Vitamin	Function	Results of deficiency*	Food sources
Thiamin (B₁)	Normal growth; coenzyme in carbohydrate metabolism; normal function of heart, nerves, and muscle	Beriberi; GI: loss of appetite, gastric distress, indigestion, deficient hydrochloric acid; CNS: fatigue, neuritis, paralysis; CV: heart failure, edema of legs especially	Pork, beef, liver, whole or enriched grains, legumes
Riboflavin (B₂)	Normal growth and vigor; coenzyme in protein and energy metabolism	Ariboflavinosis; wound aggravation, cracks at corners of mouth, glossitis (smoothness of tongue), eye irritation and sensitivity to light, skin eruptions	Milk, liver, enriched cereals
Niacin (nicotinic acid)—precursor: tryptophan	Coenzyme in energy production; normal growth, health of skin, normal activity of stomach, intestines, and nervous system	Pellagra; weakness, lack of energy, and loss of appetite; skin: scaly dermatitis; CNS: neuritis, confusion	Meat, peanuts, enriched grains
Pyridoxine (B₆)	Coenzyme in amino acid metabolism: protein synthesis, heme formation, brain activity; carrier for amino acid absorption	Anemia; CNS: hyperirritability, convulsions, neuritis	Wheat, corn, meat, liver
Pantothenic acid	Coenzyme in formation of active acetate: fat, cholesterol, and heme formation and amino acid activation	Unlikely because of widespread occurrence and intestinal bacteria synthesis	Liver, eggs, milk, beef, cheese, legumes, broccoli, kale, sweet potatoes, yellow corn; also intestinal bacteria synthesis
Folic acid	Growth and development of red blood cells	Certain types of anemia; megaloblastic (large, immature red blood cells)	Liver, green leafy vegetables, asparagus, eggs
Cobalamin (B₁₂)	Normal red blood cell formation, nerve function, and growth	Pernicious anemia (B₁₂ is necessary extrinsic factor that combines with intrinsic factor of gastric secretions for absorption)	Liver, meats, milk, eggs, cheese

*Key: GI, gastrointestinal; CNS, central nervous system; CV, cardiovascular.

Human requirements. In its 1968 revisions the National Research Council made a statement for the first time about folacin requirements and continued it in the 1980 revisions. The daily allowance for adults is 400 µg. During pregnancy this is raised to 800 µg daily and for lactation to 500 µg. Requirements for children range from 30 µg daily for infants to 400 µg daily for adolescents.

Sources. The main sources of folic acid are liver, meats, fish, nuts, yeast, green vegetables, legumes, eggs, whole grains, and mushrooms.

Stability. Storage and cooking losses are high, regardless of the method of cooking used.

VITAMIN B$_{12}$

Function. Vitamin B$_{12}$ is the extrinsic factor involved in the treatment of pernicious anemia. When administered parenterally, it relieves the many symptoms of pernicious anemia.

Human requirements. For the first time the 1968 revisions of the National Research Council also included daily allowances for vitamin B$_{12}$ and continued them in the 1988 revisions. The council recommends 3 mg daily for adults, with increases for pregnant and lactating women to 4 mg. Requirements for children range from 0.5 mg for infants to 3 mg for adolescents.

Sources. Liver, kidney, and fresh muscle meats are the richest known sources at the present time.

Stability. Since vitamin B$_{12}$ occurs as a protein complex in foods (hence mainly in foods of animal origin), it is stable in ordinary cooking processes.

A summary of the functions, deficiency results, the best food sources of the selected B-complex vitamins previously discussed is given in Table 6-3.

SUMMARY

The average healthy adult requires vitamins but usually does not require vitamin supplements. Vitamins are best purchased at the grocery counter in foods that supply the variety of nutrients needed by the body. A well-balanced diet will provide ample vitamins for usual needs. Therefore the use of supplementary vitamins in addition to an adequate diet is rarely necessary; it is expensive, and in some cases it is dangerous. Vitamins A and D can both be toxic in excessive doses.

Vitamin D taken in excess may cause anorexia, nausea, vomiting, diarrhea, weakness, and weight loss. Also, an excess of calcium may be deposited in the body. An adequate diet should provide enough vitamin A for normal persons. Evidence concerning the toxicity of an excess of vitamin A emphasizes the need for caution in the use of vitamin A and D preparations. Some of the signs of vitamin A toxicity are skin lesions, thinning hair, coarse skin, and often pains in the joints.

The other vitamins are not toxic, but if an excess is taken, it is simply excreted, hence wasted.

Vitamins are essential, but clinical preparations of them should be reserved for states of debilitation, malnutrition, and clinical disease.

Questions on vitamins

1. What are the functions of vitamins in the body?
2. How were vitamins first discovered?
3. What are the fat-soluble vitamins?
4. What are the water-soluble vitamins?
5. What is meant by deficiencies?
6. What is meant by subclinical deficiencies?
7. Which vitamins are humans able to store to any extent?
8. What are the functions of vitamin A?
9. What is the adult requirement of vitamin A?
10. Name some good sources of vitamin A.
11. Name some good sources of carotene.
12. Compare the vitamin value of carotene and of true vitamin A.
13. Discuss the stability of vitamin A.
14. How is a deficiency in vitamin A manifested?
15. What are the functions of vitamin D?
16. Does vitamin D decrease the requirement of calcium and phosphorus?
17. What parts of the body are usually most affected by rickets?
18. What is the average daily requirement of vitamin D?
19. What are the sources of vitamin D?
20. What is one source of vitamin D that will provide an adequate daily intake?
21. Is vitamin D stable?
22. How is a deficiency in vitamin D manifested?
23. What is the function of vitamin K?
24. How does bile affect the absorption of vitamin K?
25. What are the sources of vitamin K?
26. When is vitamin K therapy sometimes used?
27. What are the food sources of vitamin K?
28. What are the functions of vitamin C?
29. What is the daily requirement of vitamin C for adults?
30. What are the food sources of vitamin C?
31. Discuss the stability of vitamin C.
32. How is a deficiency in vitamin C manifested?
33. What are the functions of thiamin?
34. What is the average adult requirement of thiamin?
35. When is it necessary to increase the intake of thiamin?
36. What are some good food sources of thiamin?
37. Discuss the stability of thiamin.
38. What are the results of a deficiency in thiamin?
39. What are the functions of riboflavin?
40. What is the average adult requirement of riboflavin?
41. What are the best food sources of riboflavin?
42. Discuss the stability of riboflavin.

43. What are the results of a deficiency in riboflavin?
44. What are the functions of niacin?
45. What is the average adult requirement of niacin?
46. What are the best food sources of niacin?
47. What are the functions of folic acid?
48. What are the functions of pantothenic acid, and what are its best sources?
49. What is the function of vitamin B$_{12}$, and what are its best sources?
50. What vitamins are toxic if taken in excessive amounts?
51. What occurs if an excess of the other vitamins is taken?

True-false

Circle *T* if the statement is true. Circle *F* if it is false, and then write the correct statement.

T   F   1. A coenzyme acts alone to control a specific metabolic reaction.
T   F   2. Carotene is preformed vitamin A found in animal food sources.
T   F   3. Vitamin A is water soluble and hence is found in the nonfat part of milk.
T   F   4. Vitamin D and sufficient dietary calcium and phosphorus prevent rickets.
T   F   5. When a person is exposed to sunlight, vitamin D can be made from cholesterol in the skin.
T   F   6. There is no danger of toxic amounts of any of the fat-soluble vitamins.
T   F   7. Connective tissue such as collagen requires vitamin C for its formation.
T   F   8. Extra vitamin C is stored in the liver to meet the demands of tissue infections.
T   F   9. Freshly squeezed orange juice may be kept indefinitely in the refrigerator without any loss of vitamin C.
T   F   10. Beriberi is caused by a lack of thiamin.
T   F   11. The deficiency disease associated with the discovery of niacin is pellagra.

Multiple choice

Circle the letter in front of the correct answer.

1. Vitamin A is a fat-soluble vitamin produced by humans from its precursor carotene, a green and yellow plant pigment, or consumed as the fully formed vitamin A in animal food sources. Hence the main sources of this vitamin include:
   (1) skimmed milk
   (2) leafy green vegetables
   (3) carrots
   (4) oranges
   (5) butter
   (6) tomatoes
   a. (1), (2), and (4)
   b. (2), (3), and (5)
   c. (1), (3), and (6)
   d. (3), (4), and (5)
2. If you found that one of your patients was lacking in vitamin C, which of the following foods would you suggest that could be added or increased in the diet?
   a. potatoes, enriched cereals, and fortified margarine
   b. liver, other organ meats, and beef
   c. milk, eggs, and cheese
   d. citrus fruit, tomatoes, cabbage, green peppers, broccoli, and spinach

Suggestions for additional study

1. Prepare a chart showing the principal functions, sources, and requirements of each of the vitamins discussed in this chapter.
2. On one page of your notebook put illustrations of foods that will provide an adequate supply of these vitamins for 1 day.
3. Prepare a report on the work of Dr. Joseph Goldberger in his search for the cause of pellagra.

Suggested readings

Guthrie, H.A.: Introductory nutrition, ed. 5, St. Louis, 1983, The C.V. Mosby Co.

Williams, S.R.: Nutrition and diet therapy, ed. 4, St. Louis, 1981, The C.V. Mosby Co.

Williams, S.R.: Essentials of nutrition and diet therapy, ed. 3, St. Louis, 1982, The C.V. Mosby Co.

7

Minerals

MINERALS IN THE BODY
Amount

Body minerals are usually classified according to the amount of each in the body composition. Seven minerals found in the largest amounts are called major minerals: calcium, phosphorus, potassium, sulfur, sodium, chloride, and magnesium. A much larger number of minerals are found in the body in extremely small amounts and are thus called trace minerals. These 14 trace elements that have been established as essential for human nutrition: iron, zinc, selenium, manganese, copper, iodine, molybdenum, cobalt, chromium, fluorine, silicon, vanadium, nickel, and tin. A number of other trace elements have been found in the body but as yet have not been established as being essential.

Regardless of the amount of the mineral in the body, however, all the established essential trace minerals, as well as the major minerals, are vital to human life. Table 7-1 shows the relatively small amounts of these minerals in the body. One might compare the amount of calcium, which is necessary for bone structure, with the amount of cobalt, which is a necessary component of vitamin B_{12}. The effects of a deficiency of cobalt, which accounts for only two parts per trillion of body weight, can be just as devastating, if not more so, as a deficiency of calcium, which accounts for two parts per hundred (2%) of the total body weight. So the word *trace* used commonly for these minerals found in such very small amounts does not mean that they are any less significant to human life and health than are the major minerals. All are essential, both in the diet and in specific body functions.

Control of amount and distribution

The correct amount of these minerals needed by the body is usually controlled either at the point of absorption or at points of tissue uptake.

ABSORPTION. The amount of the mineral needed at a particular time may be controlled by the amount of the material available from its absorption for the gastrointestinal tract. These absorption substances, for the most part, are protein compounds. When the body has a good supply of the mineral, a rel-

60

Table 7-1. Relative amounts of selected essential minerals in the body

Class of mineral	Mineral elements	Body weight (%)
Major minerals	Calcium (Ca)	1.5-2.2
	Phosphorus (P)	0.8-1.2
	Potassium (K)	0.35
	Sulfur (S)	0.25
	Sodium (Na)	0.15
	Chlorine (Cl)	0.15
	Magnesium (Mg)	0.05
Trace elements	Iron (Fe)	0.004
	Zinc (Zn)	0.002
	Selenium (Se)	0.0003
	Manganese (Mn)	0.0002
	Copper (Cu)	0.00015
	Iodine (I)	0.00004

Based on data from Guthrie, H.A.: Introductory nutrition, ed. 5, St. Louis, 1983, The C.V. Mosby Co., p. 121.

atively small amount is absorbed. When the mineral is deficient, more will be absorbed. For example, the amount of iron entering the body tissues is controlled at the point of absorption by the amount of "unfilled" carrier protein complex available to "ferry" it across the mucosal tissue and into circulation. This is called the *ferritin mechanism*, since ferritin is the name of the absorbing protein compound.

TISSUE UPTAKE. Other minerals may be controlled at the point of their "target" tissue uptake by regulatory substances such as hormones, with the remainder being excreted in the urine. For example, the amount of iodine used by the thyroid gland to produce the thyroid hormone thyroxine is controlled by the thyroid-stimulating hormone (TSH) from the pituitary gland. When more thyroxine is needed, more iodine will be taken up by the thyroid gland under TSH stimulation. At other times, when adequate levels of thyroxine are present in the blood, less iodine is absorbed by the thyroid gland, and more is excreted.

Occurrence in the body

Minerals are found in the body in several forms in places related to their functions. There are three main forms in which minerals occur: (1) combined with organic compounds, such as iron in hemoglobin; (2) combined with other inorganic elements, such as calcium with phosphorus to form the calcium phosphate of bone; and (3) free particles (ionized *ions*, meaning that they carry an electrical charge) in body fluids, such as sodium in tissue fluids, which helps to control water balance.

GENERAL FUNCTIONS OF MINERALS

Individual minerals have specific functions. However, minerals as a group have several general types of functions essential to human life, both in body structure and in body metabolism.

BODY STRUCTURE. Minerals are constituents of bones and teeth, providing rigidity to their structure. The normal growth and maintenance of these body tissues depend on elements such as calcium and phosphorus in optimum amounts.

NERVE-MUSCLE ACTION. Certain minerals are necessary for the transmission of nerve impulses along nerve fibers. For example, both sodium and potassium in fluids bathing the nerve cells are responsible for the conduction of a nerve impulse, and calcium is necessary for the release of acetylcholine, the chemical "messenger" at the junction of two fibers. In turn, muscle action depends on several minerals. Normal muscle contraction depends on calcium in tissue fluids surrounding the muscle fibers, and normal muscle relaxation in turn depends on the presence of sodium, potassium, and magnesium. A constant balance among these elements is essential for proper muscle action and reaction.

WATER BALANCE. Mineral elements in the ionized form, called *electrolytes*, control water balance in the body. The two main electrolytes responsible for this vital balance are sodium, guarding the amount of water outside of cells, and potassium, guarding the water inside of cells.

ACID-BASE BALANCE. Certain elements also control the respective amounts of acid and base substances in the body fluid, thereby holding these fluids within the narrow acidity range compatible with life of the tissues. Some minerals, such as chlorine, sulfur, and phosphorus, are acid forming. Others, such as calcium, sodium, potassium, and magnesium, are basic, or alkaline, in solution. Also, the blood contains materials called *buffers*, such as carbonates and phosphates. These substances can react with either excess acid or excess base to maintain the necessary neutrality of fluids bathing the tissues.

ESSENTIAL BODY COMPOUNDS. Some mineral elements are essential components of vital body compounds that are synthesized in the body. If the required mineral is not present, the body cannot synthesize the compound. For example, the production of the thyroid hormone thyroxine depends on available iodine. The production and storage of insulin, which regulates glucose metabolism, involves zinc. The synthesis of hemoglobin, essential for carrying oxygen in the blood to the cells, depends on iron and copper. The production of hydrochloric acid, an essential component of gastric secretions for activation of certain digestive enzymes, depends on chlorine. In addition, minerals are an integral part of many enzymes throughout the body. Other minerals, such as cobalt in vitamin B_{12} and sulfur in thiamin, are necessary constituents of vitamins.

ESSENTIAL CATALYSTS IN TISSUE REACTIONS. A catalyst is a substance whose presence is necessary for a certain chemical reaction to take place but which does not become a part of the compound in the reaction or its end products. Many biological reactions throughout the body tissues depend on the presence of certain minerals to serve as catalysts for a specific reaction. For example, the presence of calcium is necessary for blood-clotting reactions to take place. Many reactions in the metabolism of carbohydrate, fat, and protein are mineral dependent.

MAJOR MINERALS
Calcium

FUNCTIONS. Most of the food and nutrition surveys conducted in the United States indicate that calcium is one of the minerals most likely to be deficient, as measured by the Recommended Dietary Allowances (RDA). According to the survey results, men and boys are much more likely to consume adequate amounts of calcium than are women and girls. Calcium functions in four basic ways in the body:

1. *Bone and tooth formation*. Most of the body's calcium, 99%, is found in bone tissues. When calcium phosphate is removed from bone, the remaining tissue is flexible cartilage tissue. If calcium in the diet is insufficient to build normal, healthy bone structure, deformities occur, such as bowed legs, enlarged ankles and wrists, and other malformations. The calcification of teeth occurs before eruption, so later dietary calcium does not affect tooth structure as it does in a continuing manner with bone tissue.
2. *Blood clotting*. Calcium must be present at each step in the series of actions needed for the formation of the fibrin making up the blood clot.
3. *Nerve and muscle action*. As described above, calcium acts to stimulate muscle contraction and to transmit impulses along nerve fibers.
4. *Metabolic reactions*. Calcium is required for many general metabolic functions in the body. These include absorption of vitamin B_{12}, activation of the fat-splitting enzyme pancreatic lipase, and secretion of insulin from special cells in the pancreas where it is synthesized. Calcium is also found in the cell membrane, where it governs the permeability of the membrane to various nutrients.

DEFICIENCY STATES. If calcium is deficient during growth, various bone deformities will occur. Rickets, the gross deficiency disease related to a lack of calcium absorption when vitamin D is not available, is characterized by such bone malformations. Also, a decrease of calcium in the blood results in tetany, which is characterized by abnormal spasms of the muscles.

FOOD SOURCES. Milk and milk products are the most important sources of readily available calcium. All of the amount of milk in the diet need not be consumed as a beverage. It may be used in cooking, as in soups, sauces, and puddings, or in milk products such as yogurt, cheese, and ice cream. Valuable secondary food sources of calcium include egg yolk, green leafy vegetables, whole grains, legumes, and nuts. The calcium in spinach, Swiss chard, and beet greens may not be available because of the presence of oxalic acid, which interferes with calcium absorption. However, other green vegetables such as broccoli, kale, mustard greens, and turnip greens contain no oxalic acid and are thus good sources of calcium.

REQUIREMENTS. The RDA for calcium is 800 mg/day for adults and 1200 mg/day for women during pregnancy and lactation. The RDA for children is 800 to 1200 mg/day to provide for the rapid bone growth that accompanies childhood growth and development. An adequate supply of vitamin D is also essential for the efficient use of calcium and phosphorus, but vitamin D can only function when adequate amounts of calcium and phosphorus are present. Thus milk enriched with vitamin D provides all three of these essential materials of bone growth.

Phosphorus

FUNCTIONS. Phosphorus serves as a partner with calcium in the major task of bone formation but also functions in other metabolic processes:

1. *Bone and tooth formation.* The calcification of bones and teeth depends on the fixing of phosphorus in the bone-forming tissue as calcium phosphate.
2. *Energy metabolism* Phosphate is necessary for the controlled oxidation of carbohydrate, fat, and protein in producing and storing available energy for the body. It also contributes to energy and protein metabolism, as well as to cell function and genetic inheritance, as an essential component of cell enzymes, thiamin, and the critical compounds in the cell, DNA and RNA, which control cell reproduction.
3. *Regulation of acid-base balance.* Phosphate is important as a buffer material to prevent changes in the acidity of body fluids.

DEFICIENCY STATES. Because of the widespread distribution of phosphorus in foods, there is little possibility of deficiency in a person consuming an average diet. The only evidences of deficiency have been observed among persons who consume large amounts of antacids, which interfere with phosphorus absorption, or in persons with conditions that cause excessive urinary losses of phosphorus. Symptoms such as fatigue, loss of appetite, and demineralization of bone result.

FOOD SOURCES. Foods rich in protein are rich in phosphorus. Hence meat, fish, poultry, eggs, and cereal grains are the primary sources of phosphorus in the average diet. Dairy products also provide a major source of phosphorus. Additional sources include nuts and legumes. The high-phosphorus content of carbonated soft drinks (as high as 75 mg per 12-oz bottle) is of some concern among nutritionists, especially for those people who consume large quantities and thus create an imbalance in the vital calcium/phosphorus ratio in the diet and in the blood serum.

REQUIREMENTS. The RDA for phosphorus is at least 800 mg/day, equal to the calcium allowance indicated for the growth period. If the diet is adequate in protein, it will have sufficient phosphorus also. Most U.S. diets provide about 475 to 625 mg/1000 calories. For infants the phosphorus requirement is somewhat lower, about two thirds that of calcium.

Magnesium

FUNCTIONS. The functions of magnesium are widespread throughout body metabolism, in tissue synthesis, and in muscle action.

1. *General metabolism.* Magnesium serves as a significant catalyst in hundreds of reactions in the cell through which energy is produced, body compounds are synthesized, or nutrients are absorbed and transported.
2. *Protein synthesis.* Magnesium activates amino acids for protein synthesis and facilitates the synthesis and maintenance of the genetic material DNA.
3. *Muscle action.* Magnesium promotes conduction of nerve impulses to muscles to allow normal contraction. In the action of muscles magnesium then acts as a relaxant substance, in balance with calcium, which acts as a stimulant to muscle contraction.
4. *Basal metabolic rate.* Magnesium influences the secretion of thyroxine and thus helps in the maintenance of a normal basal metabolic rate and adaptation of the body to cold temperatures.

DEFICIENCY STATES. Newer methods of measuring magnesium in body fluids have shown that magnesium depletion occurs more commonly than previously assumed. Some of the conditions that may bring on such depletion include (1) starvation, (2) persistent vomiting or diarrhea with loss of magnesium-rich intestinal secretions, (3) surgical trauma and prolonged postoperative use of magnesium-free fluids, and (4) excessive use of alcohol, which increases the rate of magnesium excretion. A deficiency of magnesium results in a tetany similar to that produced by a drop in the blood calcium level. This condition progresses over prolonged deficiency from early tremors to severe convulsive seizures. The action of the cardiovascular system and the renal system is also affected, with symptoms such as dilated blood vessels and skin changes occurring. Injections of magnesium sulfate relieve these symptoms.

FOOD SOURCES. Among the best sources of magnesium are vegetables, legumes, seafood, nuts, cereals, and dairy products. The high chlorophyll content of green leafy vegetables makes these foods valuable sources of magnesium, providing some 30% of the dietary amount.

REQUIREMENTS. The RDA for magnesium is 300 mg/day for women and 350 mg/day for men, or approximately 5 mg/kg of body weight. An additional 150 mg, or a total of 450 mg, is recommended for women during pregnancy and lactation.

Sodium

FUNCTIONS. Sodium functions mainly in water balance in the body but also has important tasks in acid-base balance and in muscle action.
1. *Water balance*. Sodium is the major electrolyte controlling the amount of body water outside of cells. As such, it helps to prevent either dehydration or water intoxication of the cells. It is also an integral part of all the digestive secretions into the gastrointestinal tract, most of which are then reabsorbed.
2. *Acid-base balance*. Sodium accounts for about 90% of the alkalinity of the fluids outside of cells and helps to balance acid-forming elements. Alkalosis, one of the main causes of an excess of base-forming elements, is a result of the continued use of antacid drugs containing sodium.
3. *Muscle action*. Sodium is necessary for normal transmission of nerve impulses to stimulate muscle action. The following muscle contraction also involves sodium.
4. *Glucose absorption*. Sodium is essential as a transport substance for the absorption of glucose across absorbing membranes.

DEFICIENCY STATES. Because the body sodium requirement is so low, a deficiency state rarely occurs. Exceptions occur, however, when heavy body losses of sodium accompany heavy sweating. This may be the case with heavy laborers or athletes performing strenuous physical exercise in a hot environment. Such persons may need additional salt to replace these heavy losses.

FOOD SOURCES. Sodium occurs naturally in foods, being most prevalent generally in foods of animal origin. There is an ample amount in such natural sources to meet body needs. However, the greatest amount of dietary sodium comes from added salt in foods, especially in processed foods. For example, cured ham has about 20 times as much sodium as raw pork.

REQUIREMENTS. There is no stated requirement for sodium, since needs vary with growth, sweat losses, and loss of other secretions, as in diarrhea. The usual intake in the American diet far exceeds basic body needs. About 2 g/day would meet adult needs, but the average intake is about five times that amount.

Potassium

FUNCTIONS. Potassium is a partner with sodium in water balance but also has many metabolic functions:
1. *Water balance*. Potassium is the major electrolyte controlling the water inside the cells. In this position it balances with sodium concentration in the water outside of cells.

Table 7-2. Potassium content per average serving of some selected foods

Group A (600 mg)	Group B (400 mg)	Group C (300 mg)	Group D (200 mg)
Dried apricots	Bananas	Avocados	Fruit Cocktail
Dried peaches	Grapfruit	Canteloupe	Grapes
Lima beans	Orange juice	Cherries	Peaches
Parsnips	Artichokes	Green beans	Pineapple
Spinach, fresh	Broccoli	Fresh tomatoes	Plums
Tomato juice	Brussels sprouts	Milk	Prunes, dried
Sweet potatoes	Carrots		Stawberries
	Cauliflower		Asparagus
	Corn		Cabbage
	Winter squash		Green peas
	Turnip greens		
	White potatoes		
	Liver		
	Pork		
	Beef		
	Chicken		
	Fish		
	Peanut butter		
	Cashew nuts		

2. *Metabolic reactions*. Potassium is involved in the synthesis of glycogen and protein in the cell and in energy production.
3. *Muscle action*. Potassium also plays a role in nerve impulse transmission to stimulate muscle action. Then, along with magnesium, sodium acts as a muscle relaxant in balance with calcium, which causes muscle contraction.
4. *Insulin release*. Potassium is involved in insulin release from the pancreas when it is triggered by a rise in blood glucose level.
5. *Blood pressure*. Sodium is also considered to be a dietary factor related to blood pressure. However, there is evidence that this relationship may be more involved with the sodium/potassium ratio rather than with the actual amount of dietary sodium alone. A potassium intake equal to that of sodium may be the protecting factor.

DEFICIENCY STATES. Potassium-deficiency symptoms are well defined but seldom relate to inadequate dietary intake. It is more likely to occur in such situations as prolonged vomiting or diarrhea, the use of diuretics, severe malnutrition, and surgery. Characteristic symptoms include overall muscle weakness, poor intestinal muscle tone with resulting bloating, heart muscle problems with possible cardiac arrest, and weakness of respiratory muscles with breathing difficulties. Excessive use of potassium replacement drugs by persons receiving diuretics may also be a problem. This is especially true with an elderly person having impaired kidney function and hence difficulty in excreting potassium.

FOOD SOURCES. Plant foods are the richest sources of potassium. However, because it is found in plants in a very soluble form, much of the potassium content may be lost in excessive use of cooking water. There is no evidence from surveys that the potassium content of average American diets is either too low or excessive. The potassium content of some selected foods is presented in Table 7-2.

REQUIREMENTS. Although potassium has been established as a dietary essential, there is little information on basic needs, and no stated requirement has been given. Minimum needs have been estimated at about 1.8 g/day, and the amount in the American diet has been estimated at 2 to 6 g. For adults, intakes of potassium between 1850 and 5500 mg are considered adequate.

Chlorine

FUNCTIONS. Chlorine is widely distributed throughout body tissues. Two significant functions involve digestion and respiration:
1. *Digestion.* Chlorine is a necessary element in the hydrochloric acid secreted in gastric juices. This constant secretion maintains the necessary acidity of stomach fluids for the action of gastric enzymes. This acid secretion also helps to maintain the acid-base balance in body fluids.
2. *Respiration.* Chloride ions or electrolytes help red blood cells to carry large amounts of carbon dioxide to the lungs for release in breathing. The chloride ions move easily in and out of red cells in balance with the carbon dioxide, to counteract any potential changes in the acid-base balance. This ready movement of chloride in and out of red blood cells is called the *chloride shift*.

DEFICIENCY STATES. Any deficiency encountered is not related to dietary intake but to a situation of loss, such as diarrhea or vomiting, or to heavy sweating.

FOOD SOURCES. Dietary chlorine is provided almost entirely by sodium chloride, or table salt. The kidney is very efficient in reabsorbing chloride when the dietary intake is low.

REQUIREMENTS. The safe and adequate ranges of chloride intake given by the National Research Council increase with age. However, at all ages the range is wide. The stated level for adults is 1700 to 5100 mg/day.

Sulfur

FUNCTIONS. Sulfur is present in every cell in the body. Several of its widespread metabolic and structural functions include the following actions:
1. *Hair, skin, and nails.* Sulfur is involved in the structure of these tissues through its presence in two amino acids, methionine and cystine, which are found in high concentration in the tissue protein keratin.
2. *General metabolic functions.* Combined with hydrogen, sulfur is an im-

Table 7-3. Summary of major minerals

Mineral	Metabolism	Physiological functions	Clinical application	Requirement	Food sources
Calcium (Ca)	Absorption according to body need, aided by vitamin D; favored by protein, lactose, acidity; hindered by excess fats and binding agents (phosphates, oxalates, phytate) Excretion chiefly in feces, 70% to 90% of amount ingested Deposition-mobilization in bone compartment constant; deposition aided by vitamin D Parathyroid hormone controls absorption and mobilization	Bone formation Teeth Blood clotting Muscle contraction and relaxation Heart action Nerve transmission Cell wall permeability Enzyme activation (ATPase)	Tetany—decrease in ionized serum calcium Rickets Renal calculi Hyperparathyroidism Hypoparathyroidism	Adults: 0.8 g Pregnancy and lactation: 1.2 g Infants: 360-540 mg Children: 0.8-1.2 g	Milk Cheese Green leafy vegetables Whole grains Egg yolk Legumes, nuts
Phosphorus (P)	Absorption with calcium aided by vitamin D; hindered by excess binding agents (calcium, aluminum, iron) Excretion chiefly by kidney according to renal threshold blood level Parathyroid hormone controls renal excretion balance with blood level Deposition-mobilization in bone compartment constant	Bone formation Overall metabolism: Absorption of glucose and glycerol (phosphorylation) Transport of fatty acids Energy metabolism (enzymes, ATP) Buffer system	Growth Hypophosphatemia: Recovery state from diabetic acidosis Sprue, celiac disease (malabsorption) Bone diseases (upset Ca:P balance) Hyperphosphatemia: Renal insufficiency Hypoparathyroidism Tetany	Adults: 1½ times calcium intake Pregnancy and lactation: 1.2 g Infants: 240-400 mg Children: 0.8-1.2 g	Milk Cheese Meat Egg yolk Whole grains Legumes, nuts

Continued.

Table 7-3. Summary of major minerals—cont'd

Mineral	Metabolism	Physiological functions	Clinical application	Requirement	Food sources
Magnesium (Mg)	Absorption increased by parathyroid hormone, hindered by excess fat, phosphate, calcium Excretion regulated by kidney	In bones and teeth Activator and coenzyme in carbohydrate and protein metabolism Essential intracellular fluid (ICF) cation Muscle, nerve irritability	Tremor, spasm; low serum level following gastrointestinal losses	300-350 mg Deficiency in humans unlikely	Whole grains Nuts Meat Milk Legumes
Sodium (Na)	Readily absorbed Excretion chiefly by kidney, controlled by aldosterone, acid-base balance	Major extracellular fluid (ECF) cation Water balance; osmotic pressure Acid-base balance Cell permeability; absorption of glucose Muscle irritability; transmission of electrochemical impulse and resulting contraction	Fluid shifts and control Buffer system Losses in gastrointestinal disorders	About 0.5 g Diet usually has more: 2-6 g	Table salt (NaCl) Milk Meat Egg Baking soda Baking powder Carrots, beets, spinach, celery
Potassium (K)	Secreted and reabsorbed in digestive juices Excretion guarded by kidney according to blood levels; increased by aldosterone	Major ICF cation Acid-base balance Regulates neuromuscular excitability and muscle contraction	Fluid shifts Losses in: Starvation Diabetic acidosis Adrenal tumors	About 2-4 g Diet adequate in protein, calcium, and iron contains adequate potassium	Whole grains Meat Legumes Fruits Vegetables

Mineral	Metabolism	Physiological functions	Clinical applications	Requirement	Food sources
		Glycogen formation Protein synthesis	Heart action—low serum potassium (tachycardia, cardiac arrest) Treatment of diabetic acidosis (rapid glycogen production reduces serum potassium) Tissue catabolism—potassium loss		
Chlorine (Cl)	Absorbed readily Excretion controlled by kidney	Major ECF anion Acid-base balance—chloride-bicarbonate shift Water balance Gastric hydrochloric acid—digestion	Hypochloremic alkalosis in prolonged vomiting, diarrhea, tube drainage	About 0.5 g Diet usually has more: 2-6 g	Table salt
Sulfur (S)	Absorbed as such and as constituent of sulfur-containing amino acid methionine Excreted by kidney in relation to protein intake and tissue catabolism	Essential constituent of cell protein Activates enzymes High-energy sulfur bonds in energy metabolism Detoxification reactions	Cystine renal calculi Cystinuria	Diet adequate in protein contains adequate sulfur	Meat Egg Cheese Milk Nuts, legumes

portant high-energy bonding in building many compounds. In this way it helps to transfer energy as needed in various tissue.

3. *Vitamin structure*. Sulfur is a part of several vitamins—thiamin, pantothenic acid, biotin, and lipoic acid—which in turn act as coenzymes in cell metabolism.

4. *Collagen structure*. Sulfur is necessary for collagen synthesis in the body and thus is important in building connective tissues.

DEFICIENCY STATES. No deficiency states have been documented. Such conditions would only relate to general protein malnutrition and absence of the sulfur-carrying amino acids methionine and cystine.

FOOD SOURCES. Sulfur is available to the body primarily as the organic sulfur in the amino acids methionine and cystine. Thus protein foods of animal sources would be the main contributors.

REQUIREMENTS. There are no stated requirements for dietary sulfur as such, since it is supplied by protein foods containing the amino acids methionine and cystine, as indicated.

A summary of the major minerals is presented in Table 7-3.

TRACE MINERALS
Iron

FUNCTIONS. Iron functions both in the synthesis of hemoglobin and in general body metabolism.

1. *Hemoglobin synthesis*. Iron is a necessary component of the nonprotein heme part of the hemoglobin structure. Hemoglobin in the red blood cell is the oxygen-carrying unit of the blood that transports oxygen to the cells for cell oxidation and metabolism. Iron is also a necessary constituent of a similar compound, myoglobin, in muscle tissue. The largest portion of body iron, about 75%, is found in hemoglobin.

2. *General metabolism*. A number of general metabolic functions require the presence of iron: glucose metabolism in the cell, antibody production, detoxification of drugs in the liver, the conversion of carotene to vitamin A, collagen synthesis, and purine synthesis. The amount of iron in the body is regulated according to the body's need, specifically to accomplish these various functions. A summary of iron metabolism, showing its absorption, transport, main use in hemoglobin formation, and storage forms, is shown in Fig. 7-1.

DEFICIENCY STATES. The major condition indicating a deficiency of iron is *anemia*, a condition characterized by a decrease in the number of red blood cells in the blood or in the amount of hemoglobin in the cells, or both. This lack of iron or inability to use it may result from several causes: (1) an inadequate supply of dietary iron; (2) excessive blood loss; (3) inability to form hemoglobin in the absence of other necessary factors such as vitamin B_{12} (pernicious anemia); (4) lack of gastric hydrochloric acid, which is necessary to liberate iron for

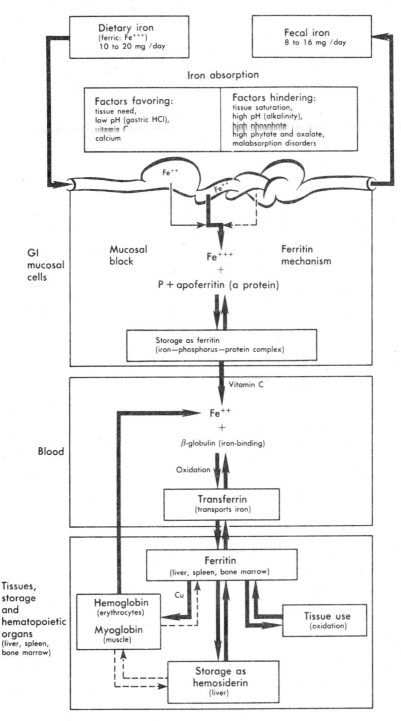

Fig. 7-1. Summary of iron metabolism, showing its absorption, transport, main use in hemoglobin formation, and storage forms (ferritin and hemosiderin).

absorption; (5) the presence of various inhibitors of iron absorption, such as phosphate or phytate; or (6) mucosal lesions that affect the absorbing surface area.

FOOD SOURCES. By far the best sources of iron are organ meats, especially liver, since this is a major storage tissue for iron in the animal body. Other food sources include meats, egg yolk, whole grains, seafood, green leafy vegetables, nuts, and legumes.

REQUIREMENTS. Adult requirements for iron differ between men and women. The RDA suggests a general intake of 10 mg/day of iron for men and 18 mg/day for women during childbearing years. The greater amount for women is needed to cover menstrual losses and the demands of pregnancy. Usually during pregnancy an iron supplement is required, since it is doubtful that the woman's ordinary diet can supply the larger quantity of iron demanded at that time. Iron needs vary with age and situation, and these allowances are designed to provide margins for safety.

Iodine

FUNCTIONS. The only known function of iodine in human metabolism is that of participating in the synthesis of the thyroid hormone thyroxine. The uptake of iodine by the thyroid gland is controlled by TSH. When the level of throxine circulating in the blood is reduced, TSH stimulates the thyroid gland to absorb more iodine so that more thyroxine may be synthesized in turn. The transport form of iodine in the blood is called serum *protein-bound iodine*. After thyroxine is used to stimulate metabolic processes in the cells, it is broken down in the liver, and the iodine portion is excreted in bile as inorganic iodine. A summary of iodine metabolism in the body is shown in Fig. 7-2. The basic overall function of iodine therefore is that of providing the thyroid gland with a necessary component in its synthesis of thyroxine, the basic hormone that controls the body's basal metabolic rate.

DEFICIENCY STATES. A lack of iodine in the diet produces goiter. This is a classic condition characterized by enlargement of the thyroid gland. It occurs in areas where the water and soil contain little iodine. The thyroid gland then is starved for iodine and cannot produce a normal quantity of thyroxine. With this low level of thyroxine in the bloodstream, therefore, the pituitary gland continues to produce TSH. In turn these large quantities of TSH continue to stimulate the thyroid gland, causing it to increase greatly in size. Such an iodine-starved thyroid gland may attain a tremendous size, weighing as much as 1 to 1½ pounds (0.45 to 0.67 kg) or more.

Cretinism is a condition encountered among children who are born to mothers who have had limited iodine intake during adolescence and pregnancy. During pregnancy the mother's need for iodine takes precedence over that of the developing child, and the baby suffers from an iodine deficiency during

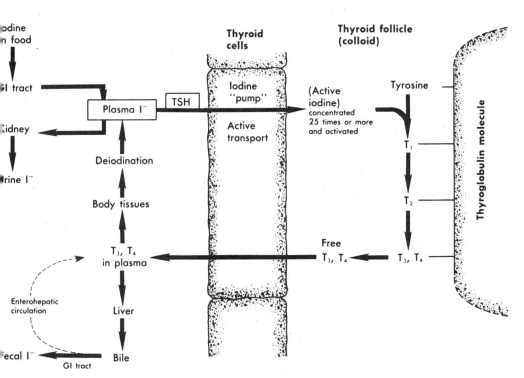

Fig. 7-2. Summary of iodine metabolism, showing active iodine pump in the thyroid cells and synthesis of thyroxine in the colloid tissue of the thyroid follicles. *TSH,* thyroid-stimulating hormone; *T₁,* monoiodotyronine; *T₂,* diiodotyrosine; *T₃,* triiodothyronine; *T₄,* tetraiodothyronine.

fetal life, as well as in continuing development following birth. These children are retarded in both physical and mental development. However, if the condition is discovered at birth and treatment is started immediately, many of the symptoms of cretinism are reversible. If the condition continues beyond early childhood, the mental and physical retardation becomes permanent.

An adult form of hypothyroidism is called *myxedema*. The symptoms of this condition are thin coarse hair, dry skin, poor tolerance for cold, and a low husky voice. An opposite condition, hyperthyroidism, in which the basal metabolic rate is elevated greatly, may also occur in adults. It is known as Graves' disease, or *exophthalmic goiter*. Symptoms resulting from such an overactive thyroid gland include weight loss, hand tremors and general nervousness, increased appetite, intolerance of heat, and protruding eyeballs.

FOOD SOURCES. The amount of iodine in natural food sources varies considerably depending on the iodine content of the soil. Foods from the sea would provide a considerable amount of iodine. However, the major dietary source of iodine is iodized table salt, achieved through the commercial addition of iodine in producing the salt. Iodized salt contains 1 mg of iodine to every 10 g of salt.

Recently some questions have been raised concerning the use of iodized salt on the basis of changes in the environment. Some of these changes include food technology associated with the bread industry, in which various iodine compounds are used as dough conditioners; and agricultural practices, especially in the dairy industry, which increase the iodine content of milk products. However, several reasons have caused nutritionists to consider the continued use of iodized salt as a wise practice: (1) moderately excessive iodine is relatively harmless, (2) persons living in certain regions may be at extreme risk of goiter, and (3) an individual's iodine intake is highly variable and may at times be insufficient depending on geographical location and food supply.

REQUIREMENTS. The RDA of iodine for adult men is 140 μg/day and for women 100 μg/day. These needs normally decrease with age during adulthood. The demand for iodine is increased, however, during periods of accelerated growth, such as in adolescence and pregnancy.

Copper

FUNCTIONS. The role of copper as an associate of iron in preventing anemia is attributed to its action in aiding iron absorption, in stimulating the synthesis of heme or the globin fraction of the hemoglobin molecule, and in helping to release stored iron from the liver so that it may be available for hemoglobin synthesis. Copper is also associated with iron in cell oxidation systems related to energy metabolism and to protein metabolism. In addition to copper's iron-related functions, it is involved in two other major areas of tissue synthesis: (1)

bone formation and (2) brain tissue formation and the maintenance of the myelin sheath on nerve fibers in the nervous system.

DEFICIENCY STATES. Dietary deficiency states of copper in humans are unknown. However, secondary deficiencies may occur because of urinary loss in kidney disease, such as nephrosis. Malabsorption of copper may occur in adult intestinal disease, such as sprue, causing low plasma levels of copper. An excess accumulation of copper occurs in a rare inherited condition known as Wilson's disease, which is characterized by degenerative changes in brain tissue and in the liver.

FOOD SOURCES. Copper is widely distributed in natural foods. Its richest sources are liver, shellfish, whole grains, nuts, and cocoa. Additional sources are found in legumes, eggs, meat, fruits, and vegetables.

REQUIREMENTS. There is no stated RDA for copper. However, a dietary intake of about 2 mg/day appears to maintain copper balance in adults, with up to 3 mg/day considered safe. Given a sufficient caloric intake, copper will usually be amply supplied in the diet. It is of some concern, however, that current diets made up of large amounts of processed foods may provide intakes of no more than 1 mg/day of copper. The greater need of infants for copper is reflected in the high copper content of human milk.

Zinc

FUNCTIONS. The widespread nature of zinc functions in the human body is reflected in its distribution in many of the body tissues, including the pancreas, liver, kidneys, lungs, muscles, bones, eyes, endocrine glands, prostate secretions, and spermatozoa. In these tissues zinc is a part of three different types of metabolic functions:

1. *Enzyme constituent.* Zinc functions mainly throughout the body tissues as an essential constituent of cell enzyme systems. Over 70 such zinc enzymes have been identified in various living systems. In its role in protein metabolism zinc is associated with wound healing and healthy skin. It has a great influence on any rapidly growing tissues. Therefore its effect on reproduction is highly significant.
2. *Insulin storage.* Zinc combines readily with insulin in the pancreas. This zinc-insulin combination thus serves as a storage form of the hormone. The pancreas of a person with diabetes contains about half the normal amount of zinc.
3. *Leukocytes.* A considerable quantity of zinc bound to protein is present in leukocytes, the white blood cells. Zinc affects the body's immune system through its essential role in the synthesis of nucleic acids (DNA and RNA) and protein. It is also needed for lymphocyte transformation. Also, lymphoid tissue, which gives rise to lymphocytes, the major white

cell populations involved in the body's immune system, contains a large amount of zinc. The leukocytes of patients with leukemia, for example, contain about 10% less zinc than normal.

DEFICIENCY STATES. Zinc is a nutritional imperative during periods of rapid tissue growth. In some populations where dietary intake of zinc is low, retarded physical growth (dwarfism) and retarded sexual maturation (hypogonadism), especially in males, has been observed. Also, impaired taste and smell acuity (hypogeusia and hyposmia) are improved with increased zinc intake.

In the care of hospitalized patients zinc is particularly associated with wound healing. Poor wound healing in patients with a zinc deficiency seems to be common in the average hospital. Patients having surgery would benefit from having zinc supplementation, since zinc plays a significant role in tissue building. Older patients with poor appetites, who subsist on marginal diets in the face of chronic wounds and illnesses, may be particularly vulnerable to developing deficiencies of zinc.

FOOD SOURCES. The best sources of zinc are seafood (especially oysters), meat, and eggs. Additional sources, although less available to the body, are legumes and whole grains. Adult needs for zinc can usually be met through the consistent use of a well-balanced diet, but there is considerable current evidence that a diet high in processed foods may well be low in zinc.

REQUIREMENTS. The RDA for adults is 15 mg/day, with additional amounts indicated for women during pregnancy and lactation. Current surveys indicate that the typical American diet has a range of 6 to 12 mg of zinc, indicating that a large portion of the population may have only a marginal intake of zinc. This seems to be especially true in populations existing on low-income levels.

Chromium

FUNCTIONS. Chromium functions as an active component of glucose tolerance factor (GTF). GTF is synthesized from inorganic chromium, niacin, and amino acids, probably in the liver or intestinal flora. It is released in response to increased blood insulin levels and then acts to bind insulin to the cell, thus aiding in the uptake of glucose by the cell. Chromium may also have a role in lipid metabolism and hence in coronary heart disease. It has been observed that chromium is deficient in some tissues of the vascular system in persons who have heart disease.

DEFICIENCY STATES. Deficient levels of chromium have been associated with a reduced tolerance to glucose and an increasing incidence of diabetes. Both of these conditions are associated with increasing age in general. Many cases of mild glucose tolerance have been treated successfully with chromium.

FOOD SOURCES. Major food sources of chromium are found in foods of plant origin, whole grains, vegetables, and fruits. Additional sources include meat products and cheese. In general chromium is lower in refined or processed foods than in whole foods.

REQUIREMENTS. There is no stated RDA for chromium. The average American diet contains from 80 to 100 μg/day. This appears to be a sufficient amount to meet the general safe and adequate intake for adults of 50 to 200 μg. The absorbed chromium from foods consumed is stored in the tissues and is released when glucose is ingested.

Selenium

FUNCTIONS. For some time it has been observed that selenium operates in collaboration with vitamin E to protect fat substances in tissues from breaking down or oxidizing easily. The action of these two substances together has been effective in treating fatty infiltration in hepatic disease and in curing certain muscle disorders that were induced in animals. It has since been discovered that selenium functions as an essential constituent of a major cell enzyme that acts as an antioxidant in the cell. This major antioxidant enzyme is glutathione peroxidase. This enzyme inhibits other enzyme actions that cause the oxidation or breakdown of fat. Vitamin E, also an antioxidant, functions similarly by competing with fat for available oxygen needed for oxidation. Thus the two substances, selenium and vitamin E, act in a complementary manner to achieve the task of protecting fatty tissues in the body from deterioration through oxidation.

DEFICIENCY STATES. Deficiency states have been observed mainly in areas where the soil is deficient in selenium. For example, in such places various muscle disorders in animals raised on crops grown in these soils appeared. More recently disease affecting the heart muscle in children and in women of childbearing age has appeared to result from degeneration of the muscle tissue. In New Zealand, where the selenium content of the soil is low, selenium has been used successfully to treat discomfort in persons following surgery, apparently by strengthening the muscles involved.

FOOD SOURCES. As indicated, the selenium content of plant foods varies with the selenium content of the soil in which it is grown. In turn this influences the amount of selenium in the tissue, hence meat, eggs, or milk, from animals raised on crops grown in such soils. Although seafood has a high selenium content inherently, it is a poor dietary source because the selenium is not available to any great extent. Thus major sources of selenium are organ meats, muscle meats, dairy products, whole grains, fruits, and vegetables. The amount of selenium present in these food substances parallels the protein content of the food. In the case of plant sources, selenium is reduced by the milling process and is lost in cooking water from vegetables.

REQUIREMENTS. There is no selenium statement in the RDA standard. However, the general range of 50 to 200 μg has been expressed as an adequate and safe range. The RDA standard also involves an expressed concern that there may be a danger in selenium supplementation, since toxicity may result from excess intake.

Manganese

FUNCTIONS. Manganese operates as a necessary component in numerous enzyme systems throughout the body tissues. In this role it is involved in protein metabolism by activating amino acids and enzymes necessary for splitting amino acids. It is also involved in activating several reactions in glucose oxidation to produce energy. Furthermore, it is involved in fat metabolism by activating a significant fat-clearing factor, lipoprotein lipase, as well as helping to synthesize long-chain fatty acids. It also helps to prevent ammonia toxicity in kidney disease through its role in activating the enzyme necessary for urea formation and hence nitrogen excretion.

DEFICIENCY STATES. There is no demonstrated manganese deficiency in humans. Its essential nutrient nature is based on its roles, as previously indicated, in widespread metabolic systems of the body. Most of the body manganese is concentrated in the pancreas, bones, liver, and kidneys. Very little is excreted in the urine. The major pathway of excretion is in the bile, but a significant amount of this is reabsorbed constantly. Thus the body conserves its manganese content. The average American diet provides from 3 to 9 μg/day of manganese, which seems adequate.

FOOD SOURCES. Major food sources of manganese include green vegetables and whole-grain cereals. However, the amount of manganese present in a particular food depends on the part of the plant and the soil in which it was grown. Tea is also an extremely rich source. For example, it is estimated that British diets, in which tea is consumed in fairly large amounts, provide 3.3 mg/day of manganese. Other food sources include nuts and legumes.

REQUIREMENTS. There is no RDA for manganese. However, the stated safe and adequate level of manganese is estimated to be about 2.5 to 5 mg for adults.

Additional trace minerals

Several additional trace minerals are briefly described here. Although all of these have been recognized as essential nutrient factors, their functions are either less widespread in the body or less well understood.

FLUORINE. The only relationship established thus far for fluorine in human metabolism is its association with dental health. The condition of dental caries, or tooth decay, has been demonstrated to be largely preventable by the addition of a small amount of fluorine to fluorine-poor drinking water or by the topical application of fluoride solutions to young developing teeth. Public health authorities advocate the fluoridation of public drinking water in the amount of one part per million in areas where the drinking water is low in fluoride content. The mechanism by which fluorine prevents dental caries is unknown.

Recently there has been some evidence that fluorine ingestion at relatively high levels during adult life gives protection against osteoporosis in later life. Other evidence seems to indicate that fluorine also has a protective function in helping to prevent periodontal disease by strengthening the bone in the jaw area often associated with the loss of teeth. These effects may result from the action of fluorine in inhibiting bone resorption by reducing the solubility of the associated minerals in the bone. Communities using fluoridated public water supplies not only ingest more fluorine in drinking water but also fluorine in foods grown and processed in these areas. Fish products, especially mackerel and salmon, are also good natural sources of fluorine. There is no stated dietary requirement for fluorine.

COBALT. Cobalt is an essential constituent of vitamin B_{12}. As such, cobalt functions largely in red blood cell formation through its role in hemoglobin synthesis. Thus it is necessary to prevent pernicious anemia. Humans do not have the ability to synthesize vitamin B_{12} and must depend on animal sources of the nutrient. In these animal sources the vitamin has been synthesized by microorganisms in the animal intestine that have the capacity to incorporate the cobalt obtained from the plants the animals eat. Thus cobalt itself is not a dietary essential for humans, but cobalt-containing vitamin B_{12} is a necessary dietary essential. The average American diet contains about 300 mg of cobalt, mainly found in meat sources such as liver, kidney, oysters, clams, lean meats, poultry, fish, and milk. Although a large amount of cobalt is thus consumed in an average diet, the only amount required is the small amount needed in vitamin B_{12}, only about 0.04 μg/day. There is some evidence that large intakes of cobalt have toxic effects. Excess intake has led to *polycythemia*, a condition characterized by the formation of an excess number of red blood cells that contain a relatively high concentration of hemoglobin. Such a condition has been observed in some cases associated with the consumption of large amounts of beer, to which cobalt has been added to control foaming.

MOLYBDENUM. Amounts of molybdenum in the body are very minute, and deficiencies in humans are unknown. This trace mineral is present in bound form as an integral part of various enzyme systems in the cell and thus functions in the action of the specific cell enzyme involved. One of these enzymes, for example, is *xanthine oxidase*, which acts in purine catabolism or breakdown. In this action the enzyme oxidizes xanthine to uric acid for excretion. The body's content of molybdenum is found in highest concentration in metabolically active tissues such as the liver, kidneys, adrenal glands, and blood cells. Food sources include legumes such as beans and peas, meat, and whole-grain cereals. There is no stated RDA for molybdenum. However, the safe and adequate intake has been estimated to be between 0.15 and 0.5 mg/day for adults. The average American dietary intake has been estimated to average 0.3 mg and to vary between 0.1 and 0.46 mg. Thus there seems to be little likelihood of a deficiency except among vegetarians or persons whose diets are composed largely of highly processed or refined foods.

VANADIUM. Recent studies have shown that vanadium is an essential element for higher animals, related to tooth and bone development particularly. It also appears to have a role in lipid metabolism, since deficiency states have been related to lowered cholesterol levels. Much additional study is needed however to determine precise human vanadium functions and requirements, but adequate vanadium nutrition should not be taken for granted. It is found widely distributed in primary foods such as grains, root vegetables, nuts, and vegetable oils. There is no RDA for vanadium. The daily need in human nutrition has been estimated to be about 0.1 to 0.3 mg.

SILICON. Research has indicated that animals deprived of silicon have symptoms of depressed growth, pallor of mucous membranes, and skeletal alterations and deformities, especially of the skull. These skeletal changes apparently involve the cartilage development. It has been suggested therefore that silicon may function as an essential agent in developing cross-linking in the structure and resilience of connective tissue. It has been shown to be essential for bone calcification. The daily dietary need for humans is unknown. It is found widely in plant foods, especially whole grains. However, there is limited information on the specific amounts in individual food sources.

NICKEL. Nickel has been established as an essential trace element, primarily through animal studies. Additional study is needed to determine more specifically its role in human nutrition. It is found in body tissue in compound form with protein as a substance called *nickeloplasmin*. It appears to be associated mainly with thyroid hormone and with DNA and RNA in the cell. Possible clinical relationships in humans may be in plasma lipid level control, cirrhosis of the liver, and chronic uremia. There is a relatively high concentration of nickel in sweat. Although there is no stated requirement for nickel in the human diet, the dietary need has been established to be under 0.6 μg daily. It is found mainly in plant foods, especially grains and vegetables, with very little in animal food sources.

TIN. Trace amounts of tin occur in many body tissues and in dietary food sources. Until recently tin has been considered more an "environmental contamination" than the essential trace mineral it is now known to be. Its chemical properties suggest that it may contribute to the structure of proteins and may also participate in certain reactions in cell enzyme systems. Dietary need for tin have been estimated at 3 to 6 mg/day. It is found in food sources such as meats and other animal products, whole grains, legumes, vegetables, and fruits, especially in acidic juices canned in tin.

A summary of trace minerals is presented in Table 7-4.

Table 7-4. Summary of trace minerals

Mineral	Metabolism	Physiological functions	Clinical application	Requirement	Food source
Iron (Fe)	Absorption according to body need controlled by mucosal block—ferritin mechanism; aided by vitamin C, gastric hydrochloric acid. Transport—transferrin. Storage—ferritin, hemosiderin. Excretion from tissue in minute quantities; body conserves the reuses	Hemoglobin formation. Cellular oxidation (cytochrome system producing ATP)	Growth (milk anemia). Pregnancy demands. Deficiency—anemia. Excess—hemosiderosis; hemochromatosis	Men: 10 mg. Women: 18 mg. Pregnancy: 18 mg. Lactation: 18 mg. Children: 10-18 mg	Liver. Meats. Egg yolk. Whole grains. Enriched bread and cereal. Dark green vegetables. Legumes, nuts
Copper (Cu)	Transported bound to an α-globulin as ceruloplasmin. Stored in muscle, bone, liver, heart, kidney, and central nervous system	Associated with iron in Enzyme systems. Hemoglobin synthesis. Absorption and transport of iron. Involved in bone formation and maintenance of brain tissue and myelin sheath in nervous system	Hypocupremia: Nephrosis. Malabsorption. Wilson's disease—excess copper storage	2-2.5 mg. Diet provides 2-5 mg	Liver. Meat. Seafood. Whole grains. Legumes, nuts. Cocoa. Raisins. Food cooked in copper utensils
Iodine (I)	Absorbed as iodides, taken up by thyroid gland under control of thyroid-stimulating hormone (TSH). Excretion by kidney	Synthesis of thyroxine, the thyroid hormone, which regulates cell oxidation	Deficiency—endemic colloid goiter; cretinism	Men: 140 μg. Women: 100 μg. Infants: 35-45 μg. Children: 60-140 μg	Iodized salt. Seafood

Continued.

Table 7-4. Summary of trace minerals—cont'd

Mineral	Metabolism	Physiologic functions	Clinical application	Requirement	Food source
Manganese (Mn)	Absorption limited Excretion mainly by intestine	Activates reactions in Urea formation Protein metabolism Glucose oxidation Lipoprotein clearance and synthesis of fatty acids	No clinical deficiency observed in humans Inhalation toxicity in miners	2.5-7 mg (estimated) Diet provides 3-9 mg	Cereals, whole grain Soybeans Legumes, nuts Tea, coffee Vegetables Fruits
Cobalt (Co)	Absorbed chiefly as constituent of vitamin B_{12}	Constituent of vitamin B_{12}; essential factor in red blood cell formation	Deficiency associated with deficiency of vitamin B_{12}—pernicious anemia	Unknown	Supplied by preformed vitamin B_{12}
Zinc (Zn)	Transported with plasma proteins Excretion largely intestinal Stored in liver, muscle, bone, and organs	Essential enzyme constituent: Carbonic anhydrase Carboxypeptidase Lactic dehydrogenase Combined with insulin for storage of the hormone	Possible relation to liver disease Wound healing Taste and smell acuity Retarded sexual and physical development	Adults: 15 mg Children: 10 mg Infants: 3-5 mg	Widely distributed Liver Seafood, especially oysters Eggs Milk Whole grains
Molybdenum (Mo)	Minute traces in the body	Constituent of specific enzymes involved in Purine conversion to uric acid Aldehyde oxidation		450-500 μg (estimated)	Organ meats Milk Whole grains Leafy vegetables Legumes
Fluorine (Fl)	Deposited in bones and teeth Excreted in urine	Associated with dental health	Small amount prevents dental caries Excess causes endemic dental fluorosis	1-3 mg (estimated)	Water (1 ppm Fl)

Mineral			Amount	Food sources
Selenium (Se)	Active as cofactor in cell oxidation enzyme systems	Associated with fat metabolism	Constituent of "factor 3," which acts with vitamin E to prevent fatty liver	Under 100 µg (estimated)	Seafoods Meats Whole grains
Chromium (Cr)	Improves faulty uptake of glucose by body tissues	Associated with glucose metabolism; raises abnormally low fasting blood sugar levels	Infants unable to metabolize sugar, and adult diabetics show definite improvement when small amounts of chromium added to diet Possible link with cardiovascular disorders and diabetes	20-50 µg (estimated)	Animal proteins, especially meats (except fish) Whole grains
Nickel (Ni)	Binding by phytate reduces intestinal absorption	Constituent of the protein nickeloplasmin Associated with thyroid hormone High in RNA	Plasma levels decreased in cirrhosis and chronic uremia	Under 0.6 µg (estimated)	Whole grains Legumes Vegetables Fruits
Tin (Sn)		Structural element in protein synthesis Associated with cell enzyme systems in energy metabolism	Wound healing Tissue growth	Under 1 mg (estimated)	Meats Whole grains Legumes Vegetables Fruits Acid juices canned in tin
Silicon (Si)		Essential agent in formation of bone, cartilage, connective tissue	Bone calcification and healing	Unknown	All plant foods
Vanadium (V)		High in teeth; may have role in bone and tooth formation	Possible relation to lipid metabolism, blood lipid levels	0.1-0.3 mg (estimated)	Grains, breads Root vegetables Nuts Vegetable oils

Questions on minerals

1. What purposes do minerals serve in the body?
2. Where are the minerals found in the body?
3. What mineral is most likely to be deficient in the average American diet?
4. What is the most important source of calcium?
5. What are some sources of phosphorus?
6. How does the cooking process affect the amount of calcium and phosphorus in the food?
7. Where is most of the calcium and phosphorus found in the body?
8. What purpose does calcium serve in the blood?
9. What is the average daily requirement of calcium?
10. What food fulfills the requirements for calcium and phosphorus most completely and in the most readily available form?
11. What vitamin is involved in the absorption and use of calcium and phosphorus?
12. Why is iron essential?
13. What foods are the best sources of iron?
14. What is the recommended amount of iron for adults?
15. What other mineral needs to be present in the liver for proper use of iron?
16. What is the average amount of iodine required by the body?
17. Where is iodine needed in the body?
18. What is the usual method of adding iodine to the diet?
19. Plan a day's menu that is rich in calcium and one that is rich in iron.
20. Of what importance is copper? Fluoride?
21. List an important function and food sources for each of the remaining trace elements discussed.

True-false

Circle *T* if the statement is true. Circle *F* if it is false, and then write the correct statement.

T   F   1. The majority of the calcium in the diet is absorbed and used by the body for bone formation.
T   F   2. The major part of the body calcium is stored in bones and teeth.
T   F   3. The average adult dietary use of sodium is far greater than the amount the body actually requires for metabolic balance.
T   F   4. Most of the dietary iron is absorbed, and the body's iron balance is then controlled by urinary excretion.
T   F   5. Liver is the body's main iron storage site.
T   F   6. Iron is widespread in food sources, so a deficiency problem is rare.
T   F   7. Vitamin C aids iron absorption.
T   F   8. The best food source of iron is milk.
T   F   9. Iodine has many metabolic functions, the most important of which is its role in thyroxine synthesis.
T   F   10. Dental caries can be largely prevented by the use of small amounts of fluorine.

Multiple choice

Circle the letter in front of the correct choice.

1. The only known function of iodine in human nutrition is related to the synthesis of thyroid hormone. Which of the following correctly describe this function?

(1) When blood levels of thyroxine are low, the pituitary gland puts out TSH.

(2) TSH causes the thyroid gland to take up iodides from the blood.

(3) In the thyroid gland thyroxine is synthesized by incorporating the iodine.

(4) The thyroxine is released, raising the blood level and shutting off the TSH.

a. (1) and (2)

b. (1) and (4)

c. (1), (2), and (4)

d. (1), (2), and (3)

e. All of these

Suggestions for additional study

1. Put illustrations in your notebook of the foods that are richest in each of the minerals discussed in this chapter.

2. Prepare a chart showing the comparative values in calcium of several of the calcium-rich foods.

3. Using the food values listed in Table A (p. 266-293), compute the amount of iron in the following: (a) $3\frac{1}{3}$ oz beef liver, (b) 3 oz round steak, (c) 1 tbs molasses, (d) 1 tbs raisins, (e) $\frac{1}{2}$ cup cooked kale, and (f) 6 stewed prunes.

Suggested readings

Food and Nutrition Board, National Academy of Sciences–National Research Council: Recommended dietary allowances, Washington, D.C., 1980, The Academy.

Guthrie, H.A.: Introductory nutrition, ed. 5, St. Louis, 1983, The C.V. Mosby Co.

Williams, S.R.: Nutrition and diet therapy, St. Louis, ed. 4, 1981, The C.V. Mosby Co.

Williams, S.R.: Essentials of nutrition and diet therapy, ed. 3, St. Louis, 1982, The C.V. Mosby Co.

8

Water balance

BODY WATER FUNCTIONS AND REQUIREMENTS
Water: the fundamental nutrient

Water is the most fundamental and indispensable of all the nutrients. The earth is a water planet, and all life on it is maintained by a constant supply of adequate and safe water. A human being can survive far longer without food than without water. Only air is a more constant need. Therefore fulfilling the body's need for a constant supply of water and maintaining the body's water composition and distribution are major nutritional and physiological tasks.

Several basic concepts or principles are essential to an understanding of the uses of water in the human body. First is the idea of a unified whole. The human body is one continuous body of water. The "sea within" is held in shape by a protective envelope of skin. Within that enveloping and protective skin, body water moves freely to all parts and is controlled in its movement only by the water's own chemical nature. Thus in this warm, fluid, chemical environment all the processes that are necessary to life can be sustained. Second is the idea of water compartments within the whole. The word *compartment* is generally used in body physiology to indicate a collective whole in body systems, the parts of which are separated and distributed throughout the whole. These water compartments in the body are separated by membranes throughout the body, and quantities of water contained in various places in the body are balanced by forces that maintain an equilibrium among all the parts. Third, basic to an understanding of these balancing forces is the idea of particles in the water solution. It is the concentration and distribution of these particles in various places throughout the body water that determines all internal shifts and balances in the total body water.

Thus one can see a picture of a unified whole, sustained in balance to protect its life. This state of dynamic balance has been called *homeostasis*. The word homeostasis is a good choice to describe this balance in the body. It was coined by an outstanding physiologist many years ago to apply to the capacity of the body to maintain its life systems within, despite what enters the system from the outside. The first part of the word, *homeo-*, is from a Greek word meaning "similar." The second half of the word, -*stasis*, is also from a Greek root, meaning "balance." The body has a marvelous capacity to employ numerous, finely balanced homeostatic mechanisms that protect its vital water supply.

FUNCTIONS. This important water supply serves several basic life functions in the body:

1. *Solvent*. Water provides the basic liquid solvent for all the body's chemical processes. The word *hydrolysis* is used to describe this water based chemical activity within the body. The first part of the word, *hydro-*, means "water," and the second part of the word, -*lysis*, means "to break apart." Therefore with water as the basic solvent, multiple water solutions may be formed throughout the body to allow all of its life-sustaining metabolic activities to proceed.

2. *Transport*. Water circulates throughout the body, some in the form of blood and some in the form of various tissue fluids. In this circulating fluid the many nutrients, secretions, products formed in body metabolism, and other materials can be carried freely about to meet the needs of all the body cells. The body cell is the basic unit of life. Its fundamental needs for oxygen and nourishment, as well as needs for all its chemical activities, must be met at all times.

3. *Body form and structure*. Water also helps to give structure and form to the body by filling in spaces within body tissues. For example, striated muscle contains more water than any body tissue other than blood.

4. *Body temperature*. Water is necessary to help maintain a stable body temperature. As the temperature rises, sweat increases and evaporates, thus cooling the body.

5. *Body lubricant*. Water also has a lubricating effect on moving parts of the body. For example, the fluid within body joints helps to provide smooth movement of the many parts. This fluid in the body joints is called *synovial* fluid.

REQUIREMENTS. The body's requirement for water varies according to several factors:

1. *Temperature influence*. As the temperature rises in the surrounding environment, more body water is lost to help maintain the body temperature, and thus more water intake is required to offset it. This increasing temperature may be caused by the natural climate, or it may be caused by the heat of a work environment.

2. *Activity level*. Heavy work or extensive physical activity, such as in sports, increases the water requirement for two reasons: more water is lost as sweat, and the increased metabolic work requires more water.

3. *Functional losses*. When any disease process interferes with the normal functioning of the body, water requirements are affected. For example, in gastrointestinal problems such as prolonged diarrhea large amounts

of water may be lost. In such cases replacement of this water is vital to prevent dehydration.

4. *Metabolic needs.* The work of body metabolism requires water. A general rule is that about 1000 ml of water is required for every 1000 calories in the diet. On the average about two thirds of the water intake is supplied by beverages. The remaining one third is supplied by the solid foods consumed.

5. *Age.* Age plays an important role in determining body requirements, especially in the case of an infant. An infant's need for water is about 1500 ml/day. Water intake is more critical at this time than at any other age in life. This critical need is based on two facts: (1) the infant's body's content of water is from 70% to 75% of the total body weight, and (2) in an infant a relatively larger amount of the total body water is outside of the cells and thus is more easily lost.

THE HUMAN WATER BALANCE SYSTEM
Body water: the solvent

AMOUNT AND DISTRIBUTION. In the body of an adult man 55% to 65% of the total body weight is water; a woman's body is from 50% to 55% water. The higher water content in men generally results from their greater muscle mass, a tissue that contains a great deal of water. This total body water is divided into two major categories, depending on its placement in the body:

1. *Total water outside cells.* The total body water outside of the cells is called the *extracellular fluid* (ECF). This collective water throughout the body outside the cells makes up about 20% of the total body weight. About one fourth of this, 5% of the body weight, is contained in the blood plasma. The remaining three fourths, 15% of the body weight, is made up of water surrounding the cells and bathing the tissues, water in dense tissue such as bone, and water moving through the body in various tissue secretions. The water in the blood plasma includes the total fluid within the heart and all the blood vessels. The fluid surrounding the cells in the tissues is called *interstitial* fluid. This fluid helps to move materials in and out of the body cells to sustain life. Fluid in transit includes all the water in various body fluids and secretions, such as those of the salivary glands, thyroid gland, liver, pancreas, gallbladder, gastrointestinal tract, gonads, various mucous membranes, skin, kidneys, and eye spaces.

2. *Total water inside cells.* Total body water inside the cells is called the *intracellular* fluid (ICF). This total collective water inside the body cells amounts to about twice that outside the cells. This is not surprising, since the cell is the basic unit of life, and hence it is within the cells

that all life-sustaining body work is done. The ICF of the body makes up about 40% of the total body weight.

These relative total amounts of body water in the different "compartments" are compared in Fig. 8-1.

OVERALL WATER BALANCE. The average adult metabolizes from 2½ to 3 L/day of water in a turnover balanced between intake and output:

1. *Intake*. Water enters the body in three main forms: (a) as preformed water in liquids that are drunk, (b) as preformed water in foods that are eaten, and (c) as a product of cell oxidation when nutrients are burned in the body.

2. *Output*. Water leaves the body through the kidneys, skin, lungs, and feces. Of these output routes, the largest amount of water output from the body is through the kidneys. A certain amount of water is necessary for urinary excretion to carry out various products of metabolism that are not needed by the body. This is called *obligatory* water loss and must occur daily for health. An additional amount of water may also be put out by the kidneys each day depending on body activities and needs. This additional or *optional* water loss will depend on climate and physical activity. On the average the daily water output from the adult body totals about 2600 ml.

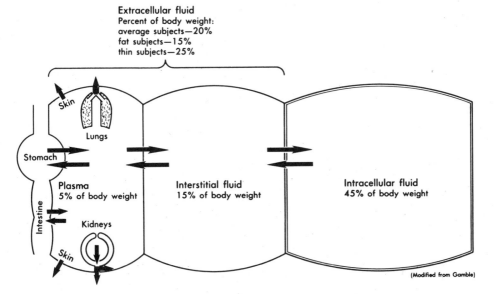

Fig. 8-1. Body fluid compartments. Note the relative total quantities of water in the intracellular compartment and the extracellular compartment.

Table 8-1. Approximate daily adult intake and output of water

	Intake (replacement) ml/day		Output (loss)	
			Obligatory (insensible) ml/day	Additional (according to need) ml/day
Preformed		Lungs	350	
Liquids	1200-1500	Skin		
In foods	700-1000	Diffusion	350	
Metabolism	200-300	Sweat	100	± 250
(oxidation of food)		Kidneys	900	± 500
		Feces	150	
TOTAL	2100-2800	TOTAL	1850	750
(approx. 2600 ml/day)			(approx. 2600 ml/day)	

This comparative intake and output water balance is summarized in Table 8-1.

Solute particles in solution

Solutes in the body water are a variety of particles in solution with varying concentrations. Two main types of particles control water balance in the body: electrolytes and plasma protein.

ELECTROLYTES. Electrolytes are small inorganic substances, either single mineral elements or small compounds, that can dissociate or break apart in a solution and carry on electrical charge. These charged particles are called *ions*, from the Greek word meaning "wanderer." Thus these charged particles are free to wander throughout a solution to maintain its chemical balance. In any chemical solution these particles are constantly in balance between the *cations*, those carrying a positive charge (e.g., sodium [Na^+], potassium [K^+], calcium [Ca^{++}], and magnesium [Mg^{++}]), and the *anions*, those carrying a negative charge (e.g., chloride [Cl^-], carbonate [HCO_3^-], phosphate [$HPO_4^=$], and sulfate [$SO_4^=$]).

The constant balance between the two electrolytes, sodium outside and potassium inside the cell, maintains water balance between these two compartments. Because of their small size, these electrolytes can diffuse freely across most membranes of the body. In this way they constantly serve to help maintain a needed balance between water outside the cell and water inside the cell.

The balance between cation and anion concentrations in the body fluids maintains a state of neutrality in these fluids that is necessary to sustain life. The measure of electrolyte concentration in body fluids is given in terms of *milliequivalents* (mEg/L). This simply refers to the number of these particles

Table 8-2. Balance of cation and anion concentrations in extracellular fluid (ECF) and intracellular fluid (ICF), which maintains electroneutrality within each compartment

		ECF (mEq/L)	ICF (mEq/L)
Cation	Na$^+$	142	35
	K$^+$	5	123
	Ca^{++}	5	15
	Mg^{++}	3	2
	TOTAL	155	175
Anion	Cl$^-$	104	5
	HPO$_4^=$	2	80
	SO$_4^=$	1	10
	Organic acids	5	
	Protein	16	70
	HCO$_3^-$	27	10
	TOTAL	155	175

in solution per unit of fluid. Table 8-2 outlines the balance between cations and anions in the two major body fluid compartments. It can be seen that the number of particles in each of the two compartments exactly balance.

PLASMA PROTEIN. Plasma protein, mainly in the form of albumin, is an organic compound of large molecular size. As such, it does not move as freely across membranes as do electrolytes, which are much smaller. Thus plasma protein molecules are retained in the blood vessel. Because of this, these molecules make up a major substance in circulating blood that controls water movement in the body and preserves blood volume. In a similar manner cell protein helps to preserve cell water.

SMALL ORGANIC COMPOUNDS. In addition to the two major particles in body fluids, electrolytes and plasma protein, other organic compounds of small size are in solution in body water. However, they do not ordinarily influence shifts of water because their concentration is too small. In some instances, however, they are found in abnormally large concentrations and do influence water movement. For example, glucose is one of these small particles in body fluids. Only when it is in abnormal concentrations, such as in uncontrolled diabetes, does it influence water loss from the body.

Separating membranes

CAPILLARY WALL. The walls of the capillaries are fairly free membranes because they are thin and porous. Thus water molecules and small particles can move freely across these membranes. Such small particles would include electrolytes and various nutrients. However, larger particles such as plasma protein molecules cannot pass through pores in the capillary membrane. These plasma protein molecules remain in the capillary vessel and exert an important pressure control that keeps the water in circulation between capillaries and surrounding tissue cells.

CELL WALL. The walls of the cells are thicker membranes, constructed to protect the cell contents. These walls are structured in sandwich fashion, with outer layers of protein and an inner structure of fat material. Special transport mechanisms are necessary to carry substances across cell walls.

Forces moving water and solutes across membranes

As a result of the presence of these separating membranes, the capillary wall and the cell wall, certain forces are created that control the movement of body water and particles in solution.

OSMOSIS. Through the pressure created by osmosis, water molecules are moved from a space of greater concentration of water molecules to a space of lesser concentration of water molecules. The effect of this movement is to distribute water molecules more evenly throughout the body and thus provide a solvent base for materials the water must carry.

DIFFUSION. Diffusion is a force similar to osmosis but applies to the particles in solution in the water. It is the force by which these particles move outward in all directions from a space of greater concentration of particles to a space of lesser concentration of particles. The relative movements of water molecules and solute particles by osmosis and diffusion have the effect of balancing concentrations and hence pressures on both sides of a separating membrane. These balancing forces of osmosis and diffusion are shown in Fig. 8-2.

FILTRATION. Water is forced or filtered through the pores of membranes when there is a difference in pressures on the two sides of the membrane. This difference in pressure would be the result of differences in concentration of the particles in the two solutions.

ACTIVE TRANSPORT. Particles in solution that are vital to body processes must move across membranes throughout the body at all times, even when the pressures are against their flow. Thus some means of energy-driven active transport are necessary to carry these particles across the separating membranes. Usually these active transport mechanisms require some kind of carrier partner to help "ferry" them across the membrane. For example, glucose enters cells through an active transport mechanism that involves sodium as a "ferrying" partner.

PINOCYTOSIS. Sometimes larger particles, such as proteins and fats, enter cells by the interesting process of pinocytosis (Fig. 8-3). The word *pinocytosis* means "cell drinking." In this process these larger molecules attach themselves to the cell wall and are then engulfed by the cell. In this way they are carried into the center of the cell wall and across into the cell. For example, this is one of the mechanisms by which fat is absorbed from the small intestine.

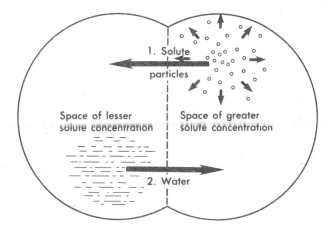

Fig. 8-2. Movement of molecules, water, and solutes by osmosis and diffusion.

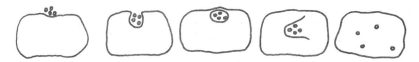

Fig. 8-3. Pinocytosis—engulfing of large molecules by the cell.

Water circulation to tissues

CAPILLARY FLUID SHIFT MECHANISM. One of the most important control mechanisms in the body that maintains overall water balance throughout is the capillary fluid shift mechanism. Water is constantly circulated through the body by the blood vessels. However, it must get out of the blood vessels to service the tissues with life-sustaining oxygen and nutrients. It must then be drawn back into circulation to maintain the normal flow. The body maintains this constant flow of water through the tissues, carrying materials to and from the cells, by means of a balance of pressures. A filtration process operates according to the differences in osmotic pressure on either side of the capillary wall.

When the blood first enters the capillary system, the blood pressure forces water and small solutes (e.g., glucose) out into the tissues to bathe and nourish the cells. This force of blood pressure is an example of *hydrostatic* pressure (*hydro*- meaning "water" and -*static* meaning "balance"). Plasma protein particles, mainly albumin, are too large to go through the pores of capillary walls. Hence the concentration of protein particles remaining in the capillary vessel exerts the necessary osmotic pressure to draw the water back into circulation after it has bathed the cells. This fluid shift mechanism, which is maintained by the balance between blood pressure and osmotic pressure of the plasma protein particles to control the flow of tissue fluid, is illustrated in Fig. 8-4.

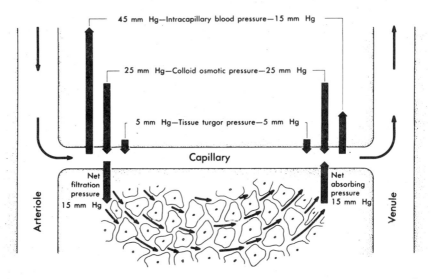

Fig. 8-4. The fluid shift mechanism. Note the balance of pressures that controls the flow of fluid.

Organ systems involved

GASTROINTESTINAL SYSTEM. Water from the blood plasma, containing vital electrolytes, is secreted constantly into the gastrointestinal tract to aid in the processes of digestion and absorption. These materials, water and electrolytes, circulate constantly between the blood plasma, the secreting cells, and the gastrointestinal tract. In the latter portion of the intestine most of the water and electrolytes are then reabsorbed into the blood to circulate over and over again. This constant movement of water and electrolytes between the blood, the secreting cells, and the gastrointestinal tract is called *gastrointestinal circulation*. The sheer magnitude of gastrointestinal circulation, as shown in Table 8-3, indicates how serious results of fluid loss from the upper or lower portion of the gastrointestinal tract can be.

Gastrointestinal fluids are held in *isotonicity* (equality of osmotic pressure resulting from ion equilibrium) with the surrounding ECF. For example, when a person drinks water, plain water without any solutes or accompanying food, electrolytes and salts enter the intestine from the surrounding blood plasma fluid. If a concentrated solution or food is ingested, additional water will then be drawn into the intestine from the surrounding fluid to dilute the intestinal contents. In each instance water and electrolytes move from compartment to compartment to maintain solutions in the gastrointestinal tract that are isotonic (equal concentration of particles) with the surrounding fluid.

This law of isotonicity has many clinical implications. For example, what would happen if a patient undergoing gastric suctioning drank water or if a

Table 8-3. Approximate total volume of digestive secretions produced in 24 hours by an adult of average size

Secretion	Volume (ml)
Saliva	1500
Gastric	2500
Bile	500
Pancreatic	700
Intestinal	3000
TOTAL	8200

Table 8-4. Approximate concentration of certain electrolytes in digestive fluids (mEq/L)

Secretion	Na^+	K^+	Cl^-	HCO_3^-
Saliva	10	25	10	15
Gastric	40	10	145	0
Pancreatic	140	5	40	110
Jejunal	135	5	110	30
Bile	140	10	110	40

patient being maintained by tube feeding were given the formula too rapidly at too concentrated a dilution? In the first case the water would cause the stomach to produce more secretions containing electrolytes. Then the electrolytes would be lost in the suctioning. In turn the plasma, from which the electrolytes are supplied, would be gradually depleted of these electrolytes and unable to supply them to tissue cells. In the second case the concentrated (hypertonic) solution being given by tube would cause a shift of water into the intestine, which would in turn rapidly shrink the surrounding blood volume. This condition would then produce symptoms of shock.

It is not surprising, because of the large amounts of water and electrolytes involved, that upper and lower gastrointestinal losses constitute the most common cause of clinical fluid and electrolyte problems. Such problems would exist, for example, in persistent vomiting or in prolonged diarrhea, in which large amounts of water and precious electrolytes are lost. The large numbers of electrolytes involved in gastrointestinal circulation are shown in Table 8-4.

KIDNEYS. The kidneys maintain appropriate levels of all the various constituents of blood by filtering the blood and then selectively reabsorbing water and needed materials to be carried throughout the body. Through this continuous "laundering" of the blood through the nephrons of the kidneys, the blood is maintained in its proper solution and water balance is continued. When disease occurs in the kidneys and this filtration process does not operate normally, water imbalances occur.

Hormonal controls. Two basic hormonal controls operate in the kidneys to maintain constant water balance in the body:

1. *ADH mechanism.* Antidiuretic hormone (ADH) is produced by the pituitary gland. It operates on the kidneys' nephrons to cause reabsorption of water. Hence it is a water-conserving mechanism. In any stress situation with threatened or real loss of body water this hormone is triggered to conserve vital body water.

2. *Aldosterone mechanism.* A second important hormonal process that governs the renal control of water and electrolyte balance is the aldosterone mechanism. The hormone aldosterone is produced by the adrenal glands. It operates on the nephrons of the kidney to cause reabsorption of sodium. This mechanism is primarily a sodium-conserving device, but it also exerts a secondary control over water. Both ADH and aldosterone may be activated by stress situations such as body injury or surgery.

These hormonal responses to stress are illustrated in Fig. 8-5.

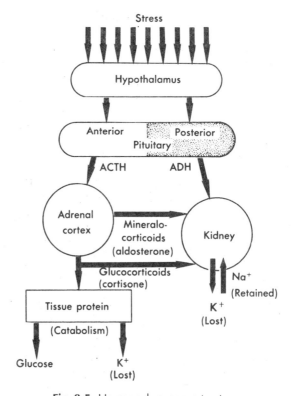

Fig. 8-5. Hormonal response to stress.

ACID-BASE BALANCE SYSTEM

Water and electrolytes are involved in a second area that has broad physiological implications: the acid-base balance system. This system is essential to the maintenance of an optimum acid-base balance throughout the body so that the processes necessary for the life of the body can be maintained.

Acids and bases

A substance is *more or less* acid, according to the degree of its concentration of hydrogen. Its degree of acidity is therefore expressed in terms of pH. The symbol pH is derived from a mathematical term. It refers to the *power* of the *H*ydrogen ion concentration. A pH of 7 is the neutral point between an acid and a base. Substances with a pH *lower* than 7 are *acid*. (Since the pH is in effect a negative mathematical factor, the higher the hydrogen ion concentration, the lower the pH.) Substances with a pH above 7 are *alkaline*.

Buffer system

The body deals with degrees of acidity by maintaining a buffer system to handle excess acid. A buffer system is a mixture of acidic and alkaline components, an acid partner and a base partner, which together protect a solution against wide variations in its pH, even when strong bases or acids are added to it. For example, if a strong acid is added to a buffered solution, the base partner reacts with the added acid to form a weaker acid. If a strong base is added to the solution, the acid partner combines with the intruder to form a weaker base. In both cases the pH is restored to its starting balance point.

THE CARBONIC ACID–SODIUM BICARBONATE BUFFER SYSTEM. Although the human body contains many buffered solutions, its main buffer system is the carbonic acid–sodium bicarbonate (H_2CO_3–$NaHCO_3$) system. The body selects this as its principal buffer system for two reasons. First, the raw materials for the production of the acid partner carbonic acid (H_2CO_3) are readily available. These materials are carbon dioxide (CO_2) and water (H_2O). Second, the lungs and kidneys can easily adjust to alterations in the acid and base partners and quickly return the body fluids to a normal pH level. The normal pH of the ECF is 7.4, with a range of 7.35 to 7.45. Maintenance of the pH within this narrow range is necessary to sustain the life of the cells.

The carbonic acid–sodium bicarbonate buffer system is able to maintain this necessary degree of acidity in the body fluids because the base bicarbonate partner in this buffer system is about 20 times as abundant as the carbonic acid partner. This 20:1 base-to-acid ratio is maintained even though the absolute amounts of the two partners may fluctuate during adjustment periods. Whether or not added base or acid enters the system, as long as the 20:1 ratio is maintained, the ECF acid-base balance is held constant (Fig. 8-6). In this way the life of the cells is protected.

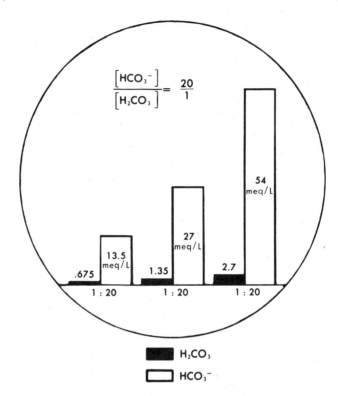

$$\frac{[HCO_3^-]}{[H_2CO_3]} = \frac{20}{1}$$

54
meq/L

27
meq/L

13.5
meq/L

.675   1.35   2.7

1 : 20   1 : 20   1 : 20

■ H_2CO_3

□ HCO_3^-

Fig. 8-6. The base/acid ratio of 20:1 maintains a constant normal blood pH of 7.4.

Questions on water balance

1. Where is the water in the body?
2. How is it distributed? Is the major portion outside or inside of cells? Why?
3. What is the balance between water intake and output? About how much water does an average healthy adult take in and put out daily? What are the sources of the water intake? What are the routes of the water output?
4. Distinguish between *obligatory* and *optional* water excretion by the kidney. Why is the latter significant in body controls of water balance?
5. What forces control the distribution of water in the body?
6. What do electrolytes do? Why are they so significant a factor in body water balance? Name two major electrolytes, one controlling water inside of cells and one controlling water outside of cells.
7. What is the important role of plasma protein (albumin) in maintaining overall body water balance throughout the tissues?
8. What happens in osmosis? Diffusion? Filtration?
9. In what other ways may molecules cross membrane when resistance is great and more metabolic work is required?
10. What is the role of gastrointestinal circulation in water distribution and use?
11. What is the role of the kidneys in maintaining water balance? How do hormones influence this function?

12. What is the difference between an acid and a base? What does the symbol pH mean?
13. What is a buffer system? How does it operate to protect a solution? What happens when an acid is added? What happens when a base is added?
14. What is the major acid-base buffer system in the body? What ratio does this system maintain between its acid and base components?

Matching

Write the correct word(s) and corresponding letter in each of the numbered blanks below.

_____ 1. Chief electrolyte guarding the water outside of cells

_____ 2. An ion carrying a negative electrical charge

_____ 3. Sodium-conserving mechanism, or control agent

_____ 4. Simple passage of water molecules (solvent) through a membrane separating solutions of different concentrations, from the side of lower concentration of solute particles to that of higher concentration of particles, thus tending to equalize the solutions

_____ 5. A substance (atom or group of atoms) that, in solution, conducts an electrical current and is dissociated into cations and anions

_____ 6. Particles, such as electrolytes and protein, in solution

_____ 7. State of dynamic equilibrium maintained by an organism among all of its parts and controlled by many finely balanced mechanisms

_____ 8. Chief electrolyte guarding the water inside of cells

_____ 9. Major plasma protein that guards and maintains the circulating blood volume

_____ 10. Abnormal increase in water held in tissue

_____ 11. An ion carrying a positive electrical charge

_____ 12. The body's means of maintaining the flow of water through tissues; accomplished by a net filtration pressure in the capillaries, resulting from the difference in opposing forces of hydrostatic pressure and colloidal osmotic pressure from plasma protein

_____ 13. Force exerted by a contained fluid, for example, blood pressure

_____ 14. Passive movement of particles throughout a solution and across membranes from the area of denser concentration of particles outward to all surrounding spaces

_____ 15. A type of fluid outside of cells

_____ 16. Movement of particles in a solution across cell walls against normal osmotic pressures, involving a carrier substance to help "ferry" them across and requiring energy to do the work

a. osmosis   d. cation
b. solutes   e. interstitial fluid
c. diffusion   f. homeostasis

g. anion
h. K$^+$
i. albumin
j. hydrostatic pressure
k. Na$^+$

l. electrolyte
m. active transport
n. aldosterone
o. capillary fluid shift mechanism
p. edema

Suggested readings

Guthrie, H.A.: Introductory nutrition, ed. 5, St. Louis, 1983, The C.V. Mosby Co.

Robinson, J.R.: Water, the indispensable nutrient, Nutr. Today **5**(1):16-29, 1970.

Williams, S.R.: Nutrition and diet therapy, ed. 4, St. Louis, 1981, The C.V. Mosby Co.

Williams, S.R.: Essentials of nutrition and diet therapy, ed. 3, St. Louis, 1982, The C.V. Mosby Co.

9

Digestion and absorption

DIGESTION
Basic principles of digestion

Digestion is the process by which food is broken up in the gastrointestinal tract, releasing its food nutrients for absorption into the body's circulation system and transport to the cells, where the varied nutrients can be used in the cell's many metabolic tasks. Before this sequence of actions can take place, however, the food that is eaten must go through a series of mechanical and chemical changes that constitute digestion (Fig. 9-1).

MECHANICAL DIGESTION: GASTROINTESTINAL MOTILITY. Mechanical digestion is made possible by the coordinated action of both muscles and nerves in the walls of the gastrointestinal tract. This coordinated activity provides the necessary *motility*—the capacity for spontaneous action—that enables the system to do its work of breaking up the food mass and moving it along at an optimum rate:

Muscles. The layers of smooth muscle making up the gastrointestinal wall interact to produce two general types of movement: (1) general muscle tone or tonic contraction, which ensures continuous passage of the food mass and valve control along the way; and (2) periodic, rhythmical contractions, which mix the food mass and move it forward. These alternating muscular contractions and relaxations that force the contents forward are known as *peristalsis*.

Nerves. Specific nerves regulate these muscular actions. A complex network of nerves within the gastrointestinal wall extends from the esophagus to the anus. These nerves control muscle tone in the wall, regulate the rate and intensity of the periodic muscle contractions, and coordinate the various movements.

CHEMICAL DIGESTION: GASTROINTESTINAL SECRETIONS. Chemical digestion is made possible by the action of a number of secretions. Generally, there are four types of secretions:

1. *Enzymes*. Digestive enzymes are proteins, specific in kind and quantity for the breaking down of specific nutrients.

2. *Hydrochloric acid and buffer ions*. These materials are needed to produce the pH required for the activity of given enzymes.

3. *Mucus*. Secretions of mucus lubricate and protect the tissues lining the gastrointestinal tract and aid in mixing the food mass.

4. *Water and electrolytes*. These components of gastrointestinal circulation are provided in sufficient quantities to carry or circulate the organic products of digestion.

Special secretory cells in the gastrointestinal tract itself or in nearby accessory organs—the pancreas and the liver—produce these special secretions for chemical digestion. The secretory action of these special cells or glands may be stimulated locally by the presence of food, by nerve stimuli, or by hormones specific for certain nutrients.

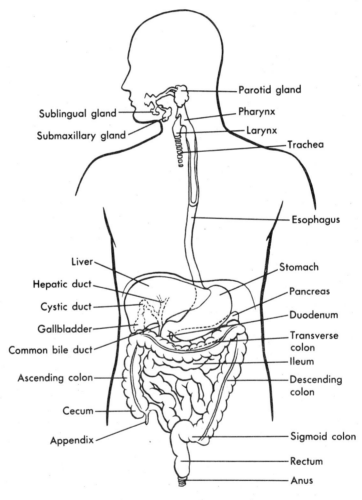

Fig. 9-1. The organs used in the digestion-absorption process.

Digestion in the mouth and esophagus

MECHANICAL DIGESTION. In the mouth, mastication (biting and chewing) begins the breaking up of the food into smaller particles. The teeth and oral structures are particularly suited for this function. Swallowing of the mixed mass of food particles and its passage down the esophagus are accomplished by peristaltic waves controlled by nerve reflexes. Gravity aids this movement down the esophagus, but for a bedridden patient in a prone position, it is much more difficult. Clinical conditions that may hinder normal food passage at this point include *cardiospasm* and *hiatus hernia*. Cardiospasm is a condition in which the muscle valve between the esophagus and the stomach fails to relax properly, closing the food passageway. Hiatus hernia is a condition in which an upper part of the stomach protrudes into the thorax through an abnormal opening in the diaphragm, which allows food to be held in the outpouched area. Both conditions cause pain or "heartburn" after eating and frequent re-gurgitation.

CHEMICAL DIGESTION. The salivary glands secrete *ptyalin*, an enzyme specific for starches, but the food remains in the mouth too brief a time for much chemical action to occur. The salivary glands also secrete a mucous material that lubricates and binds food particles to aid in swallowing each food bolus, or lump of food material. Mucous glands also line the esophagus, and their secretions aid in movement of the food mass toward the stomach.

Digestion in the stomach

MECHANICAL DIGESTION. The major parts of the stomach are shown in Fig. 9-2. Muscles in the stomach wall store, mix, and empty the food mass in slow, controlled movements. The pyloric valve at the end of the stomach releases

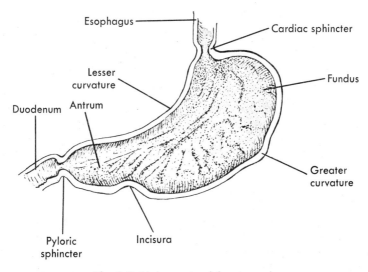

Fig. 9-2. Major parts of the stomach.

the semiliquid acid food mass, now called *chyme*, slowly enough so that it can be buffered by the alkaline intestinal secretions and not irritate the lining of the duodenum, the first section of the small intestine.

CHEMICAL DIGESTION. Special gastric cells produce hydrochloric acid and mucus. Other special cells secrete pepsinogen, which is activated by the hydrochloric acid and previously formed pepsin to form the active enzyme *pepsin*. Pepsin then begins the breakdown of proteins to smaller polypeptides. Still other secretory cells produce small amounts of a specific gastric lipase, *tributyrinase*, an enzyme that acts on tributyrin (the fat in butterfat), but this is a relatively minor activity. Nerve stimulus for these secretions is produced in response to sensation, food taken in, or emotions. For example, anger and hostility increase secretions. Fear and depression decrease secretions and inhibit blood flow and motility as well. Additional hormonal stimulus comes in response to the entrance of food into the stomach.

Digestion in the small intestine

Up to this point digestion of food consumed has been largely mechanical, delivering to the small intestine a semifluid chyme made up of fine food particles mixed with watery secretions. Chemical digestion has thus far been limited. Thus the major task of digestion, and of absorption that follows, occurs in the small intestine. Its structural parts, its synchronized movements, and its array of specific enzymes are highly developed for this all-important final task of mechanical and chemical digestion. These finely coordinated actions are presented here for study and review.

MECHANICAL DIGESTION. Under the control of nerves, or wall stretch pressure from the food mass or from hormonal stimuli, the intestinal muscles produce several types of movement, as shown in Fig. 9-3, that aid mechanical digestion:

1. *Segmentation rings* from alternate contractions of circular muscles progressively chop the food mass into successive boluses or lumps. This action constantly mixes food materials with secretions.
2. *Longitudinal rotation* by long muscles running the length of the intestine rolls the slowly moving food mass in a spiral motion, mixing it and exposing new surfaces for absorption.
3. *Pendular movements* from small local muscles sweep back and forth, stirring the chyme at the mucosal surface.
4. *Peristaltic waves* push the food mass slowly forward. The intensity of these waves may be increased by food intake or by the presence of irritants. In some cases this causes long, sweeping waves over the entire length of the intestine.
5. *Motion of the surface villi* stirs and mixes chyme in contact with the intestinal wall, exposing additional nutrient material for absorption.

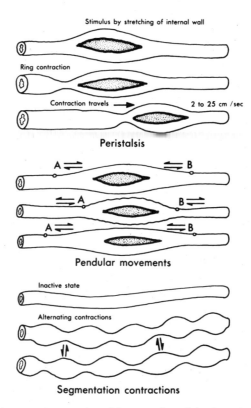

Fig. 9-3. Types of movement produced by muscles of the intestine: peristaltic waves from contraction of deep circular muscle, pendular movements from small local muscles, and segmentation rings formed by alternate contraction and relaxation of circular muscle.

CHEMICAL DIGESTION. To meet the major burden of chemical digestion, this portion of the gastrointestinal system secretes a large number of enzymes. Each one is specific for a particular nutrient. They are secreted from intestinal glands and from the pancreas, as listed below:

Enzymes from intestinal glands

1. *Fat*. Intestinal lipase converts fat to glycerides and fatty acids.
2. *Protein*. A series of enzymes complete the digestion of proteins.
    a. Enterokinase converts inactive trypsinogen (from the pancreas) to active trypsin, which in turn breaks down proteins and polypeptides to smaller peptide fragments.
    b. Amino peptidase removes the end amino acid from polypeptides.
    c. Dipeptidase converts dipeptides to amino acids.
3. *Carbohydrate*. Disaccharidases (maltase, lactase, sucrase) convert their respective disaccharides (maltose, lactose, sucrose) to the monosaccharides (glucose, fructose, galactose).

Enzymes from the pancreas

1. *Fat*. Pancreatic lipase converts fat to glycerides and fatty acids.
2. *Protein*. Additional enzymes from the pancreas also work on proteins.
   a. Active trypsin, as indicated above, breaks down proteins and polypeptides to smaller peptides. Trypsin also activates chymotrypsinogen to chymotrypsin, which in turn continues the breakdown of protein and polypeptides to smaller and smaller peptide fragments.
   b. Carboxypeptidase removes an end amino acid from polypeptides.
3. *Carbohydrate*. Pancreatic amylase converts starch to disaccharides.

Mucus secreted by intestinal glands protects the musocal lining from irritation and digestion by the highly acidic gastric juices entering the duodenum. Emotions inhibit these mucous secretions and are an important cause of duodenal ulcers.

Hormonal control of secretions

The hormone secretin, produced by mucosal glands in the first part of the intestine, controls the secretion of the enzymes from the pancreas, especially their degree of acidity. The resulting alkaline environment in the small intestine, with a pH of 8, is necessary for activity of the pancreatic enzymes.

Role of bile

Bile is not an enzyme; rather, it helps to prepare fat for enzyme action. Bile accomplishes this preparation of fat through the process of *emulsification*. In this process bile breaks the fat up into smaller bits and changes surface tension so that enzymes will have more surface area to work on and can penetrate that surface more easily. Bile is produced in the liver and is concentrated and stored by the gallbladder. When fat enters the first part of the small

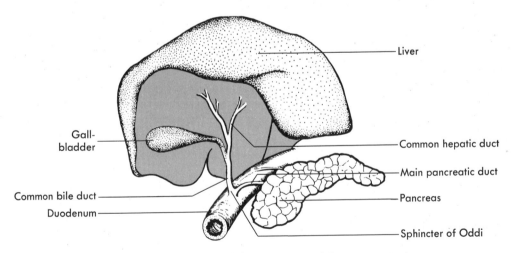

Fig. 9-4. Organs of the biliary system and the pancreatic ducts.

intestine, the specific hormone *cholecystokinin* is secreted by intestinal mucosa glands and stimulates the gallbladder to contract and release the concentrated bile into the intestine to do its important emulsifying work on fat.

The arrangement of the accessory organs to the duodenum, which comprise the biliary system, is shown in Fig. 9-4. The various nerve and hormone controls of digestion are illustrated in Fig. 9-5. A summary of the digestive processes is provided in Table 9-1.

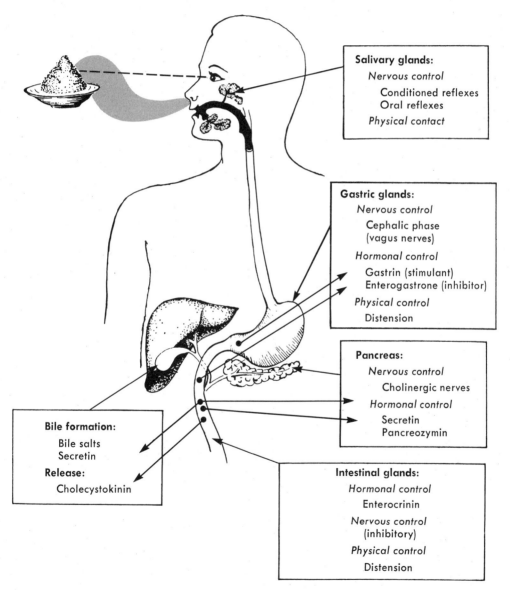

Fig. 9-5. Summary of factors influencing secretions of the gastrointestinal glands.

Table 9-1. Summary of digestive processes

Nutrient	Mouth	Stomach	Small intestine
Carbohydrate	Starch $\xrightarrow{\text{Ptyalin}}$ Dextrins		**Pancreas** Starch $\xrightarrow{\text{Amylase}}$ (Disaccharides) Starch $\longrightarrow$ Maltose and sucrose **Intestine** Lactose $\xrightarrow{\text{Lactase}}$ (Monosaccharides) Lactose $\longrightarrow$ Glucose and galactose Sucrose $\xrightarrow{\text{Sucrase}}$ Glucose and fructose Maltose $\xrightarrow{\text{Maltase}}$ Glucose and glucose
Protein		Protein $\xrightarrow[\text{Hydrochloric acid}]{\text{Pepsin}}$ Polypeptides	**Pancreas** Protein, Polypeptides $\xrightarrow{\text{Trypsin}}$ Dipeptides Protein, Polypeptides $\xrightarrow{\text{Chymotrypsin}}$ Dipeptides Polypeptides, Dipeptides $\xrightarrow{\text{Carboxypeptidase}}$ Amino acids

Intestine

Polypeptides, Dipeptides $\xrightarrow{\text{Aminopeptidase}}$ Amino acids

Dipeptides $\xrightarrow{\text{Dipeptidase}}$ Amino acids

Pancreas

Fat $\xrightarrow{\text{Lipase}}$ Glycerol
Glycerides (di-, mono-)
Fatty acids

Intestine

Fat $\xrightarrow{\text{Lipase}}$ Glycerol
Glycerides (di-, mono-)
Fatty acids

Liver and gallbladder

Fat $\xrightarrow{\text{Bile}}$ Emulsified fat

Fat

Tributyrin $\xrightarrow{\text{Tributyrinase}}$ Glycerol
(butterfat) Fatty acids

ABSORPTION
Small intestine

SPECIAL ABSORBING STRUCTURES. Three important parts of the absorbing surface structure of the intestinal wall are particularly adapted to ensure and maximize the absorption of essential nutrients freed from food in the digestive process:

1. *Mucosal folds*. The surface of the small intestine piles in folds, like so many hills and valleys in a mountain range. These folds can easily be seen with the naked eye when such tissue is examined.

2. *Villi*. Closer examination by regular light microscope reveals small, fingerlike projections, the villi, covering these piled-up folds of mucosal lining. These villi further increase the area of exposed surface. Each villus has ample blood vessels to receive protein and carbohydrate materials and a special lymph vessel to receive fat materials. This lymph vessel is called a *lacteal* because of the fatty chyme at this point looks like milk.

3. *Microvilli*. Still closer examination with an electron microscope reveals numerous smaller projections on the surface of each villus. This huge covering of microvilli on each minute villus is called the *brush border* because it looks like bristles on a brush.

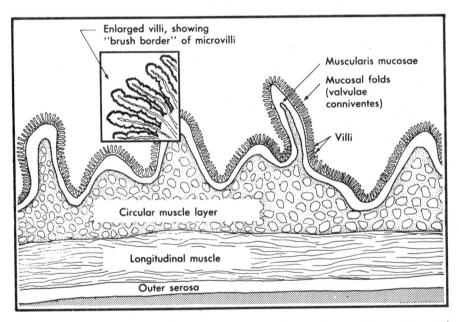

Fig. 9-6. Intestinal wall. Note the arrangement of muscle layers and the structures of the mucosa that increase the surface area for absorption—mucosal folds, villi, and microvilli.

These three structures of the inner intestinal wall, the folds, the villi, and the microvilli, combine to make the inner surface some 600 times the area of the outer surface of the intestine. Also, the length of the small intestine in a living person is about 22 feet (660 cm), and it is evident that this is a remarkable organ, well adapted to handle food and deliver its precious nutrients to the body cells. In fact as a feat in providing a tremendous absorbing surface in such a compact space, it can scarcely be equaled. It has been estimated that if this entire surface were spread out on a flat plane, the total surface area would be as large or larger than half a basketball court. Far from being the lowly "gut," this is actually one of the most highly developed, exquisitely fashioned, specialized tissues in the human body. These structures are illustrated in Fig. 9-6.

ABSORPTION PROCESSES. A number of processes accomplish the task of ensuring that all the vital nutrients can move across the absorbing wall of the intestine and into body circulation. These processes include diffusion, both passive or simple for small materials and carrier assisted for larger items, energy-driven active transport with the help of a "ferrying" substance, and penetration of large materials through engulfing pinocytosis. These processes are described in Chapter 8.

ROUTES OF ABSORPTION. Most of the products of digestion are water-soluble nutrients and so can be absorbed directly into the bloodstream. Since fatty materials are not water soluble, another route must be provided. These fat molecules pass into the lymph vessels in the villi, the lacteals, flow into the larger lymph vessels of the body, and eventually enter the blood.

Large intestine (colon)

The main absorption task remaining for the large intestine is that of taking up needed body water. The large amounts of circulating intestinal fluids handled daily by the body are presented in Table 9-2. The major portion of the water in the chyme entering the large intestine is absorbed in the first half of the

Table 9-2. Daily absorption volume in human gastrointestinal system

	Intake (L)	Intestinal absorption (L)	Elimination (L)
Food ingested	1.5		
Gastrointestinal secretions	8.5		
TOTAL	10.0		
Fluid absorbed in small intestine		9.5	
Fluid absorbed in large intestine		0.4	
TOTAL		9.9	
Feces			0.1

Table 9-3. Intestinal absorption of some major nutrients

Nutrient	Form	Means of absorption	Control agent or required cofactor	Route
Carbohydrate	Monosaccharides (glucose and galactose)	Competitive Selective Active transport via sodium pump	— — Sodium	Blood
Protein	Amino acids	Selective	—	Blood
	Some dipeptides	Carrier transport systems	Pyridoxine (pyridoxal phosphate)	Blood
	Whole protein (rare)	Pinocytosis	—	Blood
Fat	Fatty acids	Fatty acid-bile complex (micelles)	Bile	Lymph
	Glycerides (mono-, di-)		—	Lymph
	Few triglycerides (neutral fat)	Pinocytosis		Lymph
Vitamins	B_{12}	Carrier transport	Intrinsic factor (IF)	Blood
	A	Bile complex	Bile	Blood
	K	Bile complex	Bile	From large intestine to blood
Minerals	Sodium	Active transport via sodium pump	—	Blood
	Calcium	Active transport	Vitamin D	Blood
	Iron	Active transport	Ferritin mechanism	Blood (as transferritin)
Water	Water	Osmosis	—	Blood, lymph, interstitial fluid

colon. Only a small amount remains, about 100 ml, to form the feces and aid in its elimination. Dietary fiber contributes important bulk to the food mass throughout the digestion-absorption process and helps to form the feces.

A summary of some of the major features of nutrient absorption in the intestines is given in Table 9-3.

Questions on digestion and absorption

1. What is digestion?
2. What do enzymes do in the digestive process?
3. What is meant by the specific action of enzymes?
4. What changes in the food take place in the mouth?
5. What happens to the food in the fundus part of the stomach?
6. What are the active ingredients of gastric juice?
7. What are the juices that act on food in the intestine?
8. Where does most of the absorption of food nutrients take place?
9. What is the function of the villi?

10. What products of digestion pass into the blood?
11. What products of digestion pass into the lymphatic system?
12. Does the large intestine secrete any enzymes?

True-false

Circle *T* if a statement is true. Circle *F* if it is false, and then write the correct statement.

T   F   1. The digestive products of a large meal are difficult to absorb because the overall area of the intestinal absorbing surface is relatively small.

T   F   2. Some enzymes must be activated by hydrochloric acid or other enzymes before they can act.

T   F   3. Bile is a specific enzyme for fat.

T   F   4. One enzyme may work on more than one nutrient.

T   F   5. Gastrointestinal circulation provides a constant supply of water and electrolytes to carry digestive secretions and substances being produced.

T   F   6. Secretions from gastrointestinal accessory organs, the gallbladder and the pancreas, mix with gastric secretions to aid digestion.

T   F   7. Bile is released from the gallbladder in response to the cholecystokinin hormone stimulus.

Multiple choice

Circle the letter in front of the correct choice.

1. During digestion the major muscle action that moves the food mass forward by regular rhythmic waves is called:
   a. valve contraction
   b. segmentation ring motion
   c. muscle tone
   d. peristalsis
2. Gastrointestinal secretory action is triggered by:
   (1) hormones
   (2) enzymes
   (3) nerve network
   (4) senses of sight, smell, and taste
   a. (1) and (2)
   b. (2) and (4)
   c. (1), (3), and (4)
   d. (2) and (3)
3. Mucus is an important gastrointestinal secretion because it:
   a. causes chemical changes in some substances to prepare them for enzyme action
   b. helps to create the proper degree of acidity for enzymes to act
   c. lubricates and protects the gastrointestinal lining
   d. helps to emulsify fat
4. Pepsin is:
   a. produced in the small intestine to act on protein
   b. a gastric enzyme that acts on protein
   c. produced in the pancreas to act on fat
   d. produced in the small intestine to act on fat
5. Bile is an important secretion that is:
   a. produced by the gallbladder
   b. stored in the liver

      c. an aid to protein digestion
      d. an emulsifying agent for fat
   6. The route of fat absorption is:
      a. the lymphatic system via the villi lacteals
      b. directly into the portal blood circulation
      c. with the aid of bile directly into the villi blood capillaries
      d. with the aid of protein directly into the portal circulation as lipoproteins

Suggestion for additional study

   1. If possible, secure a film showing the various processes involved in the digestion of food.

Suggested readings

Guthrie, H.A.: Introductory nutrition, ed. 5, St. Louis, 1983, The C.V. Mosby Co.

Williams, S.R.: Nutrition and diet therapy, ed. 4, St. Louis, 1981, The C.V. Mosby Co.

Williams, S.R.: Essentials of nutrition and diet therapy, ed. 3, St. Louis, 1982, The C.V. Mosby Co.

PART TWO

COMMUNITY NUTRITION:
THE LIFE CYCLE

10

Nutrition for various age groups

NUTRITION FOR CHILDREN
Infants

BREAST-FEEDING. Almost any mother can breast-feed her baby if she has had the proper diet during pregnancy and if she maintains that diet during the time she wants to nurse the baby. Human milk provides the ideal first food for the human infant and is the primary recommendation of both pediatricians and nutritionists. Its content of nutrients is uniquely adapted to meet the growth needs of the infant. Moreover, the form of these materials in human milk is better used by the baby than are those corresponding constituents of cow's milk. There is more iron in human milk, which is also better absorbed and used by the baby. Human milk contains more vitamins A and K, ascorbic acid, and niacin. It also gives the infant immunity to certain diseases.

Breast-feeding gives the baby a good start in life. It may be especially important during the first month. It also helps the mother's uterus to return to normal more quickly. It assists in the important early "bonding" process, building a warm and affectionate relationship between mother and child.

The infant may be weaned from breast-feeding after the sixth month unless another pregnancy or an illness of the mother occurs sooner. The average age for weaning the baby under usual circumstances is about 9 months.

WEIGHT GAIN. Infants will more or less establish their own rate of weight gain. As long as they make a steady gain in weight and appear to be satisfied, one can assume that they are getting enough to eat. During the first 6 months babies will usually make an average gain of 6 ounces (168 g) a week. They should have doubled their birth weight by the time they are 6 months of age. The gain in weight is slower during the second 6 months, but most babies triple their birth weight by the time they are 1 year of age. Of course, there are variations to this that are perfectly normal.

Feeding schedules should be elastic to a degree, although there should be an attempt to have a reasonably regular schedule. Usually the feedings will be about 3 hours apart at first and, later, 4 hours apart. The 2 AM feeding can usually be omitted after the first 2 months, and after the first 5 months the 10 PM one will no longer be needed.

BOTTLE FEEDING. If for some reason the mother finds breast-feeding inappropriate to her situation, she may choose bottle-feeding as an alternative. A commercial formula is usually used. A number of products, such as Similac, are available.

In special clinical conditions special commercial formulas are used. For example, in milk allergy, a soy milk product, such as Isomil, may be used. In the genetic condition phenylketonuria a special product, Lofenalac, is used. Then as solid foods are added to the child's diet, a low phenylalanine food guide is used.

Occasionally, a home-prepared formula may be used. The milk most generally used in home-prepared infant formulas is canned evaporated milk. Other types of milk that are used are fresh, pasteurized, homogenized milk; dry milk; lactic acid milk; and goat's milk. When the infant is allergic to cow's milk, soybean milk is sometimes used with good results. If canned or dried milk is used, it must be refrigerated after the can or package is opened.

Cow's milk is higher in protein, fat, and most minerals and lower in sugar than human milk. For this reason, water and sugar are added to cow's milk in making a formula. Sugar is usually added in the form of corn syrup or Dextrimaltose. Most of the calories required by the infant are supplied by the milk itself; the additional needed calories are supplied by the sugar. Water is added to dilute the protein and to meet the fluid requirements of the infant, which are 75 ml per pound of body weight.

In calculating the home-prepared formula for an infant, one must consider the calories and the amount of protein needed, as well as the amount of fluids the infant should have.

For example, a formula for a 14-pound baby, 5 months of age, is calculated as follows:

Number of feedings: 5 (if at 4-hour intervals)
Size of feedings: 7 oz
Daily total: 5 × 7 oz = 35 oz
Whole milk: 14 × 1.75 oz = 24.5 oz
Water: 35 oz − 24.5 oz = 10.5 oz
Sugar: 1 oz

This formula contains 24.5 g of protein, or 1.7 g for each pound of body weight.

NUTRIENT NEEDS. Babies require more protein per pound of body weight than adults. Whereas adults' protein needs are 0.4 g per pound, those of babies are 0.9 to 1.4 g of protein in human milk or 1.4 to 1.9 g of protein in cow's milk per pound of body weight. The protein of human milk is better adapted to the needs of infants than the protein of cow's milk.

Table 10-1. Guideline for addition of solid foods to infant's diet during the first year*

When to start	Foods added	Feeding
First month	Vitamins A, D, and C in multi-vitamin preparation (according to prescription)	Once daily at a feeding time
Fifth to sixth month, in gradual small additions	Cereal and strained cooked fruit Egg yolk (at first hard-boiled and sieved, later soft-boiled or poached)	10 AM and 6 PM
	Strained, cooked vegetable and meat	2 PM
	Zwieback or hard toast	At any feeding
Seventh to ninth month	Meat: beef, lamb, or liver (broiled or baked and finely chopped) Potato: baked or boiled, mashed or sieved	10 AM or 6 PM

Suggested meal plan for age 8 months to 1 year or older

7 AM	Milk	8 oz
	Cereal	2-3 tbs
	Strained fruit	2-3 tbs
	Zwieback or dry toast	
Noon	Milk	8 oz
	Vegetables	2-3 tbs
	Chopped meat or one whole egg	
	Puddings or cooked fruit	2-3 tbs
3 PM	Milk	4 oz
	Toast, zwieback, or crackers	
6 PM	Milk	8 oz
	Whole egg or chopped meat	
	Potato, baked or mashed	2 tbs
	Pudding or cooked fruit	2-3 tbs
	Zwieback or toast	

*Semisolid foods should be given immediately after breast- or bottle-feeding. At first 1 or 2 tsp should be given. If food is accepted and tolerated well, the amount should be increased to 1 to 2 tbs per feeding.
Note: Banana may be substituted for fruit and cottage cheese for meat or egg in any meal.

Infants also require more calories per pound than adults, the requirement being 54 calories per pound from 1 to 3 months of age, 50 calories per pound from 4 to 9 months of age, and 45 calories per pound from 10 to 12 months of age, whereas adults require only 18 to 20 calories per pound. Infants need more calories because they have more body surface in proportion to their weight and because of growth and activity.

A baby will probably be given vitamin supplements as early as 1 week of age. The dosage will depend on the vitamin preparation being used and the pediatrician's prescription for the individual baby's needs.

SOLID FOODS. Breast milk from a healthy mother who has had a good diet meets the nutritional requirements of the infant for the first 6 months. Thus it is currently recommended by pediatricians and nutritionists that solid foods not be added to the baby's diet until 5 or 6 months of age. The infant's system cannot use them very well before then, they are not needed yet, and more often they lay the foundation for infant and childhood obesity patterns from overeating.

PREMATURE BABIES. Premature babies require special care. The stomach is smaller than that of the normal baby, and the digestive system is less developed. The fluid requirements of premature babies are higher than those of normal babies. Premature babies do not tolerate fats very well. They need more calcium and more protein than full-term babies because almost 50% of the calcium and phosphorus is deposited during the last month of pregnancy. Premature babies, however, do better on a formula of cow's milk (usually low or nonfat because of poor fat tolerance) than on human milk because cow's milk is higher in calcium and protein. The cow's milk formula may be supplemented by human milk if the mothers desire. Mothers may express the milk by hand or with a common hand breast pump and then give it to the babies by bottle until they are strong enough to suck well. The bottle nipple should be soft with larger-than-usual holes.

Table 10-1 is a summary of the additions that may be made to the formula or to a breast-feeding for the normal full-term baby.

Above all, the meal hour should be a happy time. The attitude toward the meal hour, either happy or unhappy, will carry over into the later years of a child's life.

Preschool children

During the latent growth period of childhood the growth rate is slower and more erratic than that of infancy, and the child's appetite and food intake will vary accordingly. A variety of foods should be offered to the child, with an avoidance of too many refined sweets.

During the preschool years the child begins to eat an increasing variety of foods served to the rest of the family. The child at this age likes food that can be eaten with the hands, such as raw carrot sticks and chicken drumsticks. Meat should be cut in bite-sized pieces, and vegetables and raw fruits may be used regularly.

Foods should be served attractively and in small amounts. If the child wants more, a second serving may be used. Servings of food that are too large discourage a child from eating. A new food can be introduced in small portions and at a time when the child is hungry. If it is refused, it can be introduced again in a few days. The child should not be bribed or coaxed to eat. The performance will only be repeated to gain more attention.

Schoolchildren (5 to 12 years)

New problems arise when children start school. If children are not awakened early enough in the morning, they may not have time to eat a good breakfast without hurrying or worrying about being late. Association with other children who do not have good nutritional habits may cause children to question their home routine.

Schoolchildren usually have good appetites. Meals should be kept simple but adequate. The best way to influence children to establish good nutritional habits is for the parents to set a good example by eating the correct foods themselves.

Good mental development goes hand in hand with good nutrition. Children who are well nourished will be more alert in the classroom than malnourished children. The school-lunch program has helped to improve nutrition, especially of children in underprivileged areas. However, current program cuts have somewhat curtailed its use.

Adolescents

Many adolescents eat a less well-balanced diet than persons in any other age group except possibly elderly persons. Teenagers, for the most part, choose their own food. The consumption of soft drinks, hot dogs, and candy bars often reduces the intake of milk and other valuable foods. Adolescents are at an age when it is important to conform with friends in eating habits, as well as in the social amenities.

Boys usually eat a sufficient amount of food but not always the right kind. Girls are inclined to eat less than they need because of their desire to keep thin. If they are a little overweight, they may try to reduce in a foolish manner. Poor food selection is responsible for much of the obesity among teenage girls. Overweight girls can learn that they may eat a balanced diet and at the same time reduce safely.

Teenage girls may not realize that good looks and good nutrition go together. Moreover, many girls marry while still in their teens, and with a background of an inadequate diet, they are very poorly prepared for the demands of pregnancy. These girls must complete their own growth and development and at the same time supply the extra needs of the baby. It is necessary to have a very carefully planned diet to accomplish this. A teenage girl who is poorly prepared nutritionally for pregnancy may experience more of the complications incident to pregnancy, such as abortion, premature labor, and eclampsia. A girl who has maintained good nutrition throughout her teenage years and who continues a well-balanced diet throughout pregnancy will be more likely to deliver a normal, healthy, full-term infant.

NUTRITION FOR ADULTS

Both heredity and nutrition are major factors in determining the length of normal lives. Adults should, during their younger adult years, give optimum care to their bodies. A car is not expected to run for years without any care; yet many people seem to expect their bodies to do just that. The organs and tissues of the body do their respective jobs for many years if they are well nourished and protected. By giving the body intelligent care, a person can have a much healthier and more satisfying old age. The signs of old age may be postponed, but one cannot expect to wait until old age to give the body scientific care. Good nutrition is only one of the health practices that help to maintain health and vigor, but it is one that can be practiced more readily and yet is abused more frequently than any other.

Life expectancy has increased from 47 years in 1900 to about 77 years currently because of modern science. Much of this increase is a result of better prenatal and infant care, better care of chronic diseases of middle-aged and older persons, and more complete control of infectious and communicable diseases.

In addition to prolonging life, modern scientific health care has resulted in a definite increase in the years of usefulness during middle age and a postponement of the diseases incident to old age.

People may eat either too much or too little food, or they may make the wrong choice of food. Eating too much food seems to present a problem for many persons in the United States, and obesity results. For others, however, caught in the morass of poverty, food is scarce or at times nonexistent, and hunger or malnutrition results.

When seeking to maintain a good body weight, one should choose food wisely. A person on a limited financial budget is careful to spend each dollar to good advantage, and the same should hold true for a person who is trying to control excess eating. Adequate proteins, minerals, and vitamins are as important in a reducing diet as in a normal one, even though it is more difficult in a reducing diet to secure the protective foods in adequate amounts.

Vitamin preparations are usually not needed by healthy adults. If they eat a balanced diet, they will usually receive sufficient vitamins.

Pregnant women

It is very important to the health of both mother and child that a prospective mother eat a well-balanced diet with increased amounts of all the essential nutrients. The woman who has always eaten a well-balanced diet has a better chance of having a healthy baby and of remaining in good health herself than the woman who has been undernourished.

DANGERS OF CALORIE AND SODIUM RESTRICTION. A report by the National Research Council has established important changes in the nutritional care provided for women during pregnancy.* Contrary to prior belief, weight should *not* be restricted during pregnancy nor should salt be restricted. Studies indicate that women deliver healthy babies over a wide range of weight gain; it is not the *amount* of weight gain but the *quality* of that weight gain and the *quality* of the diet the woman eats to produce the gain that determines the health of the baby and the mother.

The average weight of the products of a normal pregnancy are given in the following list:

Products	*Weight (lb)*
Fetus	7.5 (3.3 kg)
Placenta	1 (0.45 kg)
Amniotic fluid	2 (0.9 kg)
Uterus (increase)	2.5 (1.1 kg)
Breast tissue (increase)	3 (1.3 kg)
Blood volume (increase)	4 (1.8 kg) (1500 ml)
Maternal stores	4-8 (1.8-3.6 kg)
	24-28 (10.8-12.6 kg)

It is clearly evident therefore that calorie restriction during pregnancy is unphysiological and potentially harmful to the developing baby and to the mother. A calorie-restricted diet cannot supply all the increased nutrient demands essential to the growth process going on during pregnancy. Thus weight reduction should *never* be undertaken during pregnancy. To the contrary, adequate weight gain should be supported with the use of a nourishing, well-balanced diet as outlined in this discussion.

About 2 to 4 pounds (0.9 to 1.8 kg) is an average weight gain during the first trimester. Thereafter about a pound (0.45 kg) a week during the remainder of the pregnancy is usual.

Just as with restriction of calories, routine restriction of sodium is unphysiological and unfounded. Physicians who prescribe diets low in calories and salt are placing pregnant women and their offspring at a distinct disadvantage and at an unnecessary risk. A number of studies have indicated the need for sodium during pregnancy and the harm to maternal-fetal health that results from salt restriction. Combined with the added injury of a routine use of diuretics, such a program places the pregnant woman and her baby in double jeopardy. The National Research Council report labels such routine use of salt-free diets and diuretics as potentially dangerous.

NUTRITIONAL REQUIREMENTS. Instead of a restricted diet approach, the National Research Council emphasizes a positive approach based on an increased demand for key nutrients during pregnancy. The major focus is on

*National Research Council: Maternal nutrition and the course of pregnancy, Washington, D.C., 1970, National Academy of Sciences.

protein. Protein is the primary need because it is the growth element for body tissues. The new recommended dietary allowances of the National Research Council indicate a need for 80 to 85 g/day of protein during pregnancy. This amount represents an increase of about 50% over the normal adult diet. Moreover, a large number of high-risk or active pregnant women need even more protein, 80 to 100 g/day, or about double their previous intake.

A number of reasons for this increased protein need during pregnancy reflect the tremendous growth period involved:

1. *Rapid growth of the baby.* The mere increase in size of the infant from one cell to millions of cells in a 7-pound (3.1 kg) child indicates how much protein is required for such rapid growth.
2. *Development of the placenta.* The mature placenta requires sufficient protein for its complete development as a vital organ to sustain, support, and nourish the baby during growth.
3. *Growth of maternal tissues.* Increased development of breast and uterine tissue is required to support pregnancy.
4. *Increased maternal circulating blood volume.* The mother's blood volume increases during pregnancy 20% to 50% over her normal volume. This increased amount of circulating blood is necessary to nourish the child and support the increased metabolic work load involved. With this increased amount of blood comes a need for increased synthesis of the components of blood, especially hemoglobin and plasma protein. Both of these substances are proteins vital to the support of the pregnancy. Increased hemoglobin is needed to supply oxygen to the growing cells. Increased plasma protein (albumin) is needed to keep the increased blood volume circulating. Albumin in the blood provides the osmotic force constantly needed to pull the tissue fluids back into circulation after they have bathed and nourished the cells, thus preventing abnormal accumulation of water in the tissues (edema).
5. *Formation of amniotic fluid.* The fluid surrounding the baby is designed to guard against shock or injury. This fluid contains proteins, and hence its formation requires still more protein.
6. *Storage reserves.* Increased tissue storage reserves are needed in the mother's body to prepare for labor, delivery, the immediate postpartum period, and lactation.

The second major focus of the diet during pregnancy is on *calories*. The amount of calories should be sufficient to meet the increased demands for energy and nutrients and to spare protein for the tissue-building requirements listed earlier. The current revisions of the National Research Council recommend a 15% to 20% increase over the usual intake of calories in an adult woman. Nutritionally deficient women or those more physically active would easily need more. The average need is about 2400 calories, with some pregnant women requiring more calories. The emphasis should always be a positive one on ample calories to secure the necessary nutrient and energy needs.

The key minerals, calcium and phosphorus, along with vitamin D, are essential for a mother's own body needs and for the bones and teeth of the fetus. Calcium is also necessary for proper clotting of the blood. A diet that includes 1 quart of milk and generous amounts of green vegetables, whole-grain cereals, and eggs will supply sufficient calcium for the needs of both the mother and the fetus.

Two additional minerals needed in increased amounts during pregnancy are iron and iodine. An adequate supply of iron is essential for the production of hemoglobin and for the necessary prenatal storage of iron in the body of the infant. Iron supplements are usually used to ensure that these needs are met. An intake of iodine is essential to meet the increased thyroid activity associated with the greater need for thyroxine, the hormone controlling the increased basal metabolic rate. This increase of iodine is ensured by the use of iodized salt.

Vitamins are also needed in increased amounts during pregnancy. These include vitamins A and C, important elements in tissue growth, and the B vitamins needed for energy production and protein synthesis. One B vitamin, folic acid, is especially needed to build mature red blood cells. A vitamin and mineral supplement including folic acid is usually used during pregnancy.

FUNCTIONAL PROBLEMS. Vomiting, which sometimes occurs during the first 3 months of pregnancy, may usually be relieved by one or more of the following dietary changes:

1. A lower intake of fat
2. A dry diet at the meal hour, with fluids between meals
3. An emphasis on foods high in carbohydrate
4. Eating dry toast or crackers on awakening in the morning

COMPLICATIONS. Complications do not usually occur in women whose diets have been adequate throughout pregnancy. They are more likely to occur when the diet is low in protein, energy, and vitamins. A woman who is underweight is more likely to have problems such as premature labor. The dietary treatment consists of a diet rich in protein, sufficient calories, minerals, and vitamins as described in Table 10-2.

Lactating women

There is even greater need for increased nutrients during lactation. A normal baby will require 2 to 2½ ounces of the mother's milk per pound of body weight. A 7-pound (3.1-kg) infant will take approximately 18 ounces, so it is easy to understand why additional food is required by the mother. One ounce of breast milk contains 20 calories. The diet of the mother who is breast-feeding her baby should be high in protein and calories, with an increase in fluids.

Table 10-2. Daily food plan for pregnancy and lactation

Food	Nonpregnant state	Pregnancy	Lactation
Milk (cheese, ice cream, other milk-based foods, skim milk, or butter-milk)	2 cups	4 cups	5-6 cups
Meat (lean meat, fish, poultry, cheese, occasionally dried beans or peas)	1 serving (3-4 oz)	2 servings (6-8 oz; include liver frequently)	2½ servings (8 oz)
Egg	1	1 or 2	1 or 2
Vegetable*: dark green or deep yellow	1	1	1 or 2
Vitamin C-rich food*: Good sources—citrus fruit, berries, cantaloupe Fair sources—tomatoes, cabbage, greens, potatoes in skin	1 good source or 2 fair sources	1 good source *and* 1 fair source, or 2 good sources	1 good source *and* 1 fair source, or 2 good sources
Other vegetables and fruits	1 serving	2 servings	2 servings
Breads and cereals (enriched or whole-grain; 1 slice bread = 1 serving)	3 servings	4 or 5 servings	5 servings
Butter or fortified margarine	As desired or needed for calories	As desired or needed for calories	As desired or needed for calories

*Use some raw daily.

High caloric liquids, especially those made with milk, should be taken between meals, rather than consumed with the meals, in an attempt to consume more of the necessary calories at mealtime. About 6 cups of milk should be used in some form each day.

A summary of foods in a daily plan for pregnancy and lactation is shown in Table 10-2.

NUTRITION FOR GERIATRIC PATIENTS

Nutrition and metabolism are fundamentally very similar throughout the lifespan. Good nutrition is as necessary in later life as in the early years, but the process of aging presents special problems, even as infancy and childhood have their special needs.

Geriatric medicine, to be truly effective, should be largely preventive medicine. A well-balanced diet for persons 40 to 60 years of age plays a big role in ensuring a healthy life for persons 60 to 80 years of age. People are largely what they are today because of their yesterdays. The older people become, the more yesterdays there are to affect them. Since all persons have varying types of yesterdays, with different problems, older persons become increasingly divergent in their reactions to foods and to life in general.

Planning diets

Some of the following points should be considered in planning diets for members of the older age group:

1. The diet should be well balanced and high in protein, vitamins, and minerals. To allow for the wastage during diminished absorption, it is important to give the aged person a diet higher in protein, vitamins, and minerals than would be theoretically necessary. The elderly are prone to suffer from protein deficiency more than from other forms of deficiency. Mild protein deficiency is made manifest by a sense of habitual fatigue. Severe protein deficiency results in loss of body tissue, damage to the organs of the body, impairment of body functions, and increased susceptibility to infections. Older persons also seem to lose some of the ability to absorb and use certain essential elements in food, especially calcium and iron. Calcium is needed to help prevent brittle and malformed bones, and iron is needed to combat the tendency toward anemia, especially in those persons who do not eat much meat. Many older persons do not eat enough meat because of the difficulty of chewing it. It is important that the meat be very tender or ground; stews and casseroles are good ways of serving it. Meat, fish, or poultry should be served at least once a day, and liver should be served once a week. The protein of meat should be supplemented by milk, eggs, and cheese. Milk and milk products are excellent sources of calcium and some of the necessary vitamins. Milk may also be given in the form of cream soups, other creamed dishes, and desserts. Dry milk may be added to a variety of foods. The adult need for vitamins remains the same as the years go by but may seem accentuated because the older person may be eating less food and generally using it less well. Very often there is also reduced tolerance of fat. The diet should be plentifully supplied with milk, eggs, fruit, whole-grain products, and vegetables prepared in such a manner that the maximum content of the vitamins is retained. Sweets are used, but they should not replace the foods needed to furnish the body with the necessary proteins, vitamins, and minerals.
2. There should be sufficient calories for the maintenance of energy and activity. The caloric intake should be such as to avoid or correct underweight or obesity. The most desirable weight is the ideal weight at 25 years of age. If it is necessary for a patient to reduce, it should be done slowly and with a nutritionally sound diet plan. Sometimes aged persons eat to excess to alleviate boredom, loneliness, or anxiety. However,

because metabolism slows down as they grow older, they do not need as many calories as previously.

3. Diminished secretion of mucus, which normally serves as a lubricant in the lower intestinal canal, contributes to the tendency toward constipation. Soft bulk is needed to prevent it. Cooked fruits and vegetables may be more easily chewed, swallowed, and digested than raw ones. Fruits stimulate the appetite and furnish bulk. Added fiber may be used also, along with adequate fluid intake.

4. Condiments and spices may be used according to individual taste, desire, or tolerance. Tasteless, bland food is neither appetizing nor satisfying and contributes to poor intake.

5. Meals consist of light, easily digested foods. A good breakfast should be the order of the day, and the evening meal should be substantial enough to prevent hunger during the night. A glass of milk or milk and crackers should be available in the evening if desired. Often, frequent small meals throughout the day meet needs better than regular meals.

6. Fluids are very important for the aged because a larger fluid intake, and therefore a larger urinary output, is needed to adequately eliminate the metabolic waste products. Sufficient fluids to produce at least 3 pints of urine a day are needed. This means a fluid intake of 2 quarts ordinarily and 3 quarts when the weather is very hot. Fluids can be taken as beverages, juices, and soups served at the meal. The kidneys must work harder to secrete a small amount of concentrated urine than a larger amount of dilute urine. Fluids are more readily absorbed and easier on the circulation if taken in small amounts at fairly frequent intervals, rather than in large amounts less frequently. Many older persons prefer most of the fluids to be hot.

7. Unless patients are undernourished or senile, it is not advisable to coax them to eat more food than they want. When the appetite is poor, especially if the will to live is weakened by long illness and helplessness, small, frequent feedings and foods requiring very little effort to eat are best. Much of the food may be served in liquid form. Trays attractively served in an atmosphere of relaxation and at regular hours sometimes help to cheer a depressed patient and stimulate the appetite.

8. The likes and dislikes of the aged should be respected. When eating habits are poor, they can usually be improved if the change is made very gradually. New foods or different ways of cooking familiar foods must be introduced slowly.

Questions on nutrition

1. What are the advantages of breast-feeding?
2. At what age is the average breast-fed baby weaned?

3. What kinds of milk are used in artificial feeding?
4. Compare cow's milk with human milk.
5. What are the fluid requirements of a baby?
6. What are the protein needs of a baby?
7. How many calories per pound does a baby require?
8. Calculate the formula for an 8-pound (3.6 kg) baby 2 months of age.
9. Why does a baby require more calories per pound than an adult?
10. When is it usually necessary to give supplementary vitamin D?
11. In what way are the requirements different for a premature baby?
12. What is the best kind of milk for a premature baby and why?
13. Plan a diet for a baby 4 months of age and one for a baby 8 months of age.
14. What are some of the problems in feeding a baby, and how can they be overcome?
15. What solid foods need to be added during the first year?
16. How does the growth pattern change in childhood years, and what is the result in the child's response to food?
17. How does good nutrition affect mental development?
18. What problems are involved in nutrition for an adolescent?
19. Why is it especially important for teenage girls to have a balanced diet?
20. What is responsible for the increase in life expectancy?
21. How does a well-balanced diet influence a person's years of usefulness?
22. What are three common nutritional errors among adults?
23. Even if reduction in food is necessary, what nutrients should always be supplied in adequate amounts?
24. How may sufficient protein be supplied in the diet?
25. What important changes in nutritional care during pregnancy have been recommended by the National Research Council?
26. What is an average gain in weight during pregnancy?
27. Why must the protein intake of a pregnant woman be increased?
28. What is the relationship of sufficient calories in the diet to protein in the diet?
29. How may sufficient protein be supplied in the pregnant woman's diet?
30. Why are additional calcium, phosphorus, and vitamin D needed?
31. What other food factors need to be increased during pregnancy?
32. Why does a physician usually order a mineral-vitamin supplement during pregnancy?
33. What type of diet should be followed when vomiting is present during early pregnancy?
34. How many calories are in 1 ounce of human milk?
35. Why does an older person tend to have a protein deficiency?
36. Why does an older person need to receive a larger amount of protein, minerals, and vitamins than is theoretically necessary?
37. How may protein deficiency in an elderly person be avoided?
38. Why would it sometimes be necessary to give fat-soluble vitamins synthetically?
39. What is the best policy to use in reducing the weight of an obese older person?
40. Why does an older person sometimes have a tendency toward constipation, and how can this be prevented?
41. What is a reasonable guide for using seasonings in an older person's diet?
42. Why are fluids important?
43. Plan a 2-day diet for an older person.

Suggestions for additional study

1. Prepare a 2-day menu for an 8-month-old infant.
2. Plan 2-day meals for each of the following: a 3-year-old child, a 6-year-old child, and an adolescent boy.
3. Make a complete study of the actual likes and dislikes of the average child 6 to 10 years of age.
4. Plan a diet for a pregnant woman.
5. Plan a diet for a nursing mother.
6. Visit an aged relative and discuss his or her eating habits. Chart the intake of food for 3 days and check it for adequacy.

Pregnancy: Tissue building on a vegetarian diet

Leah, a neighbor of yours, is 20 years old and has just discovered that she is pregnant with her first child. She and her husband are vegetarians. She asks your advice about her diet.

1. What is her basic nutritional need during her pregnancy?
2. What further information would you want about her dietary habits to help her meet this need?
3. What foods would you try first to have her use in increased amounts? Why?
4. If you learned that she is a true vegetarian using only plant foods, how would you help her get enough growth materials?
5. Why would adequate carbohydrate foods also be important in her prenatal diet?

Suggested readings

Brewer, G.S.: What every pregnant woman should know, New York, 1977, Random House, Inc.

Committee on Maternal Nutrition, Food and Nutrition Board, National Research Council: Maternal nutrition and the course of pregnancy, Washington, D.C., 1970, National Academy of Sciences.

Food and Nutrition Board, National Academy of Sciences–National Research Council: Recommended dietary allowances, Washington, D.C., 1980, The Academy.

Guthrie, H.A.: Introductory nutrition, ed. 5, St. Louis, 1983, The C.V. Mosby Co.

Williams, S.R.: Nutrition and diet therapy, ed. 4, St. Louis, 1981, The C.V. Mosby Co.

Williams, S.R.: Essentials of nutrition and diet therapy, ed. 3, St. Louis, 1982, The C.V. Mosby Co.

Worthington, B.S., Vermeersch, J., and Williams, S.R.: Nutrition in pregnancy and lactation, ed. 2, St. Louis, 1981, The C.V. Mosby Co.

11

The community food supply and its relation to health

The health of any community directly depends on the food supply available to its people and their personal choices from that supply. Thus the community food environment and individual food habits of persons living in that environment become primary concerns basic to the well-being and happiness of all.

FOOD SAFETY

Over the past few years the American food environment has been rapidly changing. Knowledge of food science and technology has greatly expanded. As a result, the number of processed foods in modern supermarkets, as well as the number of "fast-food" chains, has increased markedly, replacing many primary food items in the diets of many people. These changes bring both promise and problems—the promise of abundance and variety in the food supply and problems of increasing confusion in food identity and values, with increasing consumption of food additives and nonnutritive products.

To safeguard the community food supply, every detail of food production must always be carefully watched to protect the nutrients, to prevent contamination from harmful bacteria and other organisms, and to eliminate toxic substances. A safe water supply has been ensured in most communities. Milk and dairy products are produced under sanitary conditions. Infected cows have been eliminated, and raw milk is pasteurized for most of the population. It now remains for other food items to be made equally safe.

Role of the Food and Drug Administration

The history of public concern over the safety of its food supply goes back to 1906, when the first Pure Food and Drug Act was passed. However, not much was done until 1938, when the present law, the Federal Food, Drug, and Cosmetic Act, came into existence and created the Food and Drug Administration (FDA). The FDA, operating under the Department of Health, Education, and Welfare (Health and Human Services), is now the federal agency that is charged with the responsibility of protecting the public from contaminated or inferior products, inaccurate labeling, and harmful additives.

It was not until 1958 that increasing consumer concern caused Congress to pass the first amendment to this basic food safety law. This regulation, the Food Additives Amendment, was passed in September 1958 and became fully effective in March 1959 for all new chemical additives. The law provided for the first time that no additive could be used in food unless the FDA, after a careful review of the testing results, agreed that the compound was safe at the intended levels of use. The amendment made an exception for all additives in use at that time that were "generally recognized as safe" (GRAS). In addition, in the final hours of debate on the bill, Congress added the Delaney Clause, which states that no additive that is found to induce cancer in humans or animals by ingestion or testing shall be allowed as safe. It was under this clause that cyclamates were banned in 1969.

The result of the Food Additives Amendment of 1958-1959 has been the establishment of what is now known as the GRAS list. This list contains a large number of food additives that are "generally recognized as safe" but have not undergone rigid testing requirements. Problems, however, exist with this GRAS list. The number of food additives on the list is uncertain, and the use of them has greatly increased as the number of processed foods has increased. As a result, the federal government has now directed the FDA to reevaluate all items on the GRAS list for safety. Food additives in general are facing increasing public awareness and concern.

Food labeling

The increasing consumer concern about food products has brought about changes in regulations controlling food labels. In 1967 regulations were adopted that required more complete and more prominent information on the labels of packaged foods. These "truth in packaging" laws sought to regulate "special diet" foods, especially vitamin and mineral supplements and so-called low-calorie foods. Then in 1973 came the new nutrient-labeling regulations that were mandatory throughout the food industry by the end of 1974. In essence these laws regulate dietary supplementation by requiring that any food product making a nutrient claim must support that claim with specific nutrient information on the label. Market competition will no doubt extend the practice of including nutrient information on the labels of an increasing number of food products. Nutritional labeling is here to stay. A "nutrition revolution" has begun. Once people begin to understand the relationship between sound nutrition and good health, they will demand nutritional labeling and education, just as they demand a responsible environmental policy to control pollution.

FOODBORNE DISEASES AND CHEMICAL POISONING

After canned foods, meat, milk, and other food products have been produced under the most favorable conditions and their processing and marketing have been controlled by government regulations, there are still many possibilities of contamination with disease-producing organisms by careless food handlers. Unnecessary human contact with food should be avoided, and periodic health examinations should be required of all food handlers.

Frequent washing of the hands by food handlers is *essential*. Correct dishwashing is another important phase of food sanitation. Dishes and silverware should be allowed to drain dry. Constant attention to cleanliness and sanitation is important to health.

Various foodborne diseases result from eating contaminated food or from harmful chemicals in food:

1. Bacterial contamination of food by organisms causing tuberculosis, the common cold, dysentery, typhoid, and septic sore throat has become a serious health problem. The source of trouble is usually food improperly refrigerated or prepared under unsanitary conditions. These organisms multiply rapidly in semisoft foods, which allows them to go through the entire mass quickly. Custard pie, cream puffs, and ground-meat mixtures are rich environments for the growth of these organisms. Another frequent way in which harmful organisms are passed around is by food handlers who may be carriers of one or more diseases.
2. Food poisoning may result from eating fruits and vegetables treated with chemicals, especially lead and arsenic. All fruits and vegetables should be washed thoroughly before they are used.
3. Botulism is the most serious form of food poisoning. It usually occurs when home-canned foods have been underprocessed. The toxin can grow only in containers from which air is excluded, such as sealed cans. The foods in which it most often occurs are meats, fish, and vegetables low in acid, such as asparagus, beans, beets, and corn. The toxin is absorbed directly from the digestive tract, and within 12 to 24 hours it acts on the nervous system, causing abdominal cramps, double vision, and difficulty in swallowing. Later, nausea, vomiting, and diarrhea develop. It proves fatal in approximately 65% of patients within 3 to 7 days.
4. Certain diseases can be transmitted from animals to humans. Trichinosis results from eating raw or improperly cooked pork from an animal that was infested with the trichina organism. Tularemia may be transmitted to humans from infected rodents, especially rabbits. Undulant fever may be contracted from drinking the milk of an infected cow.
5. Mushrooms that have not been grown commercially should never be used, since certain varieties growing in the wild state are poisonous.

6. DDT and other insecticides used as surface sprays can be harmful. It is estimated that a teaspoon of DDT would be fatal. However, even more poisonous to humans is sodium fluoride powder. Neither substance should be used around food preparation areas, except with extreme caution. In fact all the newer insecticides must be used with caution around food and food preparation areas. This applies to all powders, vapors, dusts, and liquid preparations. No product should be used unless the active chemical ingredient is declared on the label. Poisonous liquids or powders should never be stored in an unlabeled container or even in the same storage area as food.

Questions on food and its relation to health

1. When was the first Food and Drug Act passed?
2. What is the significance of the Food Additives Amendment that was passed in September 1958 and the subsequent GRAS list?
3. What is the role of the FDA in relation to the food supply?
4. What are the nutrient labeling regulations?
5. Name three points that would be considered important for the sanitary handling of food.
6. What are some of the possible causes of bacterial contamination of food?
7. What is the common cause of botulism?
8. Name some diseases that may be transmitted from animals to humans.
9. What precautions should be taken in using insecticides?

Suggestions for additional study

1. If you are in a hospital, ask the laboratory to prepare a slide showing the germs on dishes that have been improperly washed or on clean dishes that have been handled by unclean hands. ·
2. Secure a film from your city health department on any of the phases of sanitation.
3. Visit a local food market and make a survey of food labels. What information do you find on them?

Suggested readings

Ross, M.L.: What's happening to food labeling? J. Am. Diet. Assoc. **64:**263, 1974.

Williams, S.R.: Nutrition and diet therapy, ed. 4, St. Louis, 1981, The C.V. Mosby Co.

Williams, S.R.: Essentials of nutrition and diet therapy, ed. 3, St. Louis, 1982, The C.V. Mosby Co.

12

Food habits and nationality food patterns

Food habits do not develop in a vacuum. They are formed from birth throughout life as a response to many influences, which include persons' culture and family, social class and setting, economic situation, and multiple psychological and emotional factors. These food habits are deeply rooted and become the basis of personal food choices. Food has many meanings, and persons' food habits are intimately tied up with their whole way of life. It is important in the health care of any person to recognize this basic fact in food behavior.

A number of nationality or cultural group food patterns are represented in American community life. Several of these are briefly listed here. One may note unusual traditional foods in each group.

ITALY

Italian foods include goat's milk, cheese, eggs, macaroni, dark breads, olive oil, garlic, green peppers, wine and other liquors, soup made from meat stock and vegetables, and polenta. The Italian diet, especially for children, could include more milk, coarse cereals, root vegetables, and potatoes and less candy and coffee.

HUNGARY

Hungarian foods include grains, potatoes, fresh and cured pork, highly seasoned foods, paprika, onions, and green and red fresh peppers. The diet also includes sour cream, sauerkraut, fish, shrimp, eggs, and fruits. Hungarians could include more raw vegetables, cereals, and milk in their diet.

POLAND

Polish foods include potatoes; rye bread; buckwheat flour; coarse cereals cooked in milk; pork (especially highly seasoned sausage); fresh, salted, or pickled fish; cabbage (raw, cooked, and as sauerkraut); vegetables cooked with meat; sour cream; and cottage cheese. More milk, raw vegetables, and fruit could be included in Polish people's diets.

TURKEY AND GREECE

Foods most characteristic of diets in Turkey and Greece are fruits, vegetables, meats rich in fat (lamb is the favorite), gravies, and yogurt, a sour milk preparation.

MEXICO

Mexican foods include the many varieties of beans, rice, potatoes, tomatoes, and some other vegetables; chili pepper; chili con carne; meat that is freshly slaughtered; tamales; and tortillas. The Mexican diet could contain more milk for children and more cheese and whole-grain breads.

PORTUGAL

Foods that are most characteristic of Portugal, together with their meats, vegetables, and fruits, are grains other than wheat, spices (especially allspice and mace), and peppers.

CHINA

Characteristic foods in the Chinese diet are fermented eggs (hen, duck, and pigeon); cereals; vegetables; sprouts, such as bean and bamboo; soybeans; rice; millet cakes in northern China; noodles; sweet potatoes; some pork, lamb, and beef (must be chopped because of an ancient law of Confucius); some buffalo milk; coagulated blood; and fish and shellfish, which are sold alive. The chief food lacking in the Chinese diet is milk.

PUERTO RICO

Foods that are most widely used in Puerto Rico are rice, beans, salted codfish, pork, sweet potatoes and other root vegetables, bananas, and oranges. The chief food lacking in the diet of the Puerto Rican people is milk.

JAPAN

The principal foods in the Japanese diet are large amounts of cereals, potatoes and other vegetables, and seafood. More milk could be used.

LEBANON

Food to an Arab is an important item. Most of the Arab dishes take hours of preparation and are mixtures of various foods. The most characteristic foods of the Lebanese are Arabic coffee in the early morning; hot boiled milk at breakfast (boiled because of the prevalence of bacteria); cheese; olives; leban, which is made from whole milk and yeast (lebni is leban with the whey removed); eggs; butter and bread; meats (preferably mutton); semnah (a heavy mutton fat); mashi, which is vegetables with meat and rice; and milk pudding.

THE JEWISH PEOPLE

The principal meats used in the Jewish people's diet are cattle, sheep, goat, deer, and antelope (animals that have cloven hooves and chew their cud). Other foods include haddock, halibut, salmon, tuna, pike, trout, buffalo, carp, whitefish, and perch (fish that have scales and fins); borscht; vegetable soup; Passover cake with potato flour; and matzo balls.

For Passover the symbols of Passover are placed at the head of the table. These symbolic food items are three matzoth, bitter herbs, a lamb bone, and kharoses, a dish made of apples, nuts, cinnamon, and wine mixed together.

Other foods in the Jewish people's diet are tomato soup, wine soup, sauerkraut soup, mixed fruit soup, gefilte fish, baked broilers, beef pot roast, roast beef with vegetables, meat and carrot tzimmes, beef with prunes and sweet potatoes, carrot sticks in honey, potato kugel, kosher dill pickles, blintzes, kreplach dough, schnecken, and strudel.

Questions on foods used by various countries

1. How are food habits formed?
2. Name at least three foods used in each of the cultural groups discussed in the chapter.

Suggested readings

Williams, S.R.: Nutrition and diet therapy, ed. 4, St. Louis, 1981, The C.V. Mosby Co.
Williams, S.R.: Essentials of nutrition and diet therapy, ed. 3, St. Louis, 1982, The C.V. Mosby Co.

PART THREE

DIET THERAPY

13

Routine hospital diets

THE PRACTICE OF DIETETICS

The primary health professional in the modern hospital who carries the major responsibility for nutritional care of the patient is the registered dietitian (R.D.), a clinical nutrition specialist. However, this nutritional care is administered in collaboration with the physician and the nurse. Only by perfect teamwork can the best results be obtained.

Early beginnings

The beginnings of dietary service to hospital patients can be traced to Florence Nightingale's work during the Crimean War in 1854. She did much to improve food service and nursing care. The nursing profession was, for many years, responsible for dietary work in hospitals. The first resident teacher of sickroom cookery, a graduate of an Eastern cooking school, was employed at Johns Hopkins Hospital in 1890 to instruct nurses in cooking. Other hospitals followed this example. At first this cooking teacher was called "superintendent of diet" and later "dietitian." Today the modern dietitian is an applied food and nutrition scientist skilled in meeting the nutritional needs of people in a variety of settings and situations.

NUTRITION AND HEALTH

Nutrition, in comparison with medicine and nursing, is an infant science. Most of the information about nutrition in relation to treatment of disease has been learned in the last 40 years. Everyone knows that good food is essential to health. This is an accepted fact, but seldom do people realize how often poor selection of food is a contributory factor in disease.

Nutrition has become a very important subject to the nursing, dietary, and medical professions. The wide interest in foods and the ready acceptance of food fads make it all the more necessary that the dietitian, nurse, and physician take every opportunity to give correct dietary information to the public.

143

Diet therapy

The normal well-balanced diet is the basis for all dietary presciptions. The therapeutic diet should be adequate if at all possible. It should be evaluated, and if any nutrient is not present in sufficient quantity, supplements should be given. If, for instance, a patient is allergic to all milk products, then certain vitamin concentrates and calcium supplements may be necessary.

The objectives of dietary treatment follow:

1. To increase or decrease weight
2. To allow a particular organ of the body to rest, such as in the restriction of fat in diseases of the gallbladder
3. To plan the diet to correspond with the body's ability to metabolize a certain nutrient, such as in diabetes
4. To remedy conditions caused by deficiencies, such as the deficiency of vitamin D in rickets
5. To eliminate certain harmful substances from the diet, such as caffeine, alcohol, and pepper in peptic ulcer disease

Diet modifications

Modifications of the normal diet may be made as necessary to meet the needs of the patient in relation to the disease. Calories may be decreased or increased. Modifications may be made in the balance of nutrients, such as high or low protein, carbohydrate, fat, minerals, or vitamins. Certain foods may be omitted, such as in cases of allergy.

Routine hospital diets

Modifications in consistency are made in the following routine hospital diets: regular, soft, mechanical soft, full liquid, and clear liquid:

1. *The regular diet* is almost unlimited in the foods that may be served.
2. *The soft diet* contains only very tender meats and tender cooked vegetables, such as carrots, asparagus, and beets. Vegetables containing much fiber should be omitted or pureed. Peaches, pears, applesauce, Royal Anne cherries, and grapfruit and orange sections that are free of membrane may be served in this diet. Coarse breads and cereals are omitted, as are highly spiced foods. Plain cake, puddings, and desserts are allowed. *The mechanical soft diet* is a modification of the soft diet, in that all foods must be very soft or ground. The mechanical soft diet is used when for various reasons a patient cannot chew or use the facial muscles.
3. *The full liquid diet* includes any food that is liquid at body temperature. Strained cereal gruel is also served in this diet. Foods in the liquid state are easier to digest because they are so finely divided. Feedings should be given six times a day in liquid diets. *The clear liquid diet* includes clear broth, tea, black coffee, and flavored gelatin.

Routine hospital diets are summarized in Table 13-1.

Table 13-1. Routine hospital diets

Food	Clear liquid	Full liquid	Soft	Light	Regular
Soup	Broth, bouillon	Same, plus strained soups	Same	All	All
Cereal		Thin cereal gruel	Refined cooked cereals, cornflakes, rice, noodles, macaroni, spaghetti	Same	All
Bread			White bread, crackers, melba toast, zwieback	Same, plus graham and rye bread	All
Protein foods		Milk, cream, milk drinks	Same, plus eggs (not fried), mild cheese, fowl, fish, sweetbreads, tender beef, veal, lamb, liver, bacon, gravy	Same	All
Vegetables			Potatoes: baked, mashed, creamed, steamed, escalloped; tender cooked whole bland vegetables (may be strained or pureed)	Same, cooked whole bland	All
Fruit and fruit juices	Apple juice	All	Same, plus bland cooked fruit: peaches, pears, applesauce, peeled apricots, white cherries, banana, orange and grapefruit sections without membrane		
Desserts and gelatin	Plain gelatin, fruit ices	Same, plus sherbet, ice cream, puddings, custard	Same, plus plain sponge cakes, plain cookies, plain cake, simple puddings	Same	All
Miscellaneous	Ginger ale, carbonated water, coffee, tea	Same	Same, plus butter, salt, pepper	Same	

Food service

The patient's tray should be attractively arranged with colorful foods. The dishes, glasses, and utensils should be gleaming, the tray cover and napkins should be immaculate, and each item should be placed on the tray in an orderly manner. Arrangement of standard items should be the same at each meal. The tray should be large enough so that it does not look crowded. The use of chipped or cracked dishes or mixed patterns should be avoided. Servings should not be too large because large servings are not as attractive as smaller portions, and they tend to discourage a patient, especially one with little desire to eat. To appeal to the patient, hot foods must be served hot and cold foods cold. Hot foods, as well as salads and desserts, should be arranged attractively on the plate. Color combinations should be considered. The person who serves the tray should be sure that everything is within reach of the patient and that everything about the tray is correct before the patient is left alone. Nothing is more exasperating to a patient, for example, than to receive a pot of hot water and no tea bag.

Fig. 13-1 shows a tray arrangement that is neat and in logical order for the patient's convenience.

Personalized care

Each patient must be treated as an individual. It should be remembered that hospitalized patients are sick persons and may not be their normal selves.

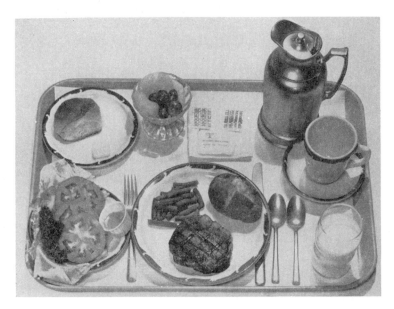

Fig. 13-1. Tray arrangement that is both attractive and convenient for the patient.

They may not want to eat. Their appetites should be tempted if possible, and they should be sympathetically treated at all times. The person who takes the tray to the patient should do so with a smile and a pleasant word. If the patient must be fed, the nurse should be very patient and not try to feed too rapidly. It is not necessary or desirable to keep up a rapid conversation, but if the patient is well enough to be interested, a little pleasant conversation will add pleasure to the meal. When a patient is happy with the food, both the physician and the nurse find treatment easier.

Questions on routine hospital diets
1. What were some of the beginnings of dietetics?
2. What is the basis of a therapeutic diet?
3. What are the objects of dietary treatment?
4. In what ways may the regular diet be modified?
5. Plan a soft diet for a patient who is allergic to milk products.
6. Plan a high-calorie medical liquid diet.

Suggestions for additional study
1. Interview the administrative dietitian or food service manager in your community hospital and observe the mode of patient food service. Report your findings to your class.
2. Interview a clinical dietitian on the hospital's clinical nutrition staff. What preparation is required and what is the nature of the work? Report your findings to your class.

Suggested readings
Williams, S.R.: Nutrition and diet therapy, ed. 4, St. Louis, 1981, The C.V. Mosby Co.
Williams, S.R.: Essentials of nutrition and diet therapy, ed. 3, St. Louis, 1982, The C.V. Mosby Co.

14

Diseases of the gastrointestinal tract

The gastrointestinal tract is composed of the stomach and the intestines and is one of the areas in which much of the treatment depends on supplying the correct diet for each particular type of gastrointestinal disturbance. The area is exposed to all kinds of dietary indiscretions, and it is affected by mental and emotional disturbances to a greater extent than are the rest of the organs involved in the processes of digestion and metabolism.

In this chapter a few of the more frequent diseases of the gastrointestinal tract are discussed. To prevent any misunderstanding, it is necessary to review the meaning of a few terms at this point. *Dietary fiber* is used to describe a variety of the undigestible portions of common foods, including several different groups of material—cellulose, hemicellulose, lignin, and pectin. *Residue* is used to describe the form of the food as it reaches the large intestine. *Roughage* is used to describe the food before it enters the body.

DISEASE OF THE UPPER GASTROINTESTINAL TRACT
Peptic ulcer disease

Peptic ulcer disease includes both the gastric ulcer, which occurs in the stomach, and the duodenal ulcer, which occurs in the duodenum.

The general objectives of diet in the treatment of an ulcer include the following:

OBJECTIVES. The objectives of diet in the treatment of an ulcer include the following:

1. To neutralize the acidic gastric juice
2. To decrease the flow of gastric juice
3. To promote healing of the ulcer by giving relief to the irritated area
4. To provide optimum nutrition as much as possible within the limitations of the diet

CURRENT LIBERAL INDIVIDUAL APPROACH. In the past a highly restrictive bland diet was used in the care of patients with peptic ulcer disease. However, it has proven to be ineffective and lacking in adequate nutritional support for the healing process. Current therapy is based on a liberal individual approach,

LIBERAL FOOD GUIDE FOR PEPTIC ULCER

General directions

1. Respect individual responses or tolerances to specific foods experienced at any given time, remembering that the same food may evoke different responses at different times depending on the stress factor.
2. Eat smaller meals more often, eat slowly, and savor your food in a calm environment as much as possible.
3. Try to avoid caffeine beverages such as coffee, cola, and tea; also avoid alcohol.
4. Cut down on or quit smoking cigarettes—not only to help the ulcer but also to help food taste better.
5. Avoid excessive pepper on food or concentrated meat broths and extractives.
6. Avoid frequent use of aspirin or other drugs that may damage the stomach lining.

Foods	Recommended foods	Controlled foods
Bread, cereals (at least 4 servings daily)	Any whole grain or enriched bread, cereals, crackers, pasta	None
Vegetables (at least 2 servings daily)	Any vegetable, raw or cooked; vegetable juices	None
Potatoes, other starches	White potatoes, sweet potatoes, yams; enriched or brown rice, corn, barley, millet, bulgur, pasta	Fried forms
Fruits (at least 2 servings daily)	Any fruit, raw or cooked; fruit juices	None
Milk, milk products (2 servings daily as desired)	Any form of milk or milk drink; yogurt; cheeses	None
Meats or substitutes (2 servings daily)	Poultry, fish and shellfish, lean meats; eggs, cheeses; legumes—dried beans and peas, lentils, soybeans; smooth peanut butter	Fried forms or too highly seasoned or fatty
Soups, stews	Mildly seasoned, less concentrated meat stock base; any cream soups	More highly seasoned or concentrated base
Desserts	Any desserts tolerated	Items containing nuts or coconut; fried pastries
Beverages	Decaffeinated coffee, cocoa, fruit drinks, mineral waters, noncola soft drinks; less strong tea with milk	Regular coffee, strong tea, colas, alcohol
Fats (use in moderation)	Margarine, butter, cream; vegetable oils; mild salad dressings, mayonnaise, oil and vinegar with herbs	Highly seasoned dressings
Sauces, gravies	Mildly flavored, less strong meat bases	Strongly seasoned, especially with pepper, hot peppers, and sauces
Miscellaneous	Salt in moderation (iodized); flavorings; herbs, spices; mustard, catsup, vinegar in moderation, as tolerated	Strongly flavored condiments; popcorn; nuts, coconut as tolerated

which recognizes variances in need and provides much more personal, psychological, physiological, and nutritional support. A food guide for use in this more effective approach is presented on p. 149.

Gastritis

Gastritis is a general inflammation of the mucous membrane of the stomach and may be either acute or chronic. It may be caused by dietary indiscretions, an excess of alcohol, overeating, or too many highly seasoned foods. If the condition is acute, a liquid diet must be given for the first 2 days, after which a small amount of cereal gruel or a small amount of milk may be given every hour. As the patient improves, the amounts may be increased and given every 2 hours. Gradually the diet may be increased by adding one low-residue food at a time until the patient is receiving a soft, bland diet.

In chronic gastritis the cause should be determined, and the offending food or drink should be eliminated from the diet. The diet should consist of easily digested foods, such as those listed in the food guide for peptic ulcer (p. 149).

DISEASE OF THE LOWER GASTROINTESTINAL TRACT
Malabsorption syndrome (sprue, celiac disease)

Sprue is a general term given to intestinal malabsorption disorders. Fat, especially, is poorly absorbed. Thus the characteristic diarrhea in sprue consists mainly of multiple foamy, bulky, greasy stools high in fat content. Adult nontropical sprue is similar in nature to childhood celiac disease.

The factor discovered to be important in the cause of sprue and celiac disease is *gluten*. Gluten is a protein found mainly in wheat, with some additional amounts in rye and oat. The gluten-free diet on pp. 151-152 has been widely used with marked improvement in symptoms.

Diarrhea

Diarrhea has various causes—the wrong foods, allergy, food poisoning, excessive use of cathartics, nervousness, or the presence of bacterial disease. It usually corrects itself if the cause is removed.

The fundamentals of the dietary treatment of diarrhea include the following:
1. Normal amounts of calories unless the patient is emaciated
2. High-calorie diet if emaciation is present
3. All of the necessary nutrients in adequate amounts
4. A diet high in vitamins to counteract lack of absorption
5. High-quality, well-prepared food attractively served
6. Food low in residue
7. Food chewed well before swallowed
8. Food intake for the day divided into six small feedings

If the feces show undigested starch, the patient should receive less starch and more protein, such as ground meat, broth soups, eggs, and milk. Pureed vegetables and a small amount of toast may also be served. Only small amounts of sweets are allowed. If there is meat fiber in the feces, the diet should be as low as possible in protein, and foods such as cereal gruels, toast, mashed potatoes, rice, bread with butter and jelly, and milk should be given. Applesauce or scraped apple may be given between meals, since the pectin in apples tends to help in the treatment of mild diarrhea.

Acute enteritis

Acute enteritis is a broad term signifying any inflammation of the bowel that is accompanied by diarrhea. It may be caused by toxins, bacteria, or anything that irritates the mucous lining of the intestines. If the case is acute,

---

GLUTEN-FREE DIET FOR NONTROPICAL SPRUE

Characteristics
1. All forms of wheat, rye, oat, buckwheat, and barley are omitted except gluten-free wheat starch (Cellu Products Co.).
2. All other foods are permitted freely, unless specified otherwise by the physician.
3. The diet should be high in protein, calories, vitamins, and minerals.

Foods	Allowed	Not allowed
Milk (2 glasses or more)	As desired	
Cheese	Any, as desired	
Eggs (1 or 2 daily)	As desired	
Meat, fish, fowl (1 or 2 servings)	Any plain meat	Breaded, creamed, or with thickened gravy; no bread dressings
Soups	All clear and vegetable soups; cream soups thickened with cream, cornstarch, or potato flour only	No wheat flour–thickened soup; no canned soup except clear broth
Vegetables (2 servings of green or yellow daily, at least)	As desired, except creamed	No cream sauce or breading
Fruits (at least 2 or 3 daily, including 1 citrus	As desired	
Bread	Only that made from rice, corn, or soybean flour or gluten-free wheat starch	All bread, rolls, crackers, cake, and cookies made from wheat and rye; Ry-Krisp; muffins, biscuits, waffles, pancake flour, and other prepared mixes; rusks, zwieback, pretzels; any product containing oatmeal, barley, or buckwheat; no breaded food or bread crumbs

CAUTION: Read labels on all packaged and prepared foods.

Continued.

GLUTEN-FREE DIET FOR NONTROPICAL SPRUE—cont'd

Foods	Allowed	Not allowed
Cereals	Cornflakes, cornmeal, hominy, rice, Rice Krispies, Puffed Rice, precooked rice cereals	No wheat or rye cereals, wheat germ, barley, buckwheat, kasha
Pasta		No macaroni, spaghetti, noodles, dumplings
Desserts	Jell-O, fruit Jell-O, ice or sherbet, homemade ice cream, custard, junket, rice pudding, cornstarch pudding (homemade)	Cakes, cookies, pastry; commercial ice cream and ice cream cones; prepared mixes, puddings; homemade puddings thickened with wheat flour
Beverages	Milk, fruit juices, ginger ale, cocoa (read label to see that no wheat flour has been added to cocoa or cocoa syrup), coffee (read labels on instant coffees to see that no wheat flour has been added), tea, carbonated beverages	Postum, malted milk, Ovaltine
Condiments and sweets	Salt; sugar, white or brown; molasses; jellies and jams; honey, corn syrup	Commercial candies containing cereal products (read labels)
Fats	Butter, margarine, oils	Commercial salad dressings, except pure mayonnaise (read labels)

---

nothing should be given orally for 24 to 48 hours except small amounts of water or cracked ice. This can be followed by a liquid diet and a gradual return to a regular diet according to individual food tolerance.

Colitis

Colitis is an inflammation of the mucous membrane of the colon. There are three types of colitis: simple colitis, mucous colitis, and ulcerative colitis.

Simple colitis is characterized by spasmodic pain and alternating constipation and diarrhea. The patient is usually under tension, and faulty food habits and the use of laxatives and enemas may be involved. The low-residue diet should be followed with an emphasis on protein foods for healing tissue. Cathartics are withdrawn, and constipation is relieved by agar, psyllium (Metamucil), or some other soft, bulk-producing agent.

Mucous colitis is characterized by constipation and the passage of large quantities of mucus, usually preceded by abdominal pain. This type of colitis is usually found in neurotic persons who have a long history of constipation and the use of purgatives. The same type of diet should be used here as in

GRADUATED LOW-RESIDUE DIET FOR ULCERATIVE COLITIS

General directions

1. Monotony in the diet should be avoided by varying the foods as much as the diet prescription allows.
2. There is an individual variation in the tolerance to certain foods. If any of the foods in this diet disagrees with the patient, some change in the diet schedule may be required.

Foods	Allowed	Not allowed
Beverages	Carbonated drinks (not iced) in small amounts, coffee or substitutes, tea, special mixtures as prescribed	Milk in any form; fruit juices
Bread	Enriched white or fine rye bread, plain or toasted; plain or salted crackers, zweiback, melba toast, plain muffins	Whole wheat, dark rye, pumpernickel, or any hot breads
Cereals	Cooked, refined, or strained—oatmeal, Cream of Wheat, Cream of Rice, Farina, Wheatena; precooked cereals—Pablum, Pabena, Cerevim Dry cereals without bran or shredded wheat; noodles, spaghetti, macaroni, plain rice	Cereals containing bran or shredded wheat; unrefined rice, hominy
Meat	Ground or tender beef, lamb, pork, veal; sweetbreads, brains, liver; may be baked, boiled, broiled, or roasted; crisp bacon	Fried, smoked, pickled, or cured meats; meat with long fibers, gristle, skin; delicatessen rare meats
Fish	Fresh fish, boiled, broiled, or baked, canned, scalded tuna or salmon; crab meat, oysters	Fried fish, lobster, other canned, smoked, pickled, preserved, or gefilte fish
Fowl	Any boiled, broiled, baked, or roasted	Gristle, skin, fat; fried fowl
Eggs	Soft- or hard-boiled, poached, coddled, plain omelet, scrambled, creamed	Fried
Cheese	Cream, cottage, mild cheddar, or American	All other cheeses
Milk	None	
Fats	Butter or margarine in limited amounts; cream for beverage or cereal; crisp bacon; plain gravies in small amounts	Any other
Soup	Bouillon, broth, meat or poultry; may add strained vegetable juices	Cream soup, vegetable soup
Vegetables	Potatoes without skins	All others
Fruits	None	All
Desserts	Plain angel food, butter, sponge, or pound cakes; plain cookies; plain sherbet or water ice; plain ice cream; plain smooth puddings (rice, tapioca, bread, starch, custard); plain Jell-O in small quantities; gelatin flavored with coffee, strained fruit juices	Nuts, coconut, raisins
Sweets	Plain jelly, sugar, honey, syrup, plain hard candies, in *limited* amounts	Large amounts of any sweets; jam or marmalade; candy with nuts or fruit; concentrated sweets; rich pastry or candy
Miscellaneous	Spices and seasonings in moderation	Nuts, olives, pickles, popcorn, horseradish, relishes

Continued.

GRADUATED LOW-RESIDUE DIET FOR ULCERATIVE COLITIS—cont'd

Additions

The following foods may be added, in order, when tolerated. Add each food in small amounts at first until tolerance is assured.

1. Banana, ripe
2. Orange juice, strained and diluted at first; begin with ¼ glass at end of a main meal and gradually increase to full glass
3. Vegetable juice, including tomato (canned) or vegetable juices prepared in a blender and strained
4. Other fruit juices, as with orange juice
5. Vegetables, cooked and strained; prepared strained baby vegetables
6. Fruits, cooked or stewed and strained; prepared strained baby fruits; canned pears; strained applesauce; baked apple without skin or seeds; no dates, figs, or other raw fruits
7. Milk, boiled for 3 minutes; may be served hot or cold; begin with ½ glass once daily; may be used in creamed soups, creamed sauce, milk toast, or plain pancakes; increase slowly to ½ glass three times daily and finally to 1 glass at a time as prescribed; may be used with flavoring nutrient powders or cream
8. Vegetables—tender, whole cooked or canned, not strained; gradually introduce asparagus tips, carrots, beets, spinach, squash, string beans, peas, and pumpkin; avoid skin and seeds; no cabbage, cauliflower, onions, radishes, and turnips
9. Raw, crisp lettuce (finely shredded); raw tomato; no other raw vegetables
10. Unboiled milk

---

simple colitis, and again, agar or some other soft, bulk-producing agent should be used to combat constipation.

Ulcerative colitis is an organic disease characterized by inflammation of the mucous membrane of the large intestine. At first the mucous membrane contains a large amount of tissue fluid and an unusual amount of blood and bleeds easily. The cause of ulcerative colitis is not known, but there are four possible factors: (1) microorganisms within the body, (2) inadequate amounts of vitamin B complex and complete proteins, (3) allergy, and (4) emotional disturbances. Once established, ulcerative colitis is usually chronic. As yet, no permanent cure has been found, but the disease can be temporarily arrested.

The dietary treatment for ulcerative colitis may be accompanied by bed rest and psychotherapy. In the acute stage a liquid diet should be given. Following the acute stage, as the patient improves, a cautious food guide such as the graduated low-residue diet (pp. 153-154) may be used. A more general low-residue diet (p. 155) giving attention to adequate protein foods, excluding milk, may be sufficient to meet needs. As soon as safety allows, a more liberal, high-protein, high-calorie diet should be given. The greater selection of foods serves to improve the patient's morale. The diet should also be high in vitamins and minerals. In addition to vitamins in the diet, vitamin supplements, es-

LOW-RESIDUE DIET

Foods	Allowed	Not allowed
Beverages	Only 2 glasses of milk, if allowed, boiled or evaporated; fruit juices, coffee, tea, carbonated beverages	Alcohol
Eggs	Prepared in any manner, except fried	Fried eggs
Cheese	Cottage, cream, mild American, Tillamook (use in small amounts)	Highly flavored cheeses
Meat or poultry	Roasted, baked, or broiled tender beef, bacon, ham, lamb, liver, veal, fish, chicken, or turkey	Tough meats, pork; no fried or highly spiced meats
Soup	Bouillon, broth, strained cream soups from the foods allowed	Any others
Fats	Butter, margarine, oils, 1 oz (30 ml) cream daily	None
Vegetables	Canned or cooked strained vegetables, such as asparagus, beets, carrots, peas, pumpkin, squash, spinach, young string beans, tomato juice	Raw or whole cooked vegetables
Fruits	Strained fruit juices, cooked or canned apples, apricots, Royal Anne cherries, peaches, pears; dried fruit puree; ripe banana and avocado; all without skins or seeds	All other raw fruits; other cooked fruits
Bread and crackers	Refined bread, toast, rolls, crackers	Pancakes, waffles, whole-grain bread or rolls
Cereals	Cooked cereal such as Cream of Wheat, Maltomeal, strained oatmeal, cornmeal, cornflakes, puffed rice, Rice Krispies, puffed wheat	Whole-grain cereals; other prepared cereals
Potatoes and substitute	Potatoes, white rice, macaroni, noodles, spaghetti	Fried potato, potato chips, brown rice
Desserts	Gelatin desserts, tapioca, angel food or sponge cake, plain custards, water ice or ice cream without fruit or nuts, rennet or simple puddings	Rich pastries, pies; anything with nuts or dried fruits
Sweets	Sugar, jelly, honey, syrups, gumdrops, hard candy, plain creams, milk chocolate	Other candy; jam, marmalade
Miscellaneous	Cream sauce, plain gravy, salt	Nuts, olives, popcorn, rich gravies, pepper, spices, vinegar

pecially vitamin B complex, should be given in double the normal amounts. Large amounts of vitamins are needed because of lack of absorption. The protein should be high because of the amount of protein lost in the feces and through hemorrhage. The diet should be low in fat, and the only fats used should be butter and cream. Supplementary iron should also be given, since anemia is frequently found in ulcerative colitis. Milk is usually not tolerated well. If the patient cannot take milk, a calcium supplement should be given.

The patient should eat three meals a day and have between-meal feedings. Adequate fluids must be taken in the amount of six to eight glasses daily. Nervous strain, emotional tension, and fatigue should be avoided. If there is constipation, corrective medication should be taken only on the advice of a physician.

Diverticulitis

Diverticulosis is the term used to indicate the presence of many small pouches, or pockets, that have formed along the intestinal tract, usually in the large colon. These diverticula usually occur in people past middle age. If one of these pockets becomes infected as a result of the accumulation of fecal matter, the condition is called diverticulitis, and there is usually pain in the affected area. Sometimes perforation occurs, in which case surgery is indicated.

After an episode of diverticulitis in which there has been no perforation, the patient should be given no food for the first day or so, followed by a liquid diet and then a low-residue diet briefly. When the infection has subsided, symptoms are relieved over the long term by a generally high-fiber diet of about 8 to 10 g of dietary fiber daily. This increase in dietary fiber is achieved by liberal use of fruits and vegetables, and of whole grains with a small amount (1 to 2 tablespoons) of added bran.

This more recent high-fiber diet, rather than the traditional low-residue diet, for treatment of diverticulitis has achieved remarkable improvement of symptoms. Residue in the colon seems to reduce the painful muscle contractions that are characteristic of the disease.

Constipation

There are two kinds of constipation, atonic and spastic. In atonic constipation, the more common of the two, the walls of the intestines lack the necessary muscular tone to promote enough peristaltic action to push the food waste through the lower intestinal tract. In spastic constipation the descending colon is subject to contractions or spasms accompanied by pain, with narrowing of the descending colon to approximately one half to one third the diameter of the normal colon.

The causes of constipation follow:
1. Repeated failure to heed the normal urge for a bowel movement
2. Faulty dietary habits in which the person does not eat a sufficient amount of food containing roughage or fiber
3. Lack of exercise, which causes muscles to become weak and to lack tone
4. The use of laxatives, which builds up a dependence on their use and produces inflammation in the colon, often rushing the food on through the intestinal tract at a pace too rapid for complete absorption to take place

5. A limited intake of fluids, which results in dry, hard feces, making defecation difficult and painful

ATONIC CONSTIPATION. In regard to roughage or fiber the foods that are of the most value in treating atonic constipation are whole grains (especially the bran portion), spinach, cabbage, cauliflower, asparagus, tomatoes, onions, and legumes. Fruits such as apples, pears, oranges, grapes, dried figs, raisins, and prunes are also valuable. Honey, too, has a mildly laxative effect. A glass of hot water with the juice of one-half lemon and 2 teaspoons of honey, taken on arising, and a 6-ounce glass of prune juice or a raw apple, taken on retiring, are beneficial. Prunes contain isatin, which is apparently a laxative factor. Milk is not a constipating food as such in most cases. Foods containing roughage should accompany protein foods such as milk, meat, poultry, fish, and eggs.

SPASTIC CONSTIPATION. A person who has spastic constipation often responds to psychotherapy. There are numerous causes of spastic constipation, including excessive use of cathartics, condiments, or tobacco; eating foods high in fiber, such as bran; and drinking too much tea, coffee, or alcoholic beverages. Nervousness and tenseness are also contributory factors.

A person with this condition is not able to eat foods that have excess fiber, such as some raw vegetables and fruits, and therefore may better tolerate vegetables and fruits that have been strained or pureed. Fruits and vegetables are important sources of vitamins and minerals. In the beginning the minimum-residue diet should be given, and as the condition improves, the low-residue diet should be prescribed.

On arising in the morning the patient may drink a glass of hot water with the juice of one-half lemon and 2 teaspoons of honey and on retiring should drink a 6-ounce glass of prune juice. Plain agar or psyllium (Metamucil) may be used if necessary to give further relief from the constipation. Plain agar is not a drug and can be taken in any reasonable amount. Through the absorption of water it gives soft bulk. It will not injure the mucous membranes of the stomach or intestines.

Questions on diseases of the gastrointestinal tract

1. Why is diet an important factor in the treatment of gastrointestinal diseases?
2. Why is a more liberal food guide now used to treat peptic ulcer disease?
3. Outline a day's food plan for a patient with peptic ulcer disease, using the liberal food guide.
4. Define residue.
5. Name the three kinds of colitis. Describe each.
6. What are some of the possible causes of ulcerative colitis?
7. Outline the dietary treatment for ulcerative colitis.
8. What is the prognosis for ulcerative colitis?
9. What are the usual causes of diarrhea?
10. Which nutrients should be increased in cases of diarrhea and why?
11. Outline the total diet requirements in the treatment of diarrhea.

12. What diet should be given in the treatment of acute enteritis?
13. What is gastritis, and what diet is used in the treatment of an acute case?
14. Name the two kinds of constipation. Describe each.
15. What are some of the causes of constipation?
16. Outline the dietary management of atonic constipation.
17. What are some of the causes of spastic constipation?
18. What type of food should be used in the diet for spastic constipation?
19. What is diverticulitis?
20. Outline the diet for diverticulitis.

Suggestions for additional study

1. Name some ways in which pureed vegetables can be made more acceptable to the patient.
2. Plan a menu for 3 days for a person with ulcerative colitis.

Ralph Gregory's ulcer

Ralph Gregory, age 40, owns and operates an interior decorating company that he has built into a successful chain of offices and display stores in several states. He has much creative, driving energy and works long hours planning innovative approaches and keeping in close touch with all his branch offices. Often this necessitates travel on extended buying trips and "trouble-shooting" visits to branch offices to settle problems that constantly arise. Lately his smoking has increased, along with his tensions, and his numerous business contacts have involved increased use of alcohol.

Ralph is married and has two teenage sons. Some discord has developed at home because of his frequent absences and what his wife interprets as lack of concern for her and their sons. She feels that the boys need their father especially now, and Ralph is rarely able to spend any time with them.

Recently Ralph began to develop a dull, gnawing pain in his upper abdomen that seemed to be relieved somewhat when he ate something. He tried to discount it as "just nerves" and used an increased amount of aspirin on his trips to relieve the accompanying headaches. Shortly after he returned home from one of his business trips the pain was unusually severe. He vomited bright red blood. His wife called their physician and, with the help of his sons, took him immediately to the hospital.

After initial treatment in the hospital with blood transfusions and intravenous fluids and electrolytes, including vitamin C, Ralph began to respond. Although he still felt weak and nauseous, he did not vomit again. However, he did pass several large "tarry" stools. Gradually he began to take sips of water, then a small amount of milk every hour with Gelusil between. The physician added orange juice and full liquids as soon as Ralph could tolerate them. Ralph continued to improve, and his diet was increased to a full soft diet according to toleration. By the end of the second week the physician told Ralph he would be able to go home. But he cautioned him that he would have to watch his diet, eat regularly, and use between-meal food with added multivitamins. He would also have to eliminate his smoking and all alcoholic beverages and rest before returning to his work. Even then he would have to greatly curtail much of his former extensive activity. He was to return to see the physician the next week.

As Ralph left the hospital with his wife, he indicated that he was glad to be up so that he could look after things with his business because a number of problems had arisen during his illness. "When are you going to learn, Ralph," his wife asked, "to let some of the other people handle a lot of that detail, and you take care of your health? You need to relax and enjoy life more."

QUESTIONS TO GUIDE YOUR INQUIRY

1. The x-ray diagnosis of Ralph's illness was a gastric ulcer in the lesser curvature. What does this mean? Where are the majority of peptic ulcers located? Why?

2. What do you think are some of the factors involved in the development of Ralph's ulcer? What effect did these factors have?

3. Identify Ralph's basic nutritional needs.

4. Outline a teaching plan you would use to help Ralph with his diet. Would you include his wife? Why?

5. What practical problems might he face when he returns to work? What solutions do you propose?

6. Ralph received medications including vitamin C and other multivitamins and iron. What is the role of this vitamin and mineral therapy in ulcer treatment?

7. Why would there be dietary emphasis on increased calories and protein with between-meal feedings?

8. Why would Ralph need to eliminate alcohol and coffee from his diet?

9. Summarize the general diet therapy principles in peptic ulcer disease and give the rationale for each principle.

Suggested readings

Williams, S.R.: Nutrition and diet therapy, ed. 4, St. Louis, 1981, The C.V. Mosby Co.

Williams, S.R.: Essentials of nutrition and diet therapy, ed. 3, St. Louis, 1982, The C.V. Mosby Co.

15

Diseases of the liver and gallbladder

LIVER FUNCTIONS

The liver is one of the largest and most important organs of the body concerned with the metabolism of food. It plays an essential role in the metabolism of carbohydrate, protein, and fat, especially during the changes the nutrients undergo after digestion:

1. It stores an appreciable amount of amino acids and releases them as they are needed. It has a part in synthesizing the plasma proteins—albumin, globulin, fibrinogen, and prothrombin. It maintains the proper ratio of albumin to globulin in the blood. It controls the concentration of amino acids in the blood. Any amino acids that are not needed for tissue building and repair are broken down by the liver. Approximately one half is converted into urea and excreted by the kidneys, and the other half is changed into glucose or fatty acids and used for heat and energy.

2. It converts the glucose resulting from the digestion of carbohydrate into glycogen and acts as a storehouse for most of the glycogen. It also converts the glycogen back to glucose as it is needed to maintain the blood sugar at its normal level.

3. It releases fatty acids through the bloodstream to the tissues of the body. Fats, which are not stored to any great extent in the healthy liver, impair the functional capacity of the liver if they are retained in excess.

4. It secretes bile, which is then carried through the main bile ducts to the hepatic duct and through the cystic duct to the gallbladder. The liver secretes 500 to 1000 ml of bile daily. Bile contains the bile salts that make the use of fat possible and retard intestinal putrefaction. Bile salts are also necessary for the absorption of fat-soluble vitamins. Bile carries waste products, which are the result of hemoglobin destruction, to the duodenum, where they proceed through the intestinal tract and are excreted in the feces.

5. It is a storehouse for about 95% of the body's supply of vitamin A and most of the vitamin D. It also stores small quantities of some of the other vitamins, principally vitamins K, E, and B_{12}.

6. It breaks down the worn-out blood cells from which iron is conserved

and reused. However, the spleen also takes an active part in the degradation of these cells. Both iron and copper are stored in the liver. The presence of copper, although it is not a component of red blood cells, is essential for their formation.

7. It is one of the organs responsible for producing antibodies that destroy harmful bacteria in the blood.

8. It synthesizes prothrombin and fibrinogen, which are necessary for blood clotting.

9. It is the chief source of plasma cholesterol, and it also plays an important part in removing cholesterol from the blood.

This list of important functions of the liver indicates the essential part this organ plays in maintaining health. The objectives in dietary treatment of liver disturbances are to protect the liver against stress and to allow it to function as efficiently as possible.

DISEASES OF THE LIVER
Infectious hepatitis

CAUSE. Infectious hepatitis is caused by a virus that is transmitted by the intestinal-oral route or by blood transfusions from a person who has had infectious hepatitis and still harbors the infection. Epidemics have been traced to contaminated food, water, and milk.

SYMPTOMS AND TREATMENT. The chief symptoms of infectious hepatitis are jaundice and enlargement of the liver. The basis of treatment is bed rest and proper diet. The diet should be high in protein and carbohydrate and low to moderate in fat, with calories ranging from 2500 to 3500 per day. An adequate or more than adequate storage of protein and carbohydrate in the liver protects it from further damage. A diet high in protein (100 to 125 g) is necessary for repair of the damaged liver tissue. A generous amount of carbohydrate (300 to 500 g) is given to provide for glycogen storage, to protect against toxins, and to raise the caloric content of the diet. A diet with a low-to-moderate fat content (50 to 90 g) is recommended. Some fat is ncessary in a high-protein diet, and fat-soluble vitamins are needed. Some fat is also needed to make the diet more palatable and therefore more acceptable to the patient. Fat should be limited largely to the more emulsified forms found in milk, cream, egg yolk, and butter.

At first the patient may not be able to eat solid food and should be given only liquids. However, the liquids given should be high in protein, carbohydrate, and calories and moderately low in fat. An example of a high-protein, high-calorie milk shake is given in Table 15-1.

As the patient improves, the diet will progress to regular foods, with an emphasis on more protein and carbohydrate and only moderate amounts of fat. A food guide for planning daily meals to meet these needs is given on p. 164.

Table 15-1. High-protein, high-calorie formula for milk shakes

Ingredients	Amount	Approximate food value	
Milk	1 cup	Protein	40 g
Eggs	2	Fat	30 g
Skimmed milk powder	6-8 tbs	Carbohydrate	70 g
or Casec	2 tbs	Calories	710
Sugar	2 tbs		
Ice cream	1 in (2.5 cm) slice or 1 scoop		
Cocoa or other flavoring	2 tbs		
Vanilla	Few drops, as desired		

HIGH-PROTEIN, MODERATE-FAT, HIGH-CARBOHYDRATE DAILY DIET

1 qt (1 L) milk
1-2 eggs
8 oz (224 g) lean meat, fish, poultry
4 servings vegetables:
  2 servings potato or substitute
  1 serving green leafy or yellow vegetable
  1-2 servings of other vegetables, including 1 raw
3-4 servings fruit (include juices often)
  1-2 citrus fruits (or other good source of ascorbic acid)
  2 servings other fruit
6-8 servings bread and cereal (whole grain or enriched)
  1 serving cereal
  5-6 slices bread, crackers
2-4 tbs butter or fortified margarine
Additional jam, jelly, honey, and other carbohydrate foods as patient desires and is able to eat
  them.
Sweetened fruit juices increase both carbohydrate and fluid.

Cirrhosis of the liver

CAUSE. Cirrhosis of the liver is caused by extreme malnutrition. Whether the condition is the result of alcoholism, chronic infectious hepatitis, or some other cause, the damage to the liver is equally serious. If a diet that supplies the essential nutrients is given, some regeneration of the liver cells will occur unless there is already too much scar tissue in the liver.

TREATMENT. During the acute stage the patient may consume light foods such as milk, cereals, milk toast, toast, cooked fruits, rice, and mashed potatoes. After the patient has shown some improvement, the diet should be high in calories, protein (100 to 125 g), and carbohydrate (300 to 500 g) and low to moderate in fat (50 to 90 g), as for infectious hepatitis. If the disease progresses to a hepatic coma, the protein is restricted to tolerance levels (about 20 to 40

LOW-PROTEIN DIETS—15 G, 30 G, 40 G, AND 50 G PROTEIN

General description
1. The following diets are used when dietary protein is to be restricted.
2. The patterns limit foods containing a large percentage of protein, such as milk, eggs, cheese, meat, fish, fowl, and legumes.
3. Avoid meat extractives, soups, broth, bouillon, gravies, and gelatin desserts.

Basic meal patterns (contains approximately 15 g of protein)

Breakfast	Lunch	Dinner
½ cup fruit or fruit juice	1 small potato	1 small potato
½ cup cereal	½ cup vegetable	½ cup vegetable
1 slice toast	salad (vegetable or fruit)	salad (vegetable or fruit)
butter	1 slice bread	1 slice bread
jelly	butter	butter
sugar	1 serving fruit	1 serving fruit
2 tb cream	sugar	sugar
coffee	coffee or tea	coffee or tea

For 30 g protein
Add: 1 cup milk
   1 oz (28 g) meat, 1 egg, or equivalent

For 40 g protein
Add: 1 cup milk
   2½ oz (70 g) meat or 1 egg and 1½ oz (42 g) meat

For 50 g protein
Add: 1 cup milk
   4 oz (112 g) meat or 2 eggs and 2 oz (56 g) meat

Examples of meat portions

1 oz (28 g) meat = 1 thin slice roast—
   1½ × 2 in (4 × 5 cm)
1 rounded tbs cottage cheese
1 slice American cheese

2½ oz (70 g) meat = Ground beef patty (5 from 1 lb [448 g])
   1 slice roast

4 oz (112 g) = 2 lamb chops
   1 average steak

g). A guide for restricting dietary protein is given above. In addition to these specifications, the diet should restrict sodium if there is any accumulation of fluids in the peritoneal cavity. It should also include foods high in vitamins, since the diet has been inadequate for some time in both vitamins and other nutrients. Fat-soluble vitamins would be low because the absorption of fat has been impaired. A complete vitamin supplement should be given, especially since the patient at first does not usually eat very well. Vitamin K is especially important because frequent hemorrhages in cirrhosis result from a lack of it. Vitamin C, or ascorbic acid, although a water-soluble vitamin, is needed in larger than normal quantities for its ability to improve the resistance of liver cells to certain toxins peculiar to the liver. The B vitamins should be added in larger than normal amounts to aid in metabolism of the increased amount of carbohydrate. Adding some brewer's yeast daily yields good results because of its high–vitamin B and high-protein content.

The person who is caring for patients must be sure that the food is eaten. Sometimes patients have anorexia and will not eat unless they are urged or fed, but without a proper dietary intake, they cannot recover. Lighter foods are usually better tolerated, and sometimes, as in infectious hepatitis, it is necessary to give all the nutrients in a liquid form. It may become necessary to resort to intravenous or tube feeding, especially for patients with swollen veins (varices) in the esophagus.

DISEASE OF THE GALLBLADDER
Cause

Disease of the gallbladder can be caused by either infection or the presence of stones. Bile, which is manufactured in the liver, is collected by many small bile ducts and then travels through the hepatic and cystic ducts to the gallbladder. In the gallbladder bile is concentrated and stored until needed. In the process of digestion, when fat enters the duodenum, it triggers the production of cholecystokinin, a hormone in the duodenum. This hormone then travels through the bloodstream to the gallbladder, causing the gallbladder to contract and send bile down through the common duct to the intestines.

When the gallbladder becomes infected, it does not concentrate bile but discharges a vastly different fluid. If stones have formed in the gallbladder, they may obstruct the outlet for the bile. There is pain when fatty foods are consumed, whether the trouble is caused by an infected gallbladder or gallstones.

Treatment

In any type of gallbladder disturbance the diet should be low in fat, especially animal fat. The average patient can usually tolerate a small amount of fat in milk and butter. During the acute stage the patient should consume only milk, cereals, toast, milk toast, cooked fruits, rice, and mashed potatoes. After the acute stage a more varied diet can be given. However, some patients with gallbladder disturbances may not tolerate spices, condiments, coffee, strong-flavored cooked vegetables, or raw vegetables. Eggs are not usually given, but sometimes they can be tolerated. All fried foods and pastries should be avoided. A low-fat or fat-free food plan is given on pp. 167-168.

When gallstones are present, surgery is usually performed to remove them. However, it is best for the patient to remain on a low-fat diet for a while after surgery to allow the inflammation in the gallbladder area to subside.

LOW-FAT AND FAT-FREE DIETS

LOW-FAT DIET
General description

1. This diet contains foods that are low in fat.
2. Foods are prepared without the addition of fat.
3. Fatty meats, gravies, oils, cream, and lard and desserts containing eggs, butter, cream, nuts, and avocados are avoided.
4. Foods should be used in amounts specified and only as tolerated.
5. The sample pattern contains approximately 85 g protein, 50 g fat, 220 g carbohydrate, and 1670 calories.

	Allowed	**Not allowed**
Beverages	Skimmed milk, coffee, tea, carbonated beverages, fruit juices	Whole milk, cream, evaporated and condensed milk
Bread and cereals	All kinds	Rich rolls or breads, waffles, pancakes
Desserts	Jell-O, sherbet, water ices, fruit whips made without cream, angel food cake, rice and tapioca puddings made with skimmed milk	Pastries, pies, rich cakes, cookies, ice cream
Fruits	All fruits, as tolerated	Avocado
Eggs	3 allowed per week, cooked any way except fried	Fried eggs
Fats	3 tsp butter or margarine daily	Salad and cooking oils, mayonnaise
Meats	Lean meat such as beef, veal, lamb, liver, lean fish and fowl; baked, broiled, or roasted without added fat	Fried meats, bacon, ham, pork, goose, duck, fatty fish, fish canned in oil, cold cuts
Cheese	Dry or fat-free cottage cheese	All other cheese
Potato or substitute	Potatoes, rice, macaroni, noodles, spaghetti; all prepared without added fat	Fried potatoes, potato chips
Soups	Bouillon or broth, without fat; soups made with skimmed milk	Cream soups
Sweets	Jam, jelly, sugar, sugar candies without nuts or chocolate	Chocolate, nuts, peanut butter
Vegetables	All kinds as tolerated	The following should be omitted if they cause distress: broccoli, cauliflower, corn, cucumber, green pepper, radishes, turnips, onions, dried peas, and beans
Miscellaneous	Salt in moderation	Pepper, spices; highly spiced food, olives, pickles, cream sauces, gravies

Continued.

LOW-FAT AND FAT-FREE DIETS—cont'd

LOW-FAT DIET—cont'd
Suggested menu pattern

Breakfast	Lunch and dinner
fruit	meat, broiled or baked
cereal	potato
toast, jelly	vegetable
1 tsp butter or margarine	salad with fat-free dressing
egg 3 times per week	bread, jelly
skimmed milk, 1 cup	1 tsp butter or margarine
coffee, sugar	fruit or dessert, as allowed
	skimmed milk, 1 cup
	coffee, sugar

FAT-FREE DIET
General description

The following additional restrictions are made to the low-fat diet to make it relatively fat free:
1. Meat, eggs, and butter or margarine are omitted.
2. A substitute for meat at the noon and evening meal is 3 oz (84 g) of fat-free cottage cheese.

Questions on diseases of the liver and gallbladder

1. Name one function of the liver in relation to amino acids.
2. What happens to the amino acids that are not needed for tissue building or repair?
3. What carbohydrate is stored in the liver, and how does the liver make use of it?
4. What happens to the fat that enters the liver?
5. What is the approximate daily secretion of bile from the liver?
6. Where does bile go from the liver and through what channels?
7. What are the functions of bile? Name three.
8. Name the two vitamins that are stored in the largest quantites in the liver.
9. What is the function of the liver in regard to red blood cells?
10. What minerals are stored in the liver, and what is the function of each?
11. What role does the liver play in destroying harmful bacteria?
12. What are the objectives in dietary treatment of diseases of the liver?
13. What is the cause of infectious hepatitis?
14. What type of diet should be used in the treatment of infectious hepatitis?
15. Explain the reason for a high-protein and high-carbohydrate diet.
16. Why is it advisable to give some fat in the diet?
17. Plan a diet for 1 day for a patient with infectious hepatitis who is past the acute stage.
18. What is the direct cause of cirrhosis of the liver?
19. Describe the diet for a patient in the acute stage of cirrhosis of the liver.
20. After the acute stage, what type of diet should a patient with cirrhosis of the liver have? When should sodium be restricted? Why should the diet be high in vitamins? Why is there a need for an increased amount of vitamins A and K, ascorbic acid, and the B vitamins? What feeding problems may arise?

21. What are the causes of gallbladder disturbances?
22. Trace the hepatic bile as formed in the liver until it reaches the intestines.
23. What hormone is involved in this process?
24. What type of diet is used in the treatment of gallbladder disturbances?

Suggestions for additional study

1. Plan a menu for 1 day for a patient in an advanced stage of cirrhosis of the liver, requiring a 40 g protein diet.
2. Make a drawing of the liver, showing the location of the gallbladder, cystic duct, and hepatic duct.

Bill's bout with infectious hepatitis

Bill is a college student who spent part of his summer vacation in Mexico. Shortly after he returned home he began to feel ill. He had little energy, no appetite, and severe headaches. Nothing he ate seemed to agree with him. He felt nauseated, began to have diarrhea, and soon developed a fever. He also began to show evidence of jaundice.

Bill was hospitalized for diagnosis and treatment. His tests indicated that he had impaired liver function and an enlarged, tender liver and spleen. The diagnosis indicated that he had infectious hepatitis.

His physician ordered a diet high in protein, carbohydrate, calories, and vitamins and moderately low in fat. However, Bill had difficulty eating. He had no appetite, and food seemed to nauseate him even more. The nurse and the dietitian told him how important his diet was in his treatment and arranged to give him foods that he could tolerate more easily.

When Bill was finally able to go home, the physician told him that he would have to rest for some time before returning to his usual activities. Before he left the hospital, the nurse and the dietitian discussed with him the importance of his diet after he was at home convalescing.

QUESTIONS TO GUIDE YOUR INQUIRY

1. What significant metabolic functions of the liver relate to its ability to handle carbohydrate?

2. What are the functions of the liver in fat metabolism?

3. What are the functions of the liver in protein metabolism?

4. What other nutrient-related functions of the liver are there?

5. What is the relationship of these normal liver functions to the effects, or clinical symptoms, that Bill experienced in his bout with infectious hepatitis?

6. Why does vigorous nutritional therapy in liver disease such as hepatitis present such a problem in planning the diet?

7. Outline a day's food plan for Bill. Calculate the amount of calories and protein to ensure that he is getting an optimum intake.

8. What vitamins and minerals would be significant aspects of Bill's nutritional therapy? Why?

Suggested readings

Williams, S.R.: Nutrition and diet therapy, ed. 4, St. Louis, 1981, The C.V. Mosby Co.

Williams, S.R.: Essentials of nutrition and diet therapy, ed. 3, St. Louis, 1982, The C.V. Mosby Co.

16

Diseases of the urinary tract

KIDNEY FUNCTIONS

The kidneys are responsible for maintaining the normal composition of the blood. Here the blood is filtered, and the waste products are excreted in the urine. Most of the waste products in the blood, except carbon dioxide, that result from the metabolism in the body are eliminated through the kidneys.

Filtration

The two kidneys together contain approximately 2 million nephrons. Each of these nephrons contains a glomerulus, the filtering device of the kidneys. The blood plasma enters the glomeruli and is filtered. This filtrate is the same composition as blood except that it contains almost no protein. The gomeruli are attached to a tubule into which the filtrate passes. It then passes on through the collecting tubules in the pelvis of the kidney. The resulting fluid is urine, and it contains about 5% solids, the rest being water.

Selective reabsorption

This phase of the kidney function is important, for it is in these tubules that the filtrate is divided and the part of the filtrate that is to be retained in the body is reabsorbed by the blood. This reabsorption into the blood is not merely a return of the filtrate to the blood plasma; many changes in composition have been brought about by the tubules. The various chemicals that are needed by the body are taken from the filtrate and put back into the blood for use by the body. In fact the final product of excretion, which is urine, is very different in both volume and composition from the filtrate as it comes from the glomerulus.

This is the means by which the body maintains the proper balance of sodium and potassium salts in the cells and in the spaces around the cells. It is also the way in which the body can discard excess salt and urea, the principal waste products of protein.

Excretion

From the pelvis of the kidney, urine is passed through the ureters into the bladder, from which it will be eliminated. The normal amount of urine excreted daily is from 1 to 2 L. Normal urine contains large amounts of urea, and if for any reason urea is not completely eliminated, it will be found in abnormal quantities in the blood. It is normal for blood to contain some urea.

NEPHRITIS

Nephritis is the term used to signify inflammation or degeneration of the kidneys and their functions. It includes both acute and chronic glomerulonephritis, nephrosclerosis, and nephrosis. Although the basal metabolic rate does not change in nephritis, many times the patient's nutritional needs do increase because of the loss of food and water that occurs in vomiting and because of the loss of protein in the urine.

There is also often considerable loss of protein as a result of toxic destruction and loss of large quantities in the urine. The amount of protein in the diet should be limited to the amount needed to replace the tissue protein and the amount of protein lost in the urine. The protein ingested should be of high biological value to be usable for tissue synthesis. Any protein in excess of the necessary amount will increase the work required of the already damaged kidneys.

The normal amounts of carbohydrate and fat are used in the diets of patients with nephritis because they put no strain on the kidneys.

Acute glomerulonephritis

CAUSE. In nephritis various parts of the nephron may be affected, but it is most often the glomeruli that are involved (Fig. 16-1). The cause of acute glomerulonephritis is believed to be bacterial invasion, usually from a streptococcal infection. It is often the result of infectious childhood diseases such as scarlet fever or pharyngitis, and it may occur some time after the initial infection. Streptococci do not lodge in the kidneys but elsewhere in the body. Evidently, they produce a circulating toxin that is the active agent in glomer-

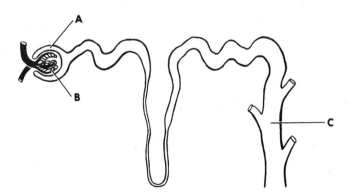

Fig. 16-1. A nephron. **A,** Glomerulus; **B,** glomerular capillaries; **C,** collecting duct.

ulonephritis. The disease generally affects young children; approximately 50% of the patients are under 10 years of age. Most of them recover completely.

TREATMENT. In the acute stage the general nutrition of the patient will be sustained within limits of individual tolerance. If there is nausea and vomiting, the patient should be given lemonade, fruit juices, ginger ale, and tea, but no more than 1 quart of fluid per day should be given. After a few days milk, cereals, toast with jelly, and fruits may be added. When the patient has improved and has no more nausea or vomiting, an essentially normal diet can be given with the protein limited to between 45 and 50 g and derived primarily from complete proteins. It is important that carbohydrate and fat be given in sufficient amounts to prevent protein from being used for energy needs. Sodium should be restricted to 500 to 1000 mg if there is edema. In general, this level of restriction may be achieved by eliminating all salt from the diet. The following diet contains 45 to 50 g of protein and 1550 calories:

2 cups milk	1 small potato
2 oz meat or 1 egg and 1 oz meat	2 servings other vegetables (1 green
4 slices bread	or yellow)
½ cup cooked cereal or ¾ cup dry	3 servings fruit (1 citrus)
cereal	2 tbs butter or fortified margarine
	7 tsp sugar or jelly

This diet is inadequate in niacin and iron. After the first 3 or 4 weeks, depending on the progress of the patient, protein may be gradually raised to the normal use level of about 60 to 70 g. If the urinary output is increased, fluids may be increased up to 1½ quarts daily. The sodium can also be increased to include a little salt in the preparation of the food. Four ounces of meat and 1 cup of milk may be added to this diet to make 65 g of protein and 1800 calories. With these additions the diet will be adequate in niacin and iron.

Chronic glomerulonephritis

CAUSE. Chronic glomerulonephritis may occasionally follow an attack of the acute form. The patient sometimes has advanced chronic glomerulonephritis before there are any symptoms. Then vague symptoms, such as headaches, polyuria, and frequent urination at night, appear, later becoming more severe.

TREATMENT. The diet should be high in protein, carbohydrate, and fat. Sodium may need to be restricted, but fluids may be given as desired. Protein is needed for the repair of body tissues. The wear and tear on the body tissues continues in a person who is ill—perhaps even more so than in the well person, since there is usually some toxic destruction of protein in severe illness. Some physicians recommend the normal amount of protein in addition to the amount lost in the urine.

The carbohydrate content of the diet should be high to prevent the protein from being used for energy needs. If either dietary protein or body protein has to be broken down to provide energy, the waste product urea is then excreted through the kidneys, which increases the work load of the kidneys.

The fat content of the diet may also be high for the same reason unless the patient is troubled with anorexia. Emulsified fats should be used, such as those found in egg yolk, butter, and cream.

If edema is present, sodium will need to be restricted to between 800 and 1000 mg. This would mean that no salted foods or foods high in sodium would be used. No salt substitutes should ever be used unless ordered by the physician.

Fluids are not restricted because the kidneys are not able to concentrate the urine. Usually 1 to 2 quarts of liquids will be sufficient to satisfy thirst and to allow the excretion of solid waste products with a minimum amount of work for the kidneys. In the case of fever or vomiting more fluids may be required.

NEPHROSCLEROSIS
Cause

Nephrosclerosis is usually found among older people. It involves the circulatory system and thus impairs the kidneys. Symptoms usually include hypertension, changes in the retina, urea nitrogen retention in the blood, and sometimes albumin in the urine.

Treatment

Protein in the diet should be maintained at the normal level if possible. When the blood urea nitrogen becomes excessively high, it indicates that the kidneys can no longer eliminate waste satisfactorily. In that case protein should be restricted to 45 to 50 g, as outlined in the diet for the treatment of acute glomerulonephritis. As much as possible of the 45 to 50 g of protein should come from complete proteins. In more advanced conditions protein may have to be limited to 25 to 35 g. Carbohydrate should furnish more than half of the total calories. A part of the fat should be in the form of butter and cream. Milk should be included. Plenty of fruits and vegetables should be included because of their vitamin and mineral content, as well as for their base-forming properties. Condiments or alcoholic beverages are usually restricted. Only 1 cup of tea or coffee a day should be permitted. A reasonable amount of salt may be added to the food when it is cooked, but no salt should be added at the table, and no extremely salty foods should be served.

NEPHROSIS
Cause

The cause of nephrosis is not definitely understood. It is distinguished by the deterioration of the glomeruli and the tubules and also by the absence of hypertension, blood in the urine, anemia, retention of nitrogen, or cardiac involvement. There is severe depletion of serum proteins, as well as a tendency toward polyuria and edema.

Treatment

In the dietary treatment of nephrosis protein should be high enough to furnish building material for body tissue and to replace protein lost in the urine. The carbohydrate intake must be high enough to prevent protein from being used to supply energy needs.

The beginning diet must provide 1500 to 1800 calories and furnish 50 to 60 g of protein. Later the diet should be increased to 80 to 125 g of protein and to 2200 calories to keep pace with he patient's activity. No salt should be added to the food after it comes to the table, and if the patient has edema, the food must be prepared without salt.

UREMIA
Cause

In uremia, urea nitrogen is retained in the blood in abnormal amounts. It can result from nephritis, heart failure, extensive burns, toxemia of pregnancy, and any other organic disturbance that can cause an injury to the kidneys. In this condition waste products are no longer excreted from the body. Nitrogenous products, especially urea, are abnormally retained in the body, and acidosis is usually present.

Treatment

Patients with uremia should be allowed to have any foods that they can tolerate, but because of anorexia and vomiting, they will usually drink only a few fruit juices or ginger ale in the beginning stage. They should be encouraged to consume only foods or beverages that are principally carbohydrate and fat, since the metabolism of carbohydrate and fat does not involve any work on the part of the kidneys. Emergency measures, such as the butter-sugar diet originated by Borst, have been used to furnish calories only. This diet consists of 200 g of unsalted butter and 200 g of sugar. The butter and sugar are made into balls and given to the patient at the meal hour.

More recently a diet for uremic patients has been outlined by an Italian physician, Giovannetti, and used successfully in modified form in England and the United States. The modified Giovannetti diet allows 20 g of protein composed of essential amino acids and ample carbohydrate for energy needs. Thus the excess urea and other nitrogenous materials are used by the body to make its needed nonessential amino acids.* However, since kidney dialysis has be-

---

*An outline of the modified Giovannetti diet (basic food plan and food exchange lists) may be found in Williams, S.R.: Nutrition and diet therapy, ed. 4, St. Louis, 1981, The C.V. Mosby Co., pp. 644-649.

come available to more persons with kidney failure, such highly restrictive diets are no longer necessary in most cases.

RENAL STONES
Cause

Renal stones are usually caused by chemical changes in the urine. Abnormal secretions from other organs in the body may affect the normal chemistry of the urine. Some persons have an obscure tendency to form stones in apparently normal urine, which is slightly acidic.

There are three main kinds of renal stones: calcium phosphate, uric acid, and calcium oxalate. A fourth rare form is that of cystine stones, caused by a genetic disease. Calcium stones develop in alkaline urine; uric acid stones develop in urine that is too acidic.

Treatment

The diet prescribed in the treatment of calcium phosphate stones should be of predominately acid ash foods, which of course would also make it low in calcium. The low-calcium, acid ash foods are eggs, meats, fish, poultry, bread, cereals, corn, cranberries, plums, prunes, and rhubarb. They should be eaten liberally, and other foods such as milk, vegetables, and fruits should be used only in such amounts as are necessary for good nutrition. Food guides for controlling dietary calcium and phosphorus are given on pp. 178-179. A listing of the acid and alkaline ash foods and a food guide for planning an acid ash diet are given on pp. 180-181.

The diet in the treatment of uric acid stones should be low in purines. This means that meats, poultry, and fish should be rigidly restricted to only 2 ounces a day. The following meats, meat products, and fish must be omitted entirely: anchovies, broth, bouillon, gravies, kidney, liver, meat extracts, roe, sardines, and sweetbreads. Only one of the following vegetables may be eaten daily: asparagus, beans (kidney, lima, or navy), lentils, mushrooms, peas, and spinach. Bread, cereals, cheese, eggs, fruit, milk, sweets, and other vegetables may be used freely. A low-purine food guide is outlined on pp. 181-183.

The dietary treatment for calcium oxalate stones consists of the restriction of all foods high in calcium and in oxalates. Spinach, potatoes, beans, endive, tomatoes, dried figs, plums, strawberries, cocoa, coffee, and tea are foods that are high in oxalates and should be omitted from the diet. Foods that contain only a small amount of oxalates and may be used in reasonable amounts are bread, muscle meats, liver, sweetbreads, and cereals. Foods containing little or no oxalate that may be used in the diet freely are milk, cheese, eggs, butter and other fats, peas, rice, cabbage, cauliflower, asparagus, mushrooms, apricots, grapes, and melons. A summary listing of oxalate food sources is given on p. 183. *Text continued on p. 182.*

LOW-CALCIUM DIET (APPROXIMATELY 400 MG CALCIUM)

	Foods allowed	Foods not allowed
Beverages*	Carbonated, coffee, tea	Chocolate-flavored drinks, milk, milk drinks
Bread	White and light rye bread or crackers	Dark breads
Cereals	Refined	Oatmeal, whole-grain cereals
Desserts	Cake, cookies, gelatin, pastries, pudding, sherbets, all made without chocolate, milk, or nuts; if egg yolk is used, it must be from 1 egg allowance	
Fat	Butter, cream, 2 tbs daily; French dressing, margarine, salad oil, shortening	Butter and cream, except in amounts allowed, mayonnaise
Fruit	Canned, cooked, or fresh fruit or juice except rhubarb	Dried fruit, rhubarb
Meat, eggs	8 oz daily of any meat, fowl, or fish except clams, oysters, or shrimp; not more than 1 egg daily, including those used in cooking	Clams, oysters, shrimp, cheese
Potato or substitute	Potato, hominy, macaroni, noodles, refined rice, spaghetti	Whole-grain rice
Soup	Broth, vegetable soup made from allowed vegetables	Bean or pea soup, cream or milk soups
Sweets	Honey, jam, jelly, sugar	
Vegetables	Any canned, cooked, or fresh vegetables or juice except those listed	Dried beans, broccoli, green cabbage, celery, chard, collards, endive, greens, lettuce, lentils, okra, parsley, parsnips, dried peas, rutabagas
Miscellaneous	Herbs, pickles, popcorn, relishes, salt, spices, vinegar	Chocolate, cocoa, milk gravy, nuts, olives, white sauce

*Depending on calcium content of local water supply; in instances of high-calcium content distilled water may be indicated.

LOW-PHOSPHORUS DIET (APPROXIMATELY 1 G PHOSPHORUS AND 40 G PROTEIN)

	Foods allowed	Foods not allowed
Milk	Not more than 1 cup daily; whole, skimmed, or buttermilk or 3 tbs powdered including the amount used in cooking	
Beverages	Fruit juices, tea, coffee, carbonated drinks, Postum	Milk and milk drinks except as allowed
Bread	White only; enriched commercial, French, hard rolls, soda crackers, rush	Rye and whole grain breads, cornbread, biscuits, muffins, waffles

LOW-PHOSPHORUS DIET (APPROXIMATELY 1 G PHOSPHORUS AND 40 G PROTEIN)—cont'd

	Foods allowed	Foods not allowed
Cereals	Refined cereals such as Cream of Wheat, Cream of Rice; rice; cornmeal; dry cereals, cornflakes; spaghetti, noodles	All whole-grain cereals
Desserts	Berry or fruit pies, cookies, cakes in average amounts; Jell-O, gelatin, angel food cake, sherbet, meringues made with egg whites; puddings if made with 1 egg or milk allowance	Desserts with milk and eggs, unless made with the daily allowance
Eggs	Not more than 1 egg daily including those used in cooking; extra egg whites may be used	
Fats	Butter, margarine, oils, shortening	
Fruits	Fresh, frozen, canned, as desired	Dried fruits such as raisins, prunes, dates, figs, apricots
Meat	1 large serving or 2 small servings daily of beef, lamb, veal, pork, rabbit, chicken, or turkey	Fish, shellfish (crab, oyster, shrimp, lobster), dried and cured meats (bacon, ham, chipped beef), liver, kidney, sweetbreads, brains
Cheese	None	Avoid all cheese and cheese spreads
Vegetables	Potatoes as desired; at least 2 servings per day of any of the following: asparagus, carrots, beets, green beans, squash, lettuce, rutabagas, tomatoes, celery, peas, onions, cucumber, corn; no more than 1 serving daily of either cabbage, spinach, broccoli, cauliflower, brussels sprouts, or artichokes	Dried vegetables such as peas, mushrooms, lima beans
Miscellaneous	Sugar, jams, jellies, syrups, salt, spices, seasonings, condiments in moderation	Chocolate, nuts, and nut products such as peanut butter; cream sauces

Sample menu pattern

Breakfast	Lunch	Dinner
Fruit juice	Meat 2 oz (56 g)	Meat 2 oz (56 g)
Refined cereal	Potato	Potato
Egg	Vegetable	Vegetable
White toast	Salad	Salad
Butter	Bread, white	Bread, white
½ cup milk	Butter	Butter
Coffee or tea	½ cup milk	Dessert
	Dessert	Coffee or tea
	Coffee or tea	

ACID AND ALKALINE ASH FOOD GROUPS

Acid ash	Alkaline ash	Neutral
Meat	Milk	Sugars
Whole grains	Vegetables	Fats
Eggs	Fruit (except cranberries,	Beverages (coffee and tea)
Cheese	Prunes, and plums)	
Cranberries		
Prunes		
Plums		

ACID ASH DIET

The purpose of this diet is to furnish a well-balanced diet in which the total acid ash is greater than the total alkaline ash each day. It lists the following:

    I. Unrestricted foods
   II. Restricted foods
 III. Foods not allowed
 IV. Sample of a day's diet

I. Unrestricted foods: you may eat all you want of the following foods

1. Breads: any, preferably whole grain; crackers; rolls
2. Cereals: any, preferably whole grain
3. Desserts: angel food or sunshine cake; cookies made without baking powder or soda; cornstarch pudding; cranberry desserts; custards; gelatin; ice cream, sherbet; plum or prune desserts; rice or tapioca pudding
4. Fats: any, such as butter, margarine, salad dressings, Crisco, Spry, lard, salad oils, olive oil
5. Fruits: cranberries, plums, prunes
6. Meat, egg, cheese; any meat, fish, or fowl, 2 servings daily; at least 1 egg daily
7. Potato substitutes: corn, hominy, lentils, macaroni, noodles, rice, spaghetti, vermicelli
8. Soup: broth as desired; other soups from foods allowed
9. Sweets: cranberry or plum jelly; sugar; plain sugar candy
10. Miscellaneous: cream sauce, gravy, peanut butter, peanuts, popcorn, salt, spices, vinegar, walnuts

II. Restricted foods: do not eat any more than the amount allowed each day

1. Milk: 1 pt daily (may be used other than as beverage)
2. Cream: $1/3$ cup or less daily
3. Fruits: 1 serving daily (in addition to those listed previously); certain fruits listed below are not allowed at any time
4. Vegetables, including potato: 2 servings daily; certain vegetables listed below are not allowed at any time

ACID ASH DIET—cont'd

III. Foods are allowed

1. Carbonated beverages, such as ginger ale, Coca-Cola, root beer
2. Cake or cookies made with baking powder or soda
3. Fruits: dried apricots, bananas, dates, figs, raisins, rhubarb
4. Vegetables: dried beans, beet greens, dandelion greens, carrots, chard, lima beans
5. Sweets: chocolate or candies other than those in group I; syrups
6. Miscellaneous: other nuts, olives, pickles

IV. Sample menu

Breakfast	Lunch	Dinner
Grapefruit	Creamed chicken	Broth
Wheatena	Steamed rice	Roast beef, gravy
Scrambled eggs	Green beans	Buttered noodles
Toast, butter, plum jam	Bread, butter	Sliced tomato
Coffee, cream, sugar	Stewed prunes	Mayonnaise
	Milk	Bread, butter
		Vanilla ice cream

LOW-PURINE DIET (APPROXIMATELY 125 MG PURINE)

General directions

1. During acute stages use only list 1
2. After acute stage subsides and for chronic conditions, use the following schedule:
    a. Two days a week but not consecutively use list 1 entirely
    b. The remaining days add foods from lists 2 and 3 as indicated
    c. Avoid list 4 entirely
3. Keep diet moderately low in fat

Typical meal pattern

Breakfast	Lunch	Dinner
Fruit	Egg or cheese dish	Egg or cheese dish
Refined cereal and/or egg	Vegetables as allowed (cooked	Cream of vegetable soup if de-
White toast	or in salad)	sired
Butter, 1 tsp	Potato or substitute	Starch (potato or substitute)
Sugar	White bread	Colored vegetable as allowed
Coffee	Butter, 1 tsp	White bread and butter, 1 tsp
Milk if desired	Fruit or simple dessert	if desired
	Milk	Salad as allowed
		Fruit or simple dessert
		Milk

Continued.

LOW-PURINE DIET (APPROXIMATELY 125 MG PURINE—cont'd

Food list 1: The following contain an insignificant amount of purine and may be used as desired

Beverages	Vegetables
Carbonated	Artichokes
Chocolate	Beets
Cocoa	Beet greens
Coffee	Broccoli
Fruit juices	Brussels sprouts
Postum	Cabbage
Tea	Carrots
Butter*	Celery
Breads: white and crackers, corn bread	Corn
Cereals and cereal products	Cucumber
Corn	Eggplant
Rice	Endive
Tapioca	Kohlrabi
Refined wheat	Lettuce
Macaroni	Okra
Noodles	Parsnips
Cheese of all kinds*	Potato, white and sweet
Eggs	Pumpkin
Fats of all kinds* (moderate amount)	Rutabagas
Fruits of all kinds	Sauerkraut
Gelatin, Jell-O	String beans
Milk: buttermilk, evaporated, malted, sweet	Summer squash
Nuts of all kinds*	Swiss chard
Peanut butter*	Tomato
Pies* (except mincemeat)	Turnips
Sugar and sweets	

Food list 2: One item 4 times a week: foods that contain a moderate amount (up to 75 mg) or purine in 100 g serving)

Asparagus	Herring	Oysters
Bluefish	Kidney beans	Peas
Bouillon	Lima beans	Salmon
Cauliflower	Lobster	Shad
Chicken	Mushrooms	Spinach
Crab	Mutton	Tripe
Finnan haddie	Navy beans	Tuna fish
Ham	Oatmeal	Whitefish

*High in fat.

An acid ash, low-purine, or low-oxalate diet is ineffective in removing stones that are already formed, but they can reduce the probability that stones will recur. The diet should be adequate and well balanced and contain sufficient protein to meet normal requirements. Water should be drunk freely to prevent urine that is too concentrated.

LOW-PURINE DIET (APPROXIMATELY 125 MG PURINE—cont'd

Food list 3: One item once a week: foods that contain a large amount (75-150 mg) or purine in 100 g serving

Bacon	Lentils	Quail
Beef	Liver sausage	Rabbit
Calf tongue	Meat soups	Sheep
Carp	Partridge	Shellfish
Chicken soup	Perch	Squab
Codfish	Pheasant	Trout
Duck	Pigeon	Turkey
Goose	Pike	Veal
Halibut	Pork	Venison

Food list 4: Avoid entirely: foods that contain large amounts (150-1000 mg) of purine in 100 g serving

Sweetbreads	825 mg	Kidneys (beef)	200 mg
Anchovies	363 mg	Brains	195 mg
Sardines (in oil)	295 mg	Meat extracts	160-400 mg
Liver (calf, beef)	233 mg	Gravies	Variable

FOOD SOURCES OF OXALATES

Fruits	Nuts	Vegetables	Beverages
Currants	Almonds	Beans, green and wax	Chocolate
Concord grapes	Cashews	Beets	Cocoa
Figs		Beet greens	Tea
Gooseberries		Chard	
Plums		Endive	
Raspberries		Okra	
Rhubarb		Spinach	
		Sweet potatoes	
		Tomatoes	

Questions on diseases of the urinary tract

1. What is the function of the kidneys?
2. How many nephrons are in the kidneys?
3. What is the function of the glomeruli?
4. How does the composition of the filtrate compare with the composition of blood?
5. What is the percentage of solids in urine?
6. Trace the filtrate from the time it leaves the glomeruli and until it becomes urine in the pelvis of the kidney.
7. What is the principal waste product of protein?

8. How does the urine reach the bladder?
9. What is the amount of urine normally excreted in a day?
10. What happens if the urea is not completely eliminated by the kidneys?
11. What is nephritis?
12. Through what channels is protein lost in nephritis?
13. What determines the amount of protein that should be in the diet in the treatment of nephritis?
14. Why is the amount of protein limited?
15. Why is the normal amount of carbohydrate and fat used in the diet for nephritis?
16. What is believed to be the cause of acute glomerulonephritis?
17. What age group does acute glomerulonephritis usually affect?
18. Discuss the diet in the treatment of acute glomerulonephritis.
19. Why should the diet for chronic glomerulonephritis be high in protein, carbohydrate, and fat? How would the presence of edema alter the diet? Why are fluids not restricted?
20. What age group does nephrosclerosis usually affect? Why should protein be restricted to 45 to 50 g a day and why? What percentage of the diet should be carbohydrate? What other specifications are included in regard to the diet?
21. What are the symptoms of nephrosis? How much protein and how many calories should be in the beginning diet, and how much should they be increased later on?
22. What are some of the causes of uremia? Why is the patient given principally carbohydrate and fat? What is the Borst diet?
23. Name the three main kinds of renal stones and describe the diet that should be given in the treatment of each.

Suggestions for additional study

1. Write a menu for 1 day for a 45- to 50-g protein, 1000-mg sodium diet.
2. Plan a menu for 1 day for the following diets: (a) an acid ash diet, (b) a low-purine diet, and (c) a diet low in oxalates.
3. Trace the route taken by the blood plasma from the glomeruli to the bladder.

The patient with kidney stones

Jim Roberts, age 25, lived in a small walk-up studio apartment in Manhattan, where he taught school with a group of other young teachers in a ghetto school. He had group medical coverage through his employment in the city school system. He had been well during the past year except for several bouts with a recurring urinary tract infection. On one occasion he had suffered some renal colic and passed several small stones.

Jim ate sporadically, getting little for breakfast before he left the apartment, having a sandwich for lunch at school, and eating irregularly in the evening at dinner time. Sometimes he would get involved in reading or studying and skip dinner altogether, getting snacks through the evening and drinking several glasses of milk. Occasionally he would have dinner at a small neighborhood restaurant near his apartment. He drank a great deal of milk, a carry-over habit from his childhood. His mother had always told him that it was "a perfect food," and besides, it was easy to keep and filling. Most days he would drink about 2 quarts at least. He was also fond of ice cream and could eat as much as a quart at a time.

During the past month or so, Jim had been feeling increasing pain through his right flank and back. He had mentioned this to Susan, his girlfriend, who had encouraged him to see a physician. However, since the pain passed, he put off checking into it. One day, however, the pain became so severe that he could not go to school. He telephoned the principal to report his illness. He began to have chills. When he took his temperature, his temperature was 100° F.

When Susan came by Bill's apartment after school to see how he was, she found him nauseous, vomiting, and in severe pain. She called his physician and drove him immediately to the hospital. After the hospital examination the physician decided to keep Jim in the hospital for several days for studies to determine what treatment would be needed. The results of the studies indicated normal kidney function and normal uric acid levels. However, there was some elevation of urinary calcium and serum calcium and phosphorus. The roentgenograms indicated the presence of a rather large stone in the kidney pelvis on the left side. The physician ordered a diet for Jim of 400 mg of calcium and 1000 mg of phosphorus, acid ash. He also asked the nurse to force fluids.

As Jim's pain diminished and he began to feel better, the physician had him walk around the ward as much as possible. After a few more days of observation, the decision was made to remove the kidney stone surgically. Jim tolerated the surgery well, and his recovery was rapid.

QUESTIONS TO GUIDE YOUR INQUIRY

1. What conditions predispose to the formation of kidney stones? Which of these factors may have been operative in Jim's case?

2. What do the test results indicate that the probable chemistry of Jim's kidney stone was? What kind of stone do the test results rule out?

3. Give the reason for the diet the doctor ordered for Jim. Indicate the reasons for each factor in the diet.

4. Outline a day's menu for Jim on his special diet. Calculate the amount of calcium and phosphorus to ensure proper amounts of each factor.

5. When Jim was ready to go home and needed instructions concerning his diet, what suggestions would you have given him? What problems would he face in carrying them out? What solutions would you propose?

6. What does "urinary ash" mean? What foods produce an alkaline ash? What foods produce an acid ash? What is the value of such a dietary modification in cases of renal calculi or urinary tract infections?

Suggested readings

Williams, S.R.: Nutrition and diet therapy, ed. 4, St. Louis, 1981, The C.V. Mosby Co.
Williams, S.R.: Essentials of nutrition and diet therapy, ed. 3, St. Louis, 1982, The C.V. Mosby Co.

17

Diseases of the blood

THE BLOOD CIRCULATION
Blood volume

The normal person has about 5 to 6 quarts of blood that travel the circuit of the vascular system in less then 30 seconds. The average number of red blood corpuscles in men is 5 million per cubic millimeter and in women 4.5 million per cubic millimeter.

Blood components

Blood consists of plasma, in which erythrocytes, leukocytes, and platelets are suspended. The life of an erythrocyte, or red blood cell, is approximately 90 to 100 days, after which the old cell is destroyed and a new one is formed. The old red blood cell is usually destroyed in the spleen; iron is saved for further use, and the remainder of the red blood cell is excreted. A red blood cell contains hemoglobin, which is made up of heme, a nonprotein iron compound, and globin, a protein. Iron is the oxygen-carrying element of the blood. Leukocytes, or white blood cells, act as scavengers and help resist infections. When invading bacteria overcome them, the dead bodies of the leukocytes, or white blood corpuscles, correct in the form of pus, which causes an abscess if there is no outlet for it. The platelets have a part in the clotting process.

Blood functions

The functions of the blood follow:

1. It transports the end products of digestion from the digestive tract to the tissues of the body. It also carries oxygen from the lungs to the body tissues.

2. It carries the waste products of the body to the kidneys, lungs, skin, and intestines.

3. It carries the hormones to their target organs.

4. The white blood cells act as protection against disease.

5. It helps to regulate the body temperature.

6. It is essential for maintaining acid-base and water balance in the body.

ANEMIA

Anemia is a condition in which there is a reduction in the number and size of red blood corpuscles or in the amount of hemoglobin, or both. The symptoms of anemia are general weakness, poor appetite, pallor, fatigue, and increased sensitivity to cold. In more advanced conditions gastrointestinal tract disturbances and difficult breathing occur.

Anemias are divided into the following three general classifications: (1) anemias caused by loss of blood, called hemorrhagic anemia; (2) anemias caused by the nutritional deficiency of iron or protein or the lack of absorption of these nutrients, called nutritional or iron deficiency anemia; and (3) anemia caused by deficient formation of red blood cells in the bone marrow, called pernicious anemia.

Hemorrhagic anemia

Loss of blood occurs in excessive bleeding from an injury or from an abnormal condition within the body that results in a loss of blood volume. The body replaces the loss in volume with water, and in a normal person the system automatically replaces lost iron and other substances from the reserve in the body. However, a better than adequate amount of protein and iron in the diet will hasten the process. If the blood loss is large, a blood transfusion is advised.

Anemia often occurs in adolescent girls who experience excessive menstruation and whose diet is insufficient in protein and iron.

Nutritional anemia

DEFICIENCY IN IRON. The adult body contains about 3 to 4 g of iron, which is slowly absorbed from the food in the small intestine and passes in the blood to the bone marrow. There it is used in the manufacture of red blood cells. If there is a reduced amount of iron in the blood, the oxygen-carrying capacity is lessened.

The best answer to the problem of iron-deficiency anemia is prevention from fetal life onward. This means that during pregnancy the mother must have an adequate intake of iron (18 mg) daily. This will ensure an adequate storage of iron in the fetus, which will meet the need for iron for the first 5 or 6 months of the infant's life, after which foods high in iron, such as egg yolk, should be added to the milk diet.

Throughout life all persons should be certain of receiving an adequate intake of iron, which is 10 mg for men and 18 mg for women. Additional iron (total of 18 mg) is necessary for adolescent girls and women throughout their reproductive years because of menstruation and childbearing demands. Adolescent boys should receive 18 mg of iron daily because of rapid growth.

DEFICIENCY IN PROTEIN. Diets high in iron but inadequate in protein will not rebuild red blood cells. When the amount of protein in the blood is reduced by hemorrhage, extensive burns, or pathological disturbances, the normal ex-

IRON-RICH FOOD GUIDE

The foods highest in iron are liver, beef, veal, lamb, pork, turkey, chicken, oysters, enriched bread and cereals, eggs, peanut butter, dried navy and lima beans, soybeans, dried apricots, peaches, prunes, figs, dates, raisins, and molasses.

Sample menu

Breakfast	Lunch	Dinner
Stewed prunes	Navy bean soup	Broiled liver with onions
Oatmeal	Chicken sandwich	Mashed potatoes
Cream	Carrot and raisin salad	Fresh broccoli
Poached egg	Citrus fruit cup	Tomato salad
Toast	Milk	Whole-wheat bread
Butter or margarine		Butter or margarine
Coffee		Date pudding
		Milk

change of fluids between the blood vessels and peritoneal cavities is lessened, and edema results.

LACK OF ABSORPTION. In certain pathological conditions iron is not properly used. Dietary iron must be changed in form through acid reduction before it can be absorbed. Thus absorption of iron is facilitated by an acid medium. Iron absorption is aided by such agents as ascorbic acid (vitamin C). Most of the iron is absorbed in the duodenum, the first portion of the small intestine. This occurs because the gastric juice is acidic and remains somewhat acidic when it first enters the intestinal tract. Therefore a person who has low gastric acidity needs both hydrochloric acid and iron supplements. The usual iron supplement given is ferrous sulfate, taken after each meal. It is less likely to upset the stomach if it is taken after a meal.

The diet should be high in iron (20 to 25 mg) and protein (100 to 150 g). A diet high in iron but low in protein will not promote regeneration of hemoglobin. Liver is the most effective food in stimulating the production of blood. Liver once a week and lean meat and eggs daily are good sources of both iron and protein. Whole-grain or enriched bread and cereals, legumes, green leafy vegetables, and dried fruits are good sources of iron. The diet should also be high in vitamins, especially B complex and ascorbic acid. Insufficient calcium and vitamin D also interfere with proper use and storage of iron. A general iron-rich food guide is summarized above. A number of these foods also contain quality protein.

Pernicious anemia

Pernicious anemia is characterized by the deficient formation of red blood cells in the bone marrow. The cells become large and fewer in number. These large, immature red blood cells are called macrocytes. Normally, red blood cells are not released from bone marrow until they are mature. However, when the bone marrow becomes crowded with abnormal immature cells, they are released into the blood.

The symptoms of pernicious anemia are gastrointestinal tract disturbances, sore mouth, low gastric acidity, loss of appetite, neurological disturbances, and pain in the abdominal region.

The cause of pernicious anemia is the lack of the intrinsic factor in the gastric juice, which is essential for the absorption of vitamin B_{12}. Vitamin B_{12} is stored in the liver until needed by the bone marrow for maturing red blood cells. However, even though there is insufficient absorption of vitamin B_{12}, the liver is a sufficiently concentrated source of the vitamin to permit some absorption to take place without the intrinsic factor, thus protecting the nervous system from further damage.

In pernicious anemia vitamin B_{12} is absorbed much better if it is given parenterally, or by injection. When it is given orally, it is not used because it has to pass through the gastrointestinal system, where there is a lack of the intrinsic factor in the gastric juices.

Formerly, liver extracts were given parenterally and achieved good results. However, the use of vitamin B_{12} has superseded the administration of liver extracts. Folic acid also helps in the treatment of pernicious anemia, but it should not be used as the only medication. It relieves some of the symptoms but does not improve the neurological disturbances.

The diet should be high in calories and protein. The diet should be high in carbohydrate to bring the weight up to normal and spare the protein for blood regeneration. The fat content should be low and made up largely of emulsified fats. Vitamins and minerals should also be increased. Iron supplements are usually given. Copper must also be present, but if an adequate diet is eaten, there will be sufficient copper. The consistency of the diet depends on the condition of the patient. If there is anorexia and soreness in the mouth, the beginning diet must be liquid. The patient will usually take liquids even though there is no desire for food. As the patient improves, the diet can be gradually changed to soft foods and a little later to regular foods.

After recovery a patient with pernicious anemia must receive maintenance therapy of vitamin B_{12} injections for life.

Questions on diseases of the blood

1. How much blood is present in the normal person?
2. What is the average red blood cell count for men? For women?
3. What three kinds of cells are found in the blood plasma?
4. What is the approximate life of an erythrocyte, and what happens when the cell is destroyed?

5. What is the composition of hemoglobin?
6. What is the function of iron in the blood?
7. What is the function of leukocytes? Of platelets?
8. List three functions of blood, excluding the individual functions of iron, leukocytes, and platelets.
9. What is anemia? List some of the symptoms.
10. Name the three types of anemia discussed in this chapter.
11. What are the possible causes of anemias resulting from loss of blood?
12. What deficiencies are responsible for nutritional anemia?
13. What is the normal content of iron in the adult body?
14. What are some of the causes of iron deficiency anemia?
15. Outline in detail the diet for nutritional anemia.
16. What vitamins and minerals, in addition to iron, are needed for regeneration of the blood?
17. What are the characteristics of pernicious anemia?
18. What is the cause of pernicious anemia?
19. What role does vitamin B_{12} have in the treatment of pernicious anemia, and how should it be administered?
20. Outline the dietary treatment for pernicious anemia.
21. Is there a permanent cure for pernicious anemia?

Suggestions for additional study

1. Plan a day's menu for nutritional anemia and the same for pernicious anemia.
2. Circle the following foods that are high in iron: milk, eggs, whole-wheat bread, watermelon, tomatoes, navy beans.
3. Check the answer that correctly describes the diet for the treatment of nutritional anemia:
   a. High-calorie, low-protein, high-fat, high-iron, high–vitamin B complex, low–ascorbic acid, low-calcium, high–vitamin D.
   b. High-calorie, high-protein, low-fat, high–vitamin B complex, high–ascorbic acid, high–vitamin D, high-calcium, high-iron.
   c. High-calorie, high-protein, low-fat, high–vitamin K, low–ascorbic acid, high–vitamin D, low-calcium.

Suggested readings

Williams, S.R.: Nutrition and diet therapy, ed. 4, St. Louis, 1981, The C.V. Mosby Co.
Williams, S.R.: Essentials of nutrition and diet therapy, ed. 3, St. Louis, 1982, The C.V. Mosby Co.

18

Diseases of the cardiovascular system

Cardiovascular diseases are responsible for approximately 50% of the deaths today, partly because people in general are living longer and reaching the age at which degenerative diseases become more prevalent. Also, many people become obese in middle age, which makes them more susceptible to cardiovascular disturbances. A number of the many risk factors in heart disease are summarized in Table 18-1.

The objectives in the dietary treatment of patients with heart disease follow:
1. To provide an adequate diet if patients' conditions permit
2. To prevent patients from eating bulky or gas-forming foods that distend the stomach and exert pressure against the heart
3. To reduce patients' weight to normal if they are overweight or to slightly below normal if they are not overweight, which permits the heart freer movement and lowers metabolism, thereby furnishing less stimulus to the heart
4. To prevent edema
5. To reduce the risk of atherosclerosis by lowering the number of circulating blood lipids

There are two types of cardiac disturbances: *functional* and *organic*. In the functional type, disturbances in the rate and regularity of the heartbeat are present. Often there are pains in the heart. The principal cause is infection; however, frequently it is caused by psychological mechanisms.

The organic types of cardiac disturbances, which include rheumatic heart disease, pericarditis, coronary occlusion, angina pectoris, cardiac failure, atherosclerosis, and hypertension, are discussed separately in this chapter.

RHEUMATIC HEART DISEASE AND PERICARDITIS

Acute cardiac infection may result from rheumatic fever, or it may occur in pericarditis, which is inflammation of the membrane that encloses the heart. The objective of the diet should be to provide adequate nourishment with the least possible exertion on the part of the patient. Liquid and semiliquid foods such as milk, milk toast, broth thickened with rice, soft-cooked egg, cereal,

Table 18-1. Multiple risk factors in cardiovascular disease

Personal characteristics	Behavior patterns	Metabolic relationships
Family history	Smoking	Diabetes
Sex (higher incidence in men)	Eating habits (use of excess fats,	Hypertension
Age (approximately 30-55	sugar, salt, and quantity)	Hyperlipemia (elevated serum
years)	Exercising (little or no physical	lipids—triglycerides, lipo-
Overweight	activity)	proteins, cholesterol)
Stress (personality type: work		
addiction, with heavy pres-		
sures and limited sleep)		

fruit juice, gelatin, and custard may be given. The feedings should be small and should be given six times a day. As the patient improves, a more liberal diet may be given.

CORONARY OCCLUSION

Coronary occlusion occurs when one of the blood vessels of the heart becomes blocked, causing a myocardial infarction or heart attack. The underlying disease of the blood vessels is *atherosclerosis* (p. 198).

The patient must have absolute quiet and bed rest. For the first 3 or 4 days usually only fluids are allowed. Water and fruit juices may be given through the day, but the amount of fluids given must not exceed 1500 ml or approximately 1½ quarts. On the fourth or fifth day, if the patient has shown improvement, a soft diet may be given. Usually, to achieve cardiac rest, the diet is relatively low in calories (800 to 1200). It may also be low in sodium, to help prevent edema, and low in fat, to help reduce the level of blood fats. The patient must eat slowly and chew food well. The low-calorie diet brings not only some loss in body weight but also a reduction in basal metabolism and hence cardiac rest. After 4 to 6 weeks the number of calories may be raised to 1500 or the individual's maintenance level, but the fat-controlled food plan (pp. 194-195) should be continued.

ANGINA PECTORIS

Angina pectoris is characterized by pain around the heart and a sudden sharp pain radiating from the heart to the shoulder and down the left arm. The attacks may occur intermittently, but with proper rest and care the patient can recover. The diet should be such that it causes the least amount of work for the digestive organs.

The diet should be low in calories, especially if the patient is obese. The diet can be more liberal than the diet for the treatment of coronary occlusion. The food must be easily digested and divided into six small meals. The patient may have one cup of coffee a day if the physician permits.

FAT-CONTROLLED DIET—HIGH POLYUNSATURATED FATTY ACIDS DIET

	Foods allowed	Foods not allowed
Soups	Made from bouillon cubes, vegetables, and broths from which fat has been removed; cream soups made with nonfat milk	Meat soups, commercial cream soups, soups made with whole milk or cream
Meat, fish, poultry	1 or 2 servings daily (not to exceed a total of 4 oz) lean muscle meat, broiled or roasted; beef, veal, lamb, pork, chicken, turkey, ham; organ meats (all visible fat should be trimmed from meat); all fish and shellfish	Bacon, pork sausage, luncheon and dried meat, and all fatty cuts; wieners; fish roe; duck, goose, skin of poultry; TV dinners
Milk and milk products	At least 1 pt nonfat milk or nonfat buttermilk daily; nonfat cottage cheese, sapsago cheese	Whole milk and cream, all cheeses (except nonfat cottage cheese), ice cream, imitation ice cream (except that containing safflower oil), ice milk, sour cream, commercial yogurt
Eggs	Egg whites	Egg yolks
Vegetables	All raw or cooked as tolerated (leafy green and yellow vegetables are good sources of vitamin A)	No restrictions
Fruits	All raw, cooked, dried, frozen, or canned; use citrus or tomatoes daily; fruit juices	Avocado, olives
Salads	All fruit, vegetable, and gelatin salads	
Cereals	All cooked and dry cereals; serve with nonfat milk or fruit; macaroni, noodles, spaghetti, rice	
Breads	Whole wheat, rye, enriched white, and French bread; English muffins; graham and saltine crackers	Commercial pancakes, waffles, coffee cakes, muffins, doughnuts, and all other quick breads made with whole milk and fat; biscuit mixes and other commercial mixes; cheese crackers; pretzels

CARDIAC FAILURE

There are two types of cardiac failure: compensated and decompensated. Any of the diseases discussed before can cause cardiac failure.

Compensated cardiac failure

In compensated cardiac failure the heart is able to maintain adequate circulation to all parts of the body, usually by some enlargement of the heart and an increased pulse rate. Patients are usually able to perform daily tasks if they take extreme care to avoid any hurry, unnecessary excitement, or strenuous work.

	Foods allowed	Foods not allowed
Desserts	Fruits; tapioca, cornstarch, rice, junket puddings, all made with nonfat milk and without egg yolks; fruit whips made with egg whites; gelatin desserts; angel food cake; sherbet, ices, and special imitation ice cream containing safflower oil; cake and cookies made with nonfat milk, oil, and egg white; fruit pie (pastry made with oil)	Omit desserts and candies made with whole milk, cream, egg yolk, chocolate, cocoa butter, coconut, hydrogenated shortenings, butter, and other animal fats
Concentrated fats	Corn oil, soybean oil, cottonseed oil, sesame oil, safflower oil, sunflower oil; walnuts and other nuts except cashew and those commercially fried or roasted Margarine made from above oils Commercial French and Italian salad dressings if not made with olive oil Gravy may be made from bouillon cubes or fat-free meat stock thickened with flour and oil added if desired Freshly ground or old-fashioned peanut butter	Butter, chocolate, coconut oil, hydrogenated fats and shortenings, cashew nuts; mineral oil, olive oil, margarine, except as specified; commercial salad dressings except as listed; hydrogenated peanut butter; gravy except as noted
Sweets	Jelly, jam, honey, hard candy, sugar	
Beverages	Tea, coffee, or coffee substitutes; tomato juices, fruit juice, cocoa prepared with nonfat milk	Beverages containing chocolate, ice cream, ice milk, eggs, whole milk, or cream

If the diet is also to be high in unsaturated fat it should include liberal amounts of the following:
1. Oils allowed that can be incorporated into salad dressings or added to soups, to nonfat milk, to cereal, to vegetables
2. Walnuts, almonds, Brazil nuts, filberts, pecans
3. Extra margarine in or on foods

Dietary treatment for compensated cardiac failure follows:

1. Patients must definitely reduce their weight if they are overweight and must adhere to a low-calorie diet even if they are not overweight.

2. Bulky meals must be avoided to prevent pressure on the heart.

3. Gas-forming vegetables should be avoided for the same reason.

4. Stimulants should be avoided or used sparingly.

5. Sodium must be restricted if edema is present.

6. The diet should be well-balanced, high in carbohydrate, moderately low in protein, and low in fat, with adequate vitamins and minerals.

7. Fluids may be taken as desired.

Decompensated cardiac failure

In decompensated cardiac failure, or congestive heart failure, the heart is unable to maintain adequate circulation to all parts of the body. The patient is

RESTRICTIONS FOR A MILD LOW-SODIUM DIET (2 TO 3 G SODIUM)

Do not use

1. Salt at the table (use salt lightly in cooking)
2. Salt-preserved foods such as salted or smoked meat (bacon and bacon fat, bologna, dried or chipped beef, corned beef, frankfurters, ham, kosher meats, luncheon meats, salt pork, sausage, smoked tongue), salted or smoked fish (anchovies, caviar, salted and dried cod, herring, sardines) sauerkraut, olives
3. Highly salted foods such as crackers, pretzels, potato chips, corn chips, salted nuts, salted popcorn
4. Spices and condiments such as bouillon cubes,* catsup,* chili sauce,* celery salt, garlic sauce, onion salt, monosodium glutamate, meat sauces, meat tenderizers,* picles, prepared mustard, relishes, Worcestershire sauce, soy sauce
5. Cheese,* peanut butter*

*Dietetic low-sodium kind may be used.

RESTRICTIONS FOR A MODERATE LOW-SODIUM DIET (1000 MG SODIUM)

Do not use

1. Salt in cooking or at the table
2. Salt-preserved foods such as salted or smoked meat (bacon and bacon fat, bologna, dried or chipped beef, brains, corned beef, frankfurters, ham, kosher meats, luncheon meats, salt pork, sausage, smoked tongue, kidneys), salted or smoked fish (anchovies, caviar, salted and dried cod, herring, sardines, frozen fish fillets, canned salmon,* tuna*), sauerkraut, olives
3. Highly salted foods such as crackers, pretzels, potato chips, corn chips, salted nuts, salted popcorn
4. Spices and condiments such as bouillon cubes,* catsup,* chili sauce,* celery salt, garlic salt, onion salt, monosodium glutamate, meat sauces, meat tenderizers,* pickles, prepared mustard, relishes, Worcestershire sauce, soy sauce
5. Cheese,* peanut butter*
6. Buttermilk (unsalted buttermilk may be used) instead of skimmed milk
7. Canned vegetables,* canned vegetable juices*
8. Frozen peas, frozen lima beans, frozen mixed vegetables, any frozen vegetables to which salt has been added
9. More than 1 serving of any of these vegetables in 1 day: artichokes, beet greens, beets, carrots, celery, dandelion greens, kale, mustard greens, spinach, Swiss chard, turnips (white)
10. Regular bread, rolls,* crackers*
11. Dry cereals,* except puffed rice, puffed wheat, and shredded wheat
12. Quick-cooking Cream of Wheat
13. Shellfish: clams, crab, lobster, shrimp (oysters may be used)
14. Salted butter, salted margarine, commercial French dressings,* mayonnaise,* other salad dressings*
15. Regular baking powder,* baking soda, or anything containing them; self-rising flour
16. Prepared mixes: pudding,* gelatin,* cake, biscuit
17. Commercial candies

*Dietetic low-sodium kinds may be used.

RESTRICTIONS FOR A STRICT LOW-SODIUM DIET (500 MG SODIUM)

Do not use

1. Salt in cooking or at the table
2. Salt-preserved foods such as salted or smoked meat (bacon and bacon fat, bologna, dried or chipped beef, brains, corned beef, frankfurthers, ham, kosher meats, luncheon meats, salt pork, sausage, smoked tongue, kidneys), salted or smoked fish (anchovies, caviar, salted and dried cod, herring, sardines, frozen fish fillets, canned salmon,* tuna*), sauerkraut, olives
3. Highly salted foods such as crackers, pretzels, potato chips, corn chips, salted nuts, salted popcorn
4. Spices and condiments such as bouillon cubes,* catsup,* chili sauce,* celery salt, garlic salt, onion salt, monosodium glutamate (MSG, Accent), meat sauces, meat tenderizers,* pickles, prepared mustard, relishes, Worcestershire sauce, soy sauce
5. Cheese,* peanut butter*
6. Buttermilk (unsalted buttermilk may be used) instead of skimmed milk
7. More than 2 cups skimmed milk a day, including that used on cereal
8. Any commercial foods made of milk (ice cream, ice milk, milk shakes)
9. Canned vegetables,* canned vegetable juices*
10. Frozen peas, frozen lima beans, frozen mixed vegetables, any frozen vegetables to which salt has been added
11. These vegetables: artichokes, beet greens, beets, carrots, celery, dandelion greens, kale, mustard greens, spinach, Swiss chard, turnips (white)
12. Regular bread,* rolls,* crackers*
13. Dry cereals,* except puffed rice, puffed wheat, and shredded wheat
14. Quick-cooking cream of wheat
15. Shellfish: clams, crab, lobster, shrimp (oysters may be used)
16. Salted butter, salted margarine, commercial French dressings,* mayonnaise,* or other salad dressings*
17. Regular baking powder,* baking soda, or anything containing them; self-rising flour
18. Prepared mixes: pudding,* gelatin, cake, biscuit
19. Commercial candies

*Dietetic low-sodium kinds may be used.

short of breath because of the retarded flow of blood and because inadequate amounts of oxygen are carried to the lungs. Any exertion causes pain in the chest. As the disease progresses, edema usually develops.

DIET PATTERN. Dietary treatment for decompensated cardiac failure follows:

1. Only water, fruit juices, and milk may be allowed at first.

2. Later, as the patient improves, the following foods, without the addition of salt, may be added to the diet: cereal, milk toast, soft-cooked egg, gelatin, mashed or baked potato, pureed vegetables and fruits, custard, and plain puddings. Ice cream may also be given if it is eaten slowly. Small meals should be served six times a day to prevent the patient from becoming overtired at any one meal.

AMERICAN HEART ASSOCIATION LOW-SODIUM FOOD GUIDES. The American Heart Association has designated four standard levels of dietary sodium restriction:

1. Mild—2 to 3 g
2. Moderate—1 g
3. Strict—500 mg
4. Severe—250 mg

A series of "do not use" food lists are provided on pp. 196-197 to guide sodium control at the mild, moderate, and strict levels. A detailed low-sodium food guide is provided on pp. 199-201.

ATHEROSCLEROSIS

Atherosclerosis is a thickening of the walls of the blood vessels. It is often characterized by a rise in the blood cholesterol level and by an increase in the blood lipoproteins, which are large molecules consisting of fat and protein. A discussion of fat metabolism is given in Chapter 4 (p. 28) and should be reviewed there.

Cause

The exact cause of atherosclerosis is not known. Most authorities agree that obesity and a sedentary life have some part in its development. The most debatable issue is the question of how much and what kind of fat intake is most effective in the prevention of atherosclerosis. It is true that in the United States in the past 30 or 35 years the dietary intake of fat has increased, physical activities have decreased, and tensions have increased.

Types of lipid disorders

In some persons various blood fats (lipids), such as cholesterol, triglycerides, and lipoproteins, become elevated and lead to fatty deposits in blood vessel walls, causing the abnormal thickening. These types of lipid disorders are outlined in Table 18-2. The most common of these are type II, in which blood cholesterol mainly is elevated, and type IV, in which blood triglycerides are increased.

Lowering the intake of cholesterol in the diet does have some effect on the lowering of the blood cholesterol level although the body is able to manufacture cholesterol within itself. However, a low-saturated fat, low-cholesterol diet has also been effective in lowering the blood cholesterol level.

In view of all the findings it is advisable to avoid overweight and to have a balanced diet that is low in animal fat and low in cholesterol. The general fat-controlled food plan given on p. 194 may be used as a guide.

HYPERTENSION

Hypertension is not a disease but a symptom of other conditions such as kidney disease, or it may be of unknown origin, so-called essential hypertension. Many times it is not discovered until a person has a routine physical exami-

LOW-SODIUM DIET (500 MG SODIUM)

General description

1. All foods are to be prepared and served without the addition of salt, baking powder, or baking soda.
2. Consume only those foods that are tolerated and in the amounts specified.
3. Read all food labels for the *addition of salt or sodium in any form*.
4. Avoid medications and laxatives unless approved by your physician.
5. The suggested menu pattern for 500 mg sodium contains approximately 275 g carbohydrate, 85 g protein, 130 g fat, and 2300 calories. All menu patterns meet the recommended allowances of vitamins and minerals.

	Daily allowance	Foods to avoid
Milk	Limit to 2 cups milk daily—frozen, powdered, or canned or as 1 cup evaporated milk, used as beverage or in cooking; 2 tbs cream (1 oz [30 ml])	Malted milk, sour cream, buttermilk, condensed milk, milk shakes, chocolate milk, fruit flavored beverage powders, whipped toppings
Eggs	1 daily	
Meat, poultry	Cooked daily, 6 oz (168 g); fresh beef, lamb, liver, pork, veal, rabbit, chicken, duck, goose, quail, turkey, cod, halibut, filet sole, tuna, salmon, meats canned without salt, frozen meat containing no salt or sodium (beef or calf liver allowed not more than once in 2 weeks)	All meat, poultry, and fish not listed; avoid meat, fish, or poultry that is smoked, cured, canned, frozen, containing salt or sodium, pickled, salted, or dried (bacon, ham, luncheon meats, sausages, salt pork, canned salmon and tuna, sardines); clams, crabs, lobsters, oysters (eastern), scallops, shrimp, anchovies, salted dried cod, frozen fish fillets; commercial meat pies, TV dinners
Cheese	Special dietetic low-sodium cheese may be used as a meat substitute as part of the daily allowance	Any other
Fruits	3 servings daily including one citrus fruit—½ cup per serving, fresh, canned, or frozen	Dried figs, raisins containing sodium sulfite
Vegetables	4 servings daily (fresh, frozen, or dietetic canned vegetables only)—½ cup per serving; asparagus, green beans, wax beans, lima beans, navy beans, broccoli, cauliflower, corn, cucumber, endive, eggplant, lentils, onions, parsnips, peppers, radishes, rutabagas, cabbage, brussels sprouts, lettuce, mushrooms, okra, soybeans, squash, tomatoes, unsalted tomato juice, turnip greens	Canned vegetables or juices containing salt (V-8 juice), sauerkraut, white turnip, beets, celery, carrot, artichoke, greens (beets, spinach, chard, dandelions, kale, mustard greens), frozen peas, frozen lima beans, frozen mixed vegetables
Potato or substitute	2 servings daily of potato, rice, macaroni, spaghetti, noodles, fresh sweet potatoes	Potato chips, corn chips

Continued.

LOW-SODIUM DIET (500 MG SODIUM)—cont'd

	Daily allowance—cont'd	Foods to avoid—cont'd
Cereals	1 serving daily shredded wheat, puffed rice, puffed wheat, or cooked cereals that contain no added salt or sodium such as regular Cream of Wheat, cornmeal, Maltomeal, rice, Wheatena, Pettijohns, Ralston, oatmeal	Quick-cooking Cream of Wheat and all other read-to-eat cereals not listed; self-rising flour
Bread	Low-sodium bread or unsalted matzoth, low-sodium crackers	Potato chips, salted crackers, salted popcorn, pretzels, regular bread, rolls, biscuits, muffins; waffles, commercial mixes
Fats	Sweet butter, lard, salad oils, shortening, low-sodium salad dressing as desired; unsalted margarine (check label and brand)	Salted nuts, salted butter, bacon fat, margarine, salted peanut butter, gravies, commercial salad dressings
Soup	Homemade soup made with allowed meat, vegetables, milk	Broth, bouillon, consommé, canned soups
Sweets	Jelly, jam, sugar, honey, gumdrops, marshmallows as desired; small amounts of brown sugar	Any commercial jam and jelly containing a sodium preservative, molasses, candy, candy bars
Desserts	Fruit, gelatin dessert made with plain gelatin and fruit juice, fruit pie made without salt; rice, tapioca, or cornstarch pudding made with low-sodium milk or fruit and fruit juices; desserts made with sodium-free baking powder	All others, ice cream, sherbet, desserts made with regular baking powder, baking soda, rennet tablets, pudding mixes; commercial gelatin desserts, pudding and cake mixes
Beverages	Tea, coffee, postum, Sanka, cocoa (except Dutch process) made with low-sodium milk allowance, fruit juices	Instant cocoa mix, prepared beverage mixes
Condiments	Allspice, bay leaves, caraway seeds, cinnamon, curry powder, garlic, mace, marjoram, mustard powder, nutmeg, paprika, parsley, pimiento, rosemary, sage, sesame seeds, thyme, turmeric, ginger, pepper, vinegar; extracts of almond, lemon, vanilla, peppermint, walnut, maple	Celery salt, garlic salt, catsup, prepared mustard, salt, meat sauces, meat tenderizers, monosodium glutamate, soy sauce, pickles, relishes, olives, prepared horseradish, Worcestershire sauce, chili sauce, seasoning salts
Miscellaneous		Baking powder, baking soda, chewing tobacco

LOW-SODIUM DIET (500 MG SODIUM)—cont'd

500 mg sodium diet suggested menu pattern

Breakfast	Lunch	Dinner
1 fruit	3 oz (84 g) unsalted meat	3 oz (84 g) unsalted meat
1 egg	unsalted potato	unsalted potato
low-sodium cereal	low-sodium vegetable	low-sodium vegetable
1 low-sodium bread	low-sodium vegetable salad	low-sodium salad
1 unsalted butter	1 low-sodium bread	1 low-sodium bread
jelly	1 unsalted butter	1 unsalted butter
½ cup milk	jelly	jelly
coffee (1 oz [30 ml])	1 fruit	1 cup milk
2 tbs cream (1 oz [30 ml])	½ cup milk	coffee
	coffee	fruit

Modifications for a 250 mg sodium diet

The 250-mg sodium diet is essentially the same as 500-mg sodium diet except
1. Use low-sodium milk (2 or more glasses) instead of regular milk
2. Use only 5 oz (140 g) of meat instead of 6 oz (168 g)
3. Omit the cream

Modifications for a 1000 mg sodium diet

One of the three following modifications may be used to raise the sodium content in the 500-mg sodium diet to 1000 mg:

Modification I

1. Two slices regular bread are allowed daily
2. Regular butter, 2 tsp only (above this amount, unsalted butter must be used)
3. One serving (½ cup) is allowed daily of spinach, celery, carrots, beets, artichoke, or white turnip

Modification II (high protein)

1. Meat, 10 oz (28 g) are allowed instead of 6 oz (168 g)
2. One serving of prepared or milk dessert, such as ice cream, custard, gelatin, or 1 cup milk
3. Two eggs instead of one
4. One serving of spinach, celery, carrots, beets, or artichoke is allowed

Modification III

1. Three slices regular bread may be used in place of the low-sodium bread (above this amount, unsalted bread must be used)

Table 18-2. Types of lipid disorders

Type	Diet	Lipid pattern	Clinical signs	Genetic defect
I				
Rare	Low fat, 25-35 g;	Increased chylomicrons	Abdominal pain	Deficient en-
Early childhood	high carbohy-		Lipemia, retinalis,	zyme: lipopro-
Familial	drate; MCT		xanthoma	tein lipase
			Hepatosplenomeg-	
			aly	
II				
Common	Low cholesterol	Increased β-lipopro-	Xanthoma (tendon)	Defective plasma
All ages	Low saturated fat	teins (50% cholester-	Corneal arcus	clearing on ca-
Genetic:	High unsaturated	ol), LDL	Vascular disease	tabolism of
autosomal,	fat	Increased cholesterol	Accelerated	LDL
dominant			atherosclerosis	
IIb or III				
Relatively un-	Weight reduction	Increased abnormal	Xanthoma (palmar)	Unclear
common	Low cholesterol	form β-lipoproteins	Vascular disease	
Adult	High unsaturated	Increased triglycerides		
When genetic,	fat	Increased cholesterol		
recessive,				
sporadic				
IV				
Most common	Weight reduction	Increased pre-β-lipo-	Usually no overt	Abnormal glu-
Adult	Low carbohy-	proteins, VLDL	symptoms	cose tolerance
Familial	drate, no alco-	Increased triglycerides	Abnormal glucose	Lipogenesis
	hol	Sometimes carbohy-	tolerance	
	Low cholesterol	drate induced	High uric acid	
	High unsaturated		Stress, obesity	
	fat		Accelerated ath-	
			erosclerosis	
V				
Uncommon	Weight reduction	Increased chylomicrons	Abdominal pain	Unclear
Early adult	Low fat and car-	Increased triglycerides	Pancreatitis	
Sporadic familial	bohydrate	Increased cholesterol	Hepatosplenomeg-	
	High protein		aly	

Based on data from Fredrickson, D.S., Levy, R.I., and Lees, R.S.: N. Engl. J. Med. **276:**34, 1967.

nation. Sometimes persons with hypertension have headaches, dizziness, and shortness of breath. Many persons feel no ill effects from hypertension.

There is a thickening of the walls of the blood vessels that alters the flow of blood to the heart and kidneys and eventually damages these organs if the hypertension is severe. Although the blood pressure may decrease in some patients, there is no convincing evidence that the progress of the disease is retarded or arrested. Persons with hypertension should develop a calm, un-hurried, and unworried attitude toward life in general.

The dietary treatment for hypertension follows:

1. Patients should reduce their weight to normal or slightly below if they are obese or to 10% below normal weight if they are not obese.

2. The energy value of the diet is limited to sufficient calories to maintain ideal body weight.

3. The protein should be the normal amount of 60 to 70 g and of high biological value.

4. Approximately 50% of the calories should come from carbohydrate

5. The diet should be moderately low in fat.

6. Adequate vitamins and minerals must be included in the diet.

7. Sodium should be restricted. The low-sodium food guides in this chapter provide outlines for diet planning. Usually, with use of current antihypertensive drugs, only a mild restriction to about 2 g of sodium daily, or in some cases the moderate level of 1 g, is required.

8. Generous amounts of fruits and vegetables should be included in the diet.

9. Milk may also be included in the diet.

Questions on the cardiovascular system

1. Why is there a larger percentage of deaths from cardiovascular diseases today?
2. What are the objectives of the dietary treatment for patients with heart disease?
3. What are the two types of cardiac disturbances? Describe each.
4. What changes in the heart occur in coronary occlusion?
5. Outline the dietary treatment for coronary occlusion.
6. How does angina pectoris manifest itself?
7. What type of diet should be given in the treatment of angina pectoris?
8. Name the two types of cardiac failure. Explain each.
9. List the modifications that should be made in the diet for a patient with compensated heart failure.
10. Outline the diet for a patient with decompensated heart failure.
11. What are the characteristic symptoms of atherosclerosis?
12. What are the probable causes of atherosclerosis?
13. What effect does lowering the dietary cholesterol have on the blood cholesterol?
14. What is the most effective diet to use in the treatment of atherosclerosis in light of present-day knowledge?
15. Plan a low-fat, low-cholesterol diet for 2 days.
16. What are some of the characteristic symptoms of hypertension?
17. What occurs in the blood vessels in hypertension?
18. What are the specifications for the dietary treatment of hypertension? Discuss fully.

The patient with a myocardial infarction

Henry Thompson is a successful business executive. He works long hours and carries the major responsibility in his corporation. At his last physical checkup the physician cautioned him to slow his pace or his health would soon suffer. Already he was having some mild hypertension. His blood cholesterol was elevated, and he was overweight. In his desk job he got little exercise and found himself smoking more under tension.

Although his annual income was high in his position, his financial pressures seemed only to increase, with keeping several children in college and trying to maintain the expensive home in the suburbs, which his wife Martha seemed to enjoy.

One day while commuting on the freeway, he experienced a pain in his chest and vague apprehension. When he arrived home, the pain persisted and became more severe. He broke out into a cold sweat and felt nauseated. He thought that it was only indigestion from eating dinner too rapidly. However, when he became more ill, his wife called their physician, and he was admitted to the hospital for care.

After emergency care and tests the physician placed him in the coronary care unit at the hospital. His test results showed elevated cholesterol, pre-β-lipoproteins, glucose, prothrombin time, SGOT and LDH, and white blood cell count. The electrocardiogram revealed an infarction of the posterior wall of the myocardium.

At first the physician allowed Henry to have only a liquid diet. As Henry began to feel better and his condition stabilized, the physician increased his diet to an 800-calorie soft diet with low saturated fat. By the end of the first week, the physician had again increased Henry's diet to 1200 calories, full diet, and low saturated fat. This time, however, he specified that the calories from the fat be only 25% of the total. Henry's nurse noted these changes in his diet and discussed them with the physician and the dietitian.

Henry gradually improved over the next few weeks and finally was able to go home. The physician discussed with him the need for care at home during a period of convalescence. He explained that Henry had an underlying lipid disorder—type IV—and was to continue his weight loss with a modified fat and carbohydrate diet.

QUESTIONS TO GUIDE YOUR INQUIRY

1. What factors can you identify in Henry's background and personal and medical history that place him in a "high-risk category" for coronary disease?

2. Account for the initial symptoms of Henry's illness. What happens in a myocardial infarction?

3. Identify as many of the laboratory tests that the physician ordered as you can. Relate these tests to cell metabolism. Why would they be elevated in Henry's case?

4. Why did Henry receive only a liquid diet at first?

5. What is the reason for each of the modifications in Henry's first diet of solid food?

6. What occurs in the disease process atherosclerosis?

7. What relation, if any, does fat metabolism have to the disease?

8. Outline a day's menu for Henry on his increased diet of 1200 calories, as specified by the physician.

9. What needs might Henry have when he goes home? What plan would you make for helping him to prepare to go home?

10. Name some community resources that you might use in helping Henry understand his illness and its care.

Suggestions for additional study

1. Plan a day's menu for a patient with hypertension.
2. Plan a day's menu for a patient with coronary occlusion for the first few days and another day's menu for the same patient 6 weeks later.

Suggested readings

Williams, S.R.: Nutrition and diet therapy, ed. 4, St. Louis, 1981, The C.V. Mosby Co.
Williams, S.R.: Essentials of nutrition and diet therapy, ed. 3, St. Louis, 1982, The C.V. Mosby Co.

19

Diabetes

Diabetes may be classified as a deficiency disease in which the ability to use glucose is impaired. This deficiency may be caused by the failure of the pancreas to secrete sufficient insulin to take care of the glucose in a normal diet or may occur because the insulin produced is bound and unavailable for use. The normal pancreas supplies sufficient insulin to metabolize carbohydrate in the body.

Sometimes a mild condition can be controlled by diet alone. In some moderate conditions an oral hypoglycemic drug may be used in addition to the diet. However, in the more severe conditions insulin is required. Insulin cannot be given orally, since it is a protein and would be digested; therefore it must be given by injection.

TYPES OF DIABETES

There are two types of diabetes. Type I, or insulin-dependent, diabetes is usually manifested before the age of 20 years. It is difficult to manage and requires both dietary restrictions and insulin for its control. Patients may experience wide fluctuations in blood sugar from day to day. Type II, or non–insulin-dependent, diabetes usually develops after age 35 and is usually controlled by diet. Sometimes there may be a need for insulin in times of stress. Type II diabetes is usually milder in form than type I diabetes.

Although diabetes can be controlled, the full cause of the disease is unknown, and it cannot be prevented. It is known that the disease is hereditary and that it has afflicted humans for centuries.

DIETARY TREATMENT

The diet of a diabetic person should be determined by age, sex, body build, body weight, and degree of activity. The maintenance requirements are the same for a diabetic person as for a normal person.

CALORIES. The energy need of the person is based on sufficient calories to maintain ideal body weight. Usually for adults an allowance of about 30 calories per kilogram of ideal body weight is used.

207

PROTEIN. Approximately 1 g of protein per kilogram of body weight, or 20% of the total calories, is a baseline allowance.

CARBOHYDRATE. The current recommendations for carbohydrate are liberalized to about 50% of the total calories, with the greater portion of this allowance (about 40%) in complex carbohydrates such as starch and the lesser portion (10%) in simple carbohydrates such as fruit.

FAT. The recommendation for fat is a moderate controlled amount, no more than 25% to 30% of the total calories, with limited use of animal fat.

DIET PLANNING
Exchange system

Usually the exchange system of dietary control is used for planning the diabetic diet. The exchange system of dietary control, developed by professional organizations such as the American Dietetic Association, is based on a simple grouping of common foods according to generally equivalent nutritional values. This system may be used for any situation requiring calorie and food value control. The diet for a person with diabetes is calculated by the clinical nutritionist or dietitian, who then develops a personalized food pattern. This pattern may then be used by the patient, staff, or family in planning meals and snacks.

In the exchange system the foods are divided into six basic groups (some with subgroups), called *exchange groups*. These six food exchange groups are outlined in Table 19-1. Each food item within a group (or subgroup) contains approximately the same food value as any other food item in that group, allowing for exchange within groups and thus providing for variety in food choices, as well as food value control. Hence the term *food exchanges* is used to refer to food choices or servings. The total number of exchanges per day depends on individual nutritional needs, based on normal nutritional standards. The individual food plan will allow for a patient's food preferences and economic status.

Meal planning

The principle of planning the diabetic diet by this simplified method is based on the plan of food exchanges. The common foods in each of the six food groups are listed on pp. 210-214. These groups are used to make food choices to fulfill the basic meal pattern developed by the clinical dietitian. The greatest advantage of the exchange system is that it gives the patient more freedom in selecting food. The diet no longer needs to be monotonous, and the patient is not burdened by long lists of food values that are difficult to understand.

So-called specialty foods for diabetic patients are unnecessary. They are expensive, and the information on the package can be misleading. They are not needed, for diabetic persons can usually eat all the natural primary foods, such as breads, cereals, unsweetened fruits, and vegetables, in the proper amounts.   *Text continued on p. 214.*

Table 19-1. Food exchange groups

Food group	Unit of exchange	Composition			Calories	Characteristic items
		Carbo-hydrate (g)	Protein (g)	Fat (g)		
Milk	1 cup					Equivalents to 1 cup whole
Skimmed		12	8	—	80	milk listed; 1 cup
Low fat		12	8	5	120	skimmed + 2 fat ex-
Whole		12	8	10	170	changes = whole milk
Vegetables	½ cup	5	2		25	Variety of low-carbohydrate vegetables (e.g., toma-toes, green beans, leafy vegetables)
Fruit	Varies	10	—	—	4	Fresh or canned without sugar
						Portion size varies with carbohydrate value of item; all portions equat-ed at 10% carbohydrate
Bread	Varies; 1 slice bread	15	2	—	70	Variety of starch items, breads, cereals, vegeta-bles; portions equal in carbohydrate value to 1 slice bread
Meat	1 oz (28 g)	—				Protein foods; exchange
Lean		—	7	2.5	50.5	units equal to protein
Medium fat		—	7	5	75	value of 1 oz (28 g) lean
Higher fat		—	7	7.5	95.5	meat (cheese, egg, sea-food)
Fat	1 tsp	—				Fat food items equal to 1
Polyunsaturated		—	—	5	45	tsp margarine (oil, may-
Monounsaturated		—	—	5	45	onnaise, olives, avoca-
Saturated		—	—	5	45	dos)

FOOD EXCHANGE GROUPS

List 1: Milk exchanges (Cream portion of whole milk equals 2 fat exchanges. Hence 1 cup whole milk equals 1 cup skimmed milk plus 2 fat exchanges.)
Group A (nonfat)

Skimmed or nonfat milk	1 cup
Buttermilk	1 cup
Canned, evaporated skimmed milk	½ cup
Powdered, nonfat dry milk (before adding liquid)	⅓ cup
Yogurt made from skimmed milk (plain, unflavored)	1 cup

Group B (low fat)

Low-fat milk (2% butterfat)	1 cup
Yogurt made from low-fat milk (plain, unflavored)	1 cup

Group C (full fat)

Whole milk	1 cup
Canned, evaporated whole milk	½ cup
Powdered, whole dry milk (before adding liquid)	⅓ cup
Yogurt made from whole milk (plain, unflavored)	1 cup

List 2: Vegetable exchanges (As served plain, without fat, seasoning, or dressing. Any fat used is taken from the fat exchange allowance. One exchange is ½ cup.)

Artichoke	Endive*	Onions
Asparagus	Green pepper, chili pepper	Parsley*
Bok choy, gai choy	Greens	Pimientos
Bamboo shoots	Beet	Radishes*
Bean sprouts	Chard	Rhubarb
Beets	Collards	Rutabaga
Broccoli	Dandelion	Sauerkraut
Brussels sprouts	Escarole*	String beans: green, yellow, wax
Cabbage	Kale	Summer squash
Carrots	Mustard	Tomato juice
Cauliflower	Spinach	Tomatoes
Celery	Turnip	Turnips
Chicory*	Lettuce: all varieties*	Vegetable juice, mixed
Chinese cabbage*	Mushrooms	Watercress*
Cucumber	Okra	Zucchini
Eggplant		

*Use as desired.

FOOD EXCHANGE GROUPS—cont'd

List 3: Fruit exchanges (Unsweetened, fresh, frozen, canned, cooked. One exchange is the portion indicated by the fruit.)

Berries

Blackberries	½ cup	
Blueberries	½ cup	
Raspberries	½ cup	
Strawberries	¾ cup	

Citrus fruits

Grapefruit	½ small
Grapefruit juice	½ cup
Orange	1 small
Orange juice	½ cup
Tangerine	1 medium

Melons

Cantaloupe	¼ medium
Honeydew	⅛ medium
Watermelon	1 cup diced (approx. ½ center slice)

Dried fruits

Apricots	4 halves
Dates	2 medium
Figs	1 medium
Peaches	2 halves
Pears	2 halves
Prunes	2 medium
Raisins	2 tbs

Other fruits

Apple	1 small
Apple cider	⅓ cup
Apple juice	⅓ cup
Applesauce	½ cup
Apricots	2 medium
Banana	½ small
Cherries	10 large, 17 small
Fig	1 large
Fruit cocktail	½ cup
Grape juice	¼ cup
Grapes	10 medium
Kiwi fruit	1 medium
Mango	½ small
Nectarine	1 small
Papaya	⅓ medium, ½ small
Peach	1 medium
Pear	1 medium
Persimmon	1 medium
Pineapple	½ cup; 1 round center slice
Pineapple juice	⅓ cup
Plums	2 medium
Prune juice	¼ cup
Prunes, fresh	2 medium

List 4: Bread exchanges (Equivalent portions indicated by each item.)

Bread

Bagel	½
Bread (load, average size slice)	1 slice
French	
Italian	
Pumpernickel	
Raisin	
Rye	
White	
Whole wheat	
Bread crumbs, dried	3 tbs
English muffin	½
Hamburger bun	½
Roll, frankfurter	1
Roll, plain	1 small
Tortilla (6 in diameter)	1

Cereal

Bulgur, cooked	½ cup
Cereal, cooked	½ cup
Cereal, dry (ready-to-eat, unsweetened)	½ cup
Bran flakes	¼ cup
Grapenuts	¾ cup
Other (flake, puff)	2 tbs
Cornmeal, dry	2½ tbs
Flour	½ cup
Grits, cooked	½ cup
Pasta, cooked (spaghetti, noodles, macaroni)	1½ cups
Popcorn (popped, no fat)	½ cups
Rice, cooked	3 tbs
Wheat germ, plain	

Continued.

FOOD EXCHANGE GROUPS—cont'd

List 4: Bread exchanges—cont'd

Crackers

Arrowroot	3
Graham, 2½ in square	2
Matzoth, 4 × 6 in	1
Oyster crackers	20
Pretzels, 3⅛ × ⅛ in	25
Round butter type crackers	6
Rye wafers, 2 × 3½ in	3
Saltines	5
Soda crackers, 2½ in square	3

Dried beans, peas, lentils

Beans, peas, lentils (dried and cooked)	⅓ cup
Baked beans, no pork	¼ cup

Starchy vegetables

Corn	⅓ cup
Corn on cob (6 in ear)	½ ear
Lima beans	½ cup
Parsnips	½ cup
Peas; green	½ cup
Potato, white	1 small
Potato, white mashed	½ cup
Pumpkin	1 cup
Sweet potato, yam	½ small; ⅓ cup
Winter squash (acorn, butternut, banana)	½ cup
Yam	½ small; ⅓ cup

Prepared foods

Angel food cake (1½ in cube or small slice)	1 slice
Biscuit, 2 in diameter (omit 1 fat exchange)	1
Chips, potato or corn (omit 2 fat exchanges)	15
Corn muffin, 2 in diameter (omit 1 fat exchange)	1
Cornbread, 2 × 2 × 1¼ in (omit 1 fat exchange)	1 square
Crepe, 6 in diameter (omit 1 fat exchange)	1
Ice milk, ½ cup scoop (omit 1 fat exchange)	1 scoop
Muffin, plain, 2 in diameter (omit 1 fat exchange)	1
Pancakes, 4 in diameter (omit 1 fat exchange)	1
Potatoes, french fried (length 2-3 in (omit 1 fat exchange)	8 pieces
Sherbet, fruit ice, ½ cup scoop	1 scoop
Waffle, 4 in diameter or (omit 1 fat exchange)	1

List 5: Meat exchanges

Group A (lean)

I. Lean meats, less tissue fat

Fish (any fresh or frozen)	1 oz (28 g)
Canned salmon, tuna, mackerel	¼ cup
Sardines, drained	3
Shellfish	
Clams, oysters, scallops	5
Crab, lobster	¼ cup
Poultry (no skin)	
Chicken, turkey, cornish hen, guinea hen, pheasant	1 oz (28 g)
Veal (any lean trimmed cut)	1 oz (28 g)

II. Lean meats, more tissue fat

Beef	1 oz (28 g)
Very lean young beef; chipped beef; lean cuts of chuck, flank steak, tender loin, plate ribs and skirt steak, round (top, bottom), rump, spare ribs, tripe	
Lamb	1 oz (28 g)
Lean cuts of leg, rib, sirloin, loin (roast, chops), shank, shoulder	

FOOD EXCHANGE GROUPS—cont'd

List 5: Meat exchanges—cont'd

Pork	1 oz (28 g)	Parmesan	3 tbsp
Lean cuts of leg (rump,		Cottage cheese, recreamed	¼ cup
center shank), ham		Cholesterol foods	
(smoked center cut)		Egg	1
III. Cheese	1 oz (28 g)	Organ meats	1 oz (28 g)
Cottage cheese	¼ cup	Liver, kidney, sweet-	
Dry curd		breads, heart	
Low fat, partially re-		Shrimp	5 large
creamed	1 oz (28 g)	Other	
Other cheeses		Peanut butter (omit 2 fat	2 tbs
Less than 5% butterfat;		exchanges)	
partially skimmed		Tofu	3½ oz (98 g)
milk			

Group B (medium fat)   1 oz (28 g)

Beef
  Ground (15% fat), corned beef (canned)
Pork
  Loin (roast, chops), shoulder arm (picnic), shoulder blade, Boston butt, Canadian bacon, boiled ham
Cheese
  Mozzarella, ricotta, Swiss, Monterey Jack, farmer's cheese, Neufchâtel

Group C (high fat)

Beef	1 oz (28 g)
Brisket (fresh or corned), ground (20% of more fat)	
Lamb breast	1 oz (28 g)
Pork	1 oz (28 g)
Spare ribs, back ribs, ground pork, sausage, country style ham, deviled ham	1 oz (28 g)
Cheese, cheddar types	1 oz (28 g)
Cold cuts	1 slice
Frankfurter	1 small
Poultry	1 oz (28 g)
Capon duck, goose	

List 6: Fat exchanges
Group A (polyunsaturated plant fats)

Margarine,* soft (stick or tub)	1 tsp
Mocha mix (cream substitute)	2 tbs
Salad dressings*	
French	1 tbs
Italian	1 tbs
Mayonnaise	1 tsp
Seeds (sunflower, sesame, pumpkin)	1 tbs
Vegetable oils (safflower, corn, soy, cottonseed, sesame)	1 tsp
Walnuts	4-5 halves

Group B (monounsaturated plant fats)

Avocado	⅛
Nuts	
Almonds	10 whole
Peanuts	20 whole
Pecans	2 whole
Olives	5 small
Vegetables oils (olive, peanut)	1 tsp

Group C (saturated animal fats)

Butter	1 tsp
Cheese spreads	1 tbs

*Made with safflower, corn, soy, cottonseed oil.

Continued.

FOOD EXCHANGE GROUPS—cont'd

List 6: Fat exchanges—cont'd
Group C (saturated animal fats)—cont'd

Cream		Pork fat	
Half and Half (10% cream)	2 tbs	Bacon crisp	1 strip
Light (20% cream)	2 tbs	Bacon fat	1 tsp
Heavy (40% cream)	1 tbs	Lard	1 tsp
Sour (light)	2 tbs	Salt pork	¾ in cube
Cream cheese	1 tbs		

Miscellaneous foods allowed as desired (negligible carbohydrate, protein, fat)

Artificial sweeteners, as permitted
Bouillon, broth, clear fat free
Catsup, mustard, horseradish, meat sauce
Coffee, tea
Cranberries, cranberry juice (unsweetened)
Garlic

Gelatin, plain or D-Zerta
Herbs and spices
Lemon, lime
Pickles, dill and sour
Salt and pepper
Vinegar

Questions on diabetes

1. What is diabetes?
2. Why is insulin usually necessary?
3. Why cannot insulin be taken orally?
4. How many calories per pound should be allowed for a diabetic patient? How many grams of protein should be allowed?
5. What is the most frequently prescribed ratio of carbohydrate, protein, and fat?
6. What are the advantages of using the exchange system?
7. Name the six groups of foods used in the exchange system.
8. Why are "specialty" foods for diabetic persons not recommended?
9. Name two foods in each exchange group.
10. Name two substitutes for each of the following: 1 slice bread, ½ cup orange juice, 1 tsp butter, 1 egg.

Suggestions for additional study

1. A patient on a diabetic diet receives chicken and asparagus and will not eat either one. What can be substituted?
2. Make substitutions for the following on a diabetic diet, listing the quantities: 4 apricot halves, 2 graham crackers, 1½ inch cube sponge cake, 3 oz roast beef, 1 strip bacon, 1 slice bread, 2 prunes, tossed salad, 1 glass whole milk, ½ cup beets.

Jimmy and his family learn to live with diabetes

Jimmy, age 7, lives with his parents and two older brothers, ages 12 and 14. Recently he has begun to lose some of his usual energy. His mother also noticed that his weight was dropping steadily, despite the fact that he seemed hungry all the time and was eating a great deal. He was also drinking more water than usual and urinating more frequently. One morning when Jimmy felt too ill to go to school, his mother decided to take him to a physician. At the office the physician examined him carefully, talked with his mother, and did some simple urine and blood tests. As he had suspected, he found sugar in the urine and an elevated level in the blood.

When he told Jimmy's mother about his findings, he asked if there had been a family history of diabetes. She answered that she was not surprised because she had suspected this all along. "Jimmy's father has diabetes," she answered. "I guess we just didn't want to face the fact that Jimmy had diabetes because we knew we had given it to him."

The physician made arrangements for Jimmy to be admitted to the hospital so that more definitive tests could be made and his diabetes could be regulated. He also wanted Jimmy and his family to have a careful plan of teaching during his hospital stay. After Jimmy was admitted to the hospital the further tests on glucose tolerance did show an abnormal curve, and the fractional urine tests that were done through the days indicated an elevated and erratic pattern. There were also some positive tests for acetone in the urine.

The physician started Jimmy's diet therapy at 1600 calories because he was not as active in the hospital. The diet would need to be built up gradually as his diabetes became more regulated and he needed more food. The physician indicated that the calories would be gradually increased to a maintenance level of about 2200 calories for the present. Jimmy was to have three meals each day with snacks between meals and in the evening. He was receiving 15 U of NPH insulin, plus 5 U of regular insulin. Gradually his urine tests, although still somewhat erratic, showed improvement.

Jimmy's nurse made plans for the necessary teaching. She conferred with the physician, the hospital dietitian, and the nutritionist in the outpatient health center. She also talked with Jimmy's mother in great detail about the family's food habits and with other members of the health team who had occasion to observe Jimmy and his reaction to food in the hospital.

Jimmy's nurse also contacted the nurse at his school and reviewed Jimmy's situation with her. Together they arranged for Jimmy to have the care he needed in any emergency that might arise.

QUESTIONS TO GUIDE YOUR INQUIRY

1. What were the reasons for the initial symptoms that Jimmy experienced at home?

2. What implications for counseling might exist because of the hereditary nature of the disease?

3. If Jimmy's mother had not been alert and taken him to the physician when she did, what progression of his symptoms might have occurred? Account for these progressive symptoms by the chain of metabolic imbalances occurring in uncontrolled diabetes.

4. In planning the overall educational program for Jimmy and his parents his nurse listed all the items important for a person with diabetes to know. What would she have included in her list? Why?

5. Outline a day's diet pattern and a sample food plan (menu) for Jimmy to use at home after he returns to school on a 2200-calorie diet. He is to continue with three meals and three snacks.

6. Why must Jimmy's insulin be given by hypodermic injection, rather than be taken as an oral medication?

7. What is the relationship of the distribution of food throughout the day to the taking of insulin at the beginning of the day? Use Jimmy's insulin dosage, a mixture of NPH and regular insulin in one syringe, as an example of the balance that he would need in his food pattern through the day. How would you explain this balance to Jimmy's mother?

8. What teaching materials or community resources could you use in an educational plan for Jimmy and his family?

Richard Smith and his diabetes

Richard Smith, 21 years old, is a diabetic. He gives himself an injection of insulin every morning. He is a student, usually active in athletics. This is final examination week, however, and he is putting in long hours of study. On the day before a particularly difficult examination, he is reviewing his study materials at home and forgets to eat lunch. About midafternoon he begins to feel faint and realizes that his blood sugar is low and an insulin reaction is approaching if he does not get a quick source of energy. He looks in the kitchen, and all that he can find is orange juice, milk, butter, a loaf of bread, and a jar of peanut butter.

QUESTIONS TO GUIDE YOUR INQUIRY

1. Which of these foods should he eat *first*, immediately?

2. Why did you make the choice you did above?

Later, when Dick is feeling better, he makes a peanut butter and butter sandwich, pours a glass of milk, and eats his snack while he continues studying.

3. What carbohydrate sources of energy are in his snack?

4. Are these sources in a form the cell can burn for energy? What changes must his body then make in these sources to get them into the necessary form? What is this usable form of body sugar?

5. What important relationship do carbohydrate and fat have in the final production of energy in the body? If Dick did not take his insulin to provide the necessary control agent for metabolizing the carbohydrate, what would happen to him as the result of improper handling of fat and the resulting accumulation of ketones?

Suggested readings

American Dietetic Association: Meal planning with exchange lists, rev. ed., Chicago, 1977, The Association.

Williams, S.R.: Nutrition and diet therapy, ed. 4, St. Louis, 1981, The C.V. Mosby Co.

Williams, S.R.: Essentials of nutrition and diet therapy, ed. 3, St. Louis, 1982, The C.V. Mosby Co.

20

Obesity

THE PROBLEM OF WEIGHT CONTROL

Obesity is one of the most common health and personal problems today. It is estimated that approximately 5 million Americans weigh at least 20% more than their ideal weight. Another 20 million may be classified as being 10% above their normal weight.

In the past a fat person was thought of as a healthy person. This was especially true in regard to babies. The present desire to avoid overweight has come into prominence largely for two reasons: cultural pressure is great, especially on women, to maintain a slender figure, and data based on scientific studies show that chronic diseases such as diabetes and hypertension are influenced to a considerable extent by body weight.

Causes

Obesity may be defined as a condition caused by excessive deposits of fat in the body that result in overweight. Obesity from glandular abnormality is rare. However, tendency toward overweight and certain factors that increase hunger may be inherited. A recently developed theory indicates that a person's weight may be genetically "programmed" or regulated around a natural "set point" and that no amount of dieting can change this personal set point. Physical activity may change the set point, but each person still has a characteristic natural weight. Whatever the underlying physiological regulation, the cause of overweight in most cases is eating too much for individual need. Overweight places an added burden on the heart, circulatory system, liver, and gallbladder. It also increases the risk in surgery.

Since overweight is for the most part the result of overeating, what, then, are the causes of overeating? A person who is bored or unhappy is more likely to overeat than a well-adjusted person. Some persons have a family history of members who consistently overate and who made no effort to limit the amount consumed. Children are sometimes rewarded for good behavior with tempting bits of food; therefore they associate obedience with overeating. A person with a psychological problem may overeat to gain a temporary sense of well-being.

219

SOUND WEIGHT MANAGEMENT
Characteristics of diet

In many cases an effort to avoid obesity leads to a better selection of food. However, there are people who harm themselves by trying to reduce unwisely. It is important that a person trying to reduce receive the necessary protein, minerals, and vitamins for adequate nutrition. The so-called fad diets for reducing should be discouraged. In the first place many of them are inadequate; in the second place they do nothing to educate the person in good eating habits. This is important because often a person who has lost weight on a fad diet will resume former eating habits after losing weight and will soon regain.

A good reducing diet should lay the foundation for a sensible diet regimen that can, with some additions, be followed indefinitely. Once the loss in weight has been achieved, a person may gradually add more foods, checking weight periodically. If weight increases, a return to the former reducing regimen should follow.

Ideal body weight

Most authorities advocate that a person's ideal weight at 25 years of age is the best weight to maintain throughout life. If this is to be accomplished, calories must be reduced 3% from 30 to 40 years of age, another 3% from 40 to 50 years of age, 7.5% from 50 to 60 years of age, and another 7.5% from 60 to 70 years of age. In fact the term "middle-aged spread" is a misnomer. There is no mysterious law of nature that states that all persons must enlarge horizontally at middle age. An excessive increase in weight at this time of life is usually the result of too many calories and too little exercise. A person's normal body weight is determined not only by age but also by height and body build. For example, a person with large bones can carry more weight without being obese than a person with small bones.

Importance of exercise

A certain amount of moderate exercise is good to maintain physical well-being. People who are physically active are less likely to be overweight. Exercise and a good diet are inseparable partners in successful healthy weight management. Regular exercise, especially for younger people, makes flabby muscles firmer and helps to achieve more attractive proportions. Even middle-aged and older persons who are on reducing diets should plan some sort of moderate, consistent exercise program.

Dangers of drugs

The use of drugs to help a person reduce should be discouraged and is not advocated by any reputable physician now. Some produce extremely toxic effects, and some have a harmful cumulative effect that may not be felt for some time. Thyroid preparations are sometimes given, but unless the thyroid gland is actually deficient, they should never be taken.

Diet planning

The best and safest plan for reducing is, as it has always been, to lower the calorie intake below the actual daily needs of the body, making it necessary for the body to draw on and use its reserve fat. The reduction in food must come primarily from fats and sweets. Complex carbohydrate (starch) should provide the major fuel for energy. Protein is necessary at all times for the repair of body tissues and should be maintained at a normal level. Protein foods such as meat, eggs, fish, and cottage cheese have a high satiety value. Low-calorie vegetables and fruits will add interest to the diet and furnish needed vitamins, minerals, and bulk. The essentials of a reducing diet, then, include the following:

1. There should be sufficient high-quality protein to prevent wasting of body tissues and to furnish adequate protein for body processes.
2. There should be sufficient complex carbohydrate to prevent protein from being used for energy needs and to prevent too rapid burning of body fat.
3. Adequate minerals and vitamins must be provided.
4. The diet should be acceptable to the patient.
5. The diet should be one that will educate the patient in correct eating habits.
6. Meals should not be skipped.

An adequate breakfast gives the person a proper start for the day. There should be some protein food in each meal, especially breakfast. Simple carbohydrate alone raises the blood sugar quickly but not for long, whereas protein and complex carbohydrate raise the blood sugar level and hold it above the hunger mark longer.

Calculating energy needs

The caloric value of the diet may be cut safely to 1200 calories. Below 1200 calories a diet is not adequate, and a person on such a diet should have close nutritional supervision.

An adult who is overweight has probably been consuming at least 3000 calories daily and often more than that amount. In a reducing diet the caloric reduction should start from a person's ideal caloric allowance and not from the number of calories normally consumed. For the person whose ideal caloric intake is 2200, a cut of 1000 calories should result in a weight loss of approximately 2 pounds (0.9 kg) a week, and a daily reduction of 500 calories from the person's ideal caloric intake will, under normal conditions, result in a weight loss of 1 pound (0.45 kg) per week.

EXAMPLE: A woman 35 years of age weighs 148 pounds (66.6 kg), but her ideal weight is 125 pounds (56.2 kg).

2200 calories needed to maintain person at 125 pounds (56.2 kg)
− 1000
1200-calorie diet necessary to lose an average of 2 pounds (0.9 kg) a week

The following general dietary suggestions are helpful controls of excess calories:

1. Vinegar, lemon juice, or a slice of lemon may be used on vegetables or salads. Mayonnaise or oil dressing should not be used.
2. Fat, cream, butter, or flour should not be used in the preparation of food.

PRACTICAL SUGGESTIONS TO DIETERS

Goals	Be realistic. Do not set your goals too high. Adapt your rate of loss to 1 to 2 lb (450 to 900 g) per week. If visible tools are helpful motivation techniques, use them.
Calories	Do not be an obsessive calorie counter. Simply become familiar with the food exchanges in your diet list and learn the general calorie values of some of your favorite home dishes so that you might occasionally make substitutions.
Plateaus	Anticipate plateaus. They happen to everyone. They are related to water accumulation as fat is lost. During these periods, increase your exercise to help you get started again.
Binges	Do not be discouraged when you break the diet and have a dietary binge. This too happens to most people. Simply keep them infrequent, and when possible, plan ahead for special occasions. Adjust the following day's diet or remaining part of the same day accordingly.
Special diet foods	There is no need to purchase special low-calorie foods. Learn to read labels carefully. Most special diet foods are expensive, and many are not much lower in calories than regular foods.
Home meals	Try to avoid a separate menu for yourself. Adapt your needs to the family meal, adjusting seasoning or method of preparing family dishes to lower caloric values of added fats and starches.
Eating away from home	Watch portions. When a guest, limit extras such as sauces and dressings and trim meat well. In restaurants select singly prepared items rather than combination dishes. Avoid items with heavy sauces or fat seasoning. Select fruit or sherbet as desserts rather than pastries.
Appetite control	Avoid dependence on appetite-depressant medications. Usually they are only crutches. Beginning efforts to control appetite may be aided by nibbling on food from the free list or by saving over meal items for use between meals, such as fruit.
Meal pattern	Eat three or more meals a day. If you are used to three meals, then leave it at that. If you are helped by snacks between meals, then plan part of your day's allowance to account for them. The main thing is that you do not take all of your calories at one sitting. Avoid the all-too-common pattern of no breakfast, little or no lunch, and a huge dinner.

3. A sugar substitute in moderation may be used instead of sugar.
4. Artificially sweetened or unsweetened gelatin may be used in making salads and desserts.
5. Fruits should not have sugar added. They may be eaten raw or cooked. Canned fruit may be packed in water or juice.
6. Alcohol should be avoided.

Further practical suggestions to dieters are given on p. 222. Desirable weights for men and women 25 years and over are given in Tables 20-1 and 20-2.

Four calorie levels of weight reduction diet plans are given in Table 20-3 using the exchange system of dietary control. A variety of foods may be selected from the exchange groups to plan individual diets.

Rate of weight loss

It should take the patient 10 weeks to lose 20 pounds (9 kg). There may be a variation in the weekly loss of weight, depending on the activity of the patient, variations in the water balance of the body, and the presence of disease. The person who is on a reducing diet may plan to weigh about once a week. Otherwise, one becomes discouraged when each day does not show a loss. At

Table 20-1. Desirable weights for men 25 years of age and over (in indoor clothing)*

Height		Small frame	Medium frame	Large frame
Feet	Inches			
5	2	128-134	131-141	138-150
5	3	130-136	133-143	140-153
5	4	132-138	135-145	142-156
5	5	134-140	137-148	144-160
5	6	136-142	139-151	146-164
5	7	138-145	142-154	149-168
5	8	140-148	145-157	152-172
5	9	142-151	148-160	155-176
5	10	144-154	151-163	158-180
5	11	146-157	154-166	161-184
6	0	149-160	157-170	164-188
6	1	152-164	160-174	168-192
6	2	155-168	164-178	172-197
6	3	158-172	167-182	176-202
6	4	162-176	171-187	181-207

Courtesy Metropolitan Life Insurance Co., New York, N.Y., rev. 1983.
*Weights at ages 25-59 based on lowest mortality. Weight in pounds according to frame (in indoor clothing weighing 5 lbs., shoes with 1-inch heels).

Table 20-2. Desirable weights for women 25 years of age and over (in indoor clothing)*

Height		Small frame	Medium frame	Large frame
Feet	Inches			
4	10	102-111	109-121	118-131
4	11	103-113	111-123	120-134
5	0	104-115	113-126	122-137
5	1	106-118	115-129	125-140
5	2	108-121	118-132	128-143
5	3	111-124	121-135	131-147
5	4	114-127	124-138	134-151
5	5	117-130	127-141	137-155
5	6	120-133	130-144	140-159
5	7	123-136	133-147	143-163
5	8	126-139	136-150	146-167
5	9	129-142	139-153	149-170
5	10	132-145	142-156	152-173
5	11	135-148	145-159	155-176
6	0	138-151	148-162	158-179

Courtesy Metropolitan Life Insurance Co., New York, N.Y., rev. 1983.
*Weights at ages 25-29 based on lowest mortality. Weight in pounds according to frame (in indoor clothing weighing 3 lbs., shoes with 1-inch heels). For girls between 18 and 25 years of age, subtract 1 lb. (0.45 kg) for each year under 25.

Table 20-3. Weight reduction diets using the exchange system of dietary control

Food exchange group*	Approximate measure	800 calories	1000 calories	1200 calories	1500 calories
Total number of exchanges per day					
Milk (nonfat)	1 cup	2	2	2	2
Vegetable	½ cup	1	1	1	1
Fruit	Varies	3	3	3	4
Bread	1 slice	1	3¾	4	6
Meat	1 oz	6	1	7	7
Fat	1 tsp	1		2	3-4
Distribution of food exchanges					
Breakfast					
Fruit		1	1	1	1
Meat		1	1	1	1
Bread		1	1	1	2
Fat		1	1	1	1
Lunch and dinner					
Meat		2-3	2-3	3	3
Vegetable		1	1	1	1
Bread		0	1	1-2	2
Fat		0	0	0-1	1
Fruit		1	1	1	1
Milk		1	1	1	1-2

*See food exchange groups, pp. ●●●-●●●.

first the fat in the tissues may be replaced by water, and the person may not show a loss. It took time to put on the extra pounds, and it will take time to lose them.

Questions on obesity

1. Why is overweight a health hazard?
2. What are some of the causes of overeating?
3. What are the characteristics of a good reducing diet?
4. Why should drugs not be used for reducing purposes?
5. What is the lowest caloric intake that will give an adequate diet?
6. What should the caloric reduction be for an approximate weight loss of 2 pounds (0.9 kg) a week?
7. Plan a 1200-calorie diet and a 1000-calorie diet for 3 days using the exchange system.

Individual project: Personal energy balance

To determine your own personal energy balance state, make the following comparisons between your energy output or requirement and your energy intake in food.

Energy output
1. Record your weight in pounds and convert it to kilograms.
2. Determine your basal energy needs with the forumla in the box below.
3. Calculate the additional calories required for your physical activity according to the box below.

General approximations for daily adult basal and activity energy needs

		Man (70 kg) calories	Woman (58 kg) calories
Basal energy needs (av. 1 cal/kg/hr)*		70 × 24 = 1680	58 × 24 = 1392
Activity energy needs			
Very sedentary	+20% basal	1680 + 336 = 2016	1392 + 278 = 1670
Sedentary	+30% basal	1680 + 504 = 2184	1392 + 418 = 1810
Moderately active	+40% basal	1680 + 672 = 2352	1392 + 557 = 1949
Very active	+50% basal	1680 + 840 = 2520	1392 + 696 = 2088

*1 kg = 2.2 lb.

---

4. What then is your total energy requirement in calories?

Energy intake
1. Record your usual food intake for one day, being sure to list portion sizes and method of seasoning and preparation.

2. Using the food value tables in the appendix, calculate the total calorie value of your day's food.

3. Now compare this total energy input (food calories) with your total energy output (energy requirement calories). What is your energy balance? Are you underweight, normal weight, or overweight? How would you change your energy balance, if needed, to achieve an ideal weight?

Suggestions for additional study

1. A person whose normal weight should be 135 pounds (60.7 kg) but who weighs 155 pounds (69.7 kg) wants to lose approximately 2 pounds (0.9 kg) a week. What should be the normal caloric intake if the ideal weight is 135 pounds (60.7 kg), and what should be the caloric intake on a reduction diet?
2. Circle the correct answers in the right column to answer the questions in the left column.

Does obesity increase the load on the heart?	Yes No
Is a breakfast of sweet roll and black coffee adequate nutritionally?	Yes No
Is the cause of overweight overactive glands in most persons?	Yes No
Is chocolate cake a wise choice on a 1000-calorie diet? Give the reason for your answer.	Yes No

John's energy balance and weight reduction plan

John is a college student now leading a more or less sedentary life with classes and study. However, he is interested in wrestling and wants to make the team. To do so he must lose some of his excess weight. He begins to look carefully at his energy balance picture: weight, 180 pounds (8.1 kg) at present; average food intake each day, about 3000 calories worth of fuel. Next he plans a means of losing weight by reversing his energy balance.

QUESTIONS TO GUIDE YOUR INQUIRY

1. What does John figure his present daily total energy requirement to be?

2. How does this total energy requirement compare with the energy value of his daily food intake?

3. To lose about 2 pounds (0.9 kg) a week, how much should John reduce the caloric value of his daily diet?

4. Besides lowering his diet calories, what else could John do to help reverse his energy balance?

Tools
1. Kilogram = 2.2 pounds
2. Basal energy requirement: 1 calorie per kilogram of body weight per hour
3. Sedentary activity energy requirement: basal needs + 30% of basal needs
4. 1 pound of fat = 3500 calories

Weight control

Rosa Carlotta is a warm, outgoing 58-year-old Italian woman. She is 5 feet 2 inches (157.4 cm) tall and weighs 210 pounds (94.5 kg). Her life is centered on her large family, and she is known for her excellent Italian cooking. The family often gathers for meals, and food plays a large part in the family life.

QUESTIONS TO GUIDE YOUR INQUIRY

1. Describe the state of Rosa's overall energy balance.

2. What factors do you think help to account for her situation?

3. How would the principle of energy balance help you plan a sound diet for her?

4. What additional suggestions couls you give her to increase her energy output?

5. Why would a fad diet that allows little or no carbohydrate foods and unrestricted amounts of meat protein and fat be harmful in the long run?

Suggested readings

Bennett, W., and Gurin, J.: The dieter's dilemma, New York, 1982, Basic Books, Inc. (A lively discussion of the "setpoint" theory of individual weight regulation.)

Stuart, R.B., and Davis, B.: Slim chance in a fat world, Champaign, Ill., 1972, Reserach Press.

Williams, S.R.: Nutrition and diet therapy, ed. 4, St. Louis, 1981, The C.V. Mosby Co.

Williams, S.R.: Essentials of nutrition and diet therapy, ed. 3, St. Louis, 1982, The C.V. Mosby Co.

21

Underweight

THE PROBLEM OF UNDERWEIGHT

Extremes in underweight, just as in overweight, tend to shorten an individual's life span. Although underweight is a much less common problem than overweight, it does occur. It is often more difficult to reach the underlying cause and subsequent cure in the underweight person than in the overweight person.

A person who is more than 10% below the normal weight is considered to be underweight. Twenty percent or more below normal weight is cause for concern because serious results may occur, especially in persons in younger age groups. Resistance to infection is lowered, general health is below par, and efficiency is reduced.

Causes

Some of the causes of underweight follow:
1. Long, wasting disease with chronic elevated temperature that raises the basal metabolism
2. Diminished food intake resulting from (a) psychological reasons that cause a patient to refuse to eat, (b) anorexia or complete loss of appetite, or (c) economic reasons that curtail available food supply
3. Diminished food absorption resulting from (a) diarrhea of long duration, (b) an abnormal condition in the gastrointestinal tract, or (c) the excessive use of laxatives
4. Hyperthyroidism or any other abnormality that would increase the caloric needs of the body
5. Greatly increased activity without a corresponding increase in food
6. Unhealthy home environment, with irregular and inadequate meals, in which eating is considered unimportant and in which an indifferent attitude toward food is fostered

Dietary treatment

The purpose of a special diet for persons who are underweight is to provide a sufficiently high caloric intake so that they will gain the required amount of weight and at the same time establish good food habits. Unless good food habits are formed, people will slip back into the former way of eating, and the problem will repeat itself.

The dietary requirements in the treatment of underweight result in the following type of diet:

1. High in calories, at least 50% above the person's normal requirement
2. High in protein, since there has probably been some loss of body protein
3. High in carbohydrate, since it is easily digested
4. Normal or a little below normal in fat, since foods too high in fat are sometimes not very well tolerated
5. Normal amounts of minerals, except calcium and iron, which should be increased
6. High in vitamins, especially thiamin, which should be increased with an increase in carbohydrate (thiamin should stimulate the appetite)
7. Adequate in all the nutrients
8. Well-prepared and attractively served food to tempt the person with a poor appetite

There should be three meals daily, with high caloric nourishment between meals and in the evening. Rest before and after meals is beneficial. Because underweight persons often have little or no appetite, it is especially important that they be served the foods they like.

Additional calories should be added to the diet gradually, since the sudden change from a reduced intake to a 3000-4000-calorie intake may upset the patient. Bulky, low-calorie foods should be kept to a minimum if the patient is having difficulty in consuming all of the food.

Moderate exercise, such as walking, should be taken when possible to stimulate the appetite, maintain general health, and improve muscle tone.

The development of good food habits and a proper gain in weight should be the determining factors in measuring the success of the treatment of the patient who is underweight.

Questions on underweight

1. What percentage below normal is considered underweight?
2. What are the results of underweight?
3. What are some of the causes of underweight?
4. Plan a diet for an underweight person.

Suggested reading

Robinson, C.H.: Normal and therapeutic nutrition, ed. 16, New York, 1982, Macmillan, Inc.

22

Allergy

THE PROBLEM OF ALLERGIES

Allergy is a condition produced by allergens. An allergen is any substance to which a person is hypersensitive. Allergy may manifest itself as asthma, eczema, hives, swelling of the eyes, headache, or gastrointestinal tract ailments. The same effect may appear in different persons but still not be caused by the same allergen. Allergens enter the body in four different ways: by being swallowed (food and drinks), by being inhaled (pollen, animal dander, and dust), by external contact (clothing, cosmetics, and poisonous plants), and by injection (drugs, serums, and insect stings).

FOOD ALLERGIES

Although not all allergic manifestations are caused by a hypersensitivity to food, only this phase of allergy is discussed in this chapter. Sometimes persons can eat food to which they are allergic without any ill effects, whereas at other times these foods affect them. Sometimes, when persons are allergic to more than one item, they can tolerate one of them at a time without incurring any unfortunate results. Tests for allergy should be taken twice because an allergy may not show up the first time.

The foods that most often cause allergic conditions are wheat, milk, eggs, tomatoes, strawberries, oranges, fish, chocolate, nuts, peas, beans, potatoes, onions, and garlic. In asthma, wheat and eggs are likely to head the list of causative allergens. In headache, wheat and chocolate may be guilty. Cooked vegetables are frequently tolerated by people who are allergic to raw ones. Many people are allergic to only the peel of peaches and can eat the peach if the peel is removed.

Causes

Fatigue, nervousness, tension, unhappiness, indigestion, or certain phases of the menstrual cycle may lower the tolerance and make a person more susceptible to an allergen. Heredity is a factor in the appearance of an allergy. The evidence of an allergy in a child may appear in a different locale in the body from that in the adult from whom the tendency was inherited. The child's allergy may even be caused by a different substance from that causing the adult's allergy.

Children seem to develop allergies more readily than adults. It usually attacks children in the form of eczema or asthma, and unless the allergy is kept under control, the condition may worsen as the children grow older. Food is usually the source of allergies in very young children. Foods to which children are most often allergic are wheat, eggs, and milk. If children are allergic to whole milk, it is usually possible for them to drink milk in some other form, such as boiled milk, dry skimmed milk, or evaporated milk, or they may be able to tolerate goat's milk or soybean milk. Heating milk reduces the allergenic effect of lactalbumin, the milk protein fraction usually responsible for milk allergy. Children usually outgrow an allergy to milk.

Treatment

The offending item may be determined by an elimination diet or, if one particular item is strongly suspected, by omitting that one item and its products from the diet. If wheat is the suspected allergen, anything made from wheat or wheat products is omitted for at least 10 days. This means that all mixed foods must be analyzed to be certain that no wheat product is used in any preparation.

The quantity of a food that will produce allergenic symptoms varies. Also, the physical condition of patients makes a difference in the appearance of the allergy. If people are under strain or are overtired, they are much more likely to develop an allergic reaction to a specific food, whereas if they are rested and relaxed, they are able to tolerate it without any reaction. Sometimes whether a food is raw or cooked makes a difference. Sometimes a person is allergic to a certain portion of the food item—for example, the white of an egg—but can tolerate the remainder. At times the mere smell of a food to which the person is allergic will cause an allergic response.

The elimination diets devised by Rowe are given in Table 22-1. Diets 1 and 2 may be used separately or together. If the patient is suspected of being sensitive to cereals, then diet 3 should be used as the beginning diet. The beginning diet should be used at least 10 days, possibly 3 or 4 weeks, since the reacting bodies sometimes disappear very slowly. The diets must be adhered to very carefully, and particular attention must be used in preparation of the food. Nutritive inadequacies should be guarded against. Unless the prescribed fruits and vegetables are eaten in sufficient amounts, supplementary vitamins should be taken. When milk is excluded, meat should be eaten twice daily to secure adequate protein. In the absence of milk, calcium should be given in supplementary form.

It is important not to go hungry on an elimination diet. Eating solid food for breakfast is also important. One should not lose weight on the diet. Adequate portions of the foods allowed should be eaten.

Following is a list of foods permitted on a diet free of wheat, corn, milk, eggs, chicken, rye products, strong seasonings, and canned fruits except dietetic fruits labeled "without sugar":

Salt	Beef
White cane, granulated or lump, sugar	Veal
Water, freshly squeezed fruit juice, coffee made of freshly ground coffee beans, fresh lemonade made with cane sugar	Lamb
	Turkey
	Pork chops, pork roast
	Ham, baked, boiled, and fried
All fruits (thoroughly washed)	Bacon, Canadian bacon
All vegetables, except corn (thoroughly washed)	Ripe olives
	Olive oil (pure)
White uncoated rice	Walnuts and almonds in the shell

Patients should not eat, drink, or prepare food with any ingredient that is not included in the allergy diet list. No chewing gum, candy, shortening, seasoning, and frozen juices are permitted. Baking soda should be used instead of tooth powder or toothpaste. One-half teaspoon of baking soda to one-half glass of lukewarm water should be used instead of mouthwash.

Breakfast could include rice, water, salt, cane sugar, banana, bacon, ham, and coffee. When eating out, one could order a vegetable plate, rice, roast beef or steaks, chops, bacon, ham, and banana or other raw fruit for dessert. For infants, as a substitute for milk, 1 cup of hot water may be added to one-half can strained beef and mixed with an egg beater. This could be taken from a baby bottle.

When the period of relief from the allergy symptoms has been of sufficient duration, other foods may be cautiously added. Thereafter, canned vegetables and fruits, other meats, spices, and nuts are gradually added. After 1 to 3 months, wheat, milk, and eggs may be added, one at a time, and the results should be observed carefully. The reaction may appear immediately or several days after an article has been added to the menu.

After individual allergies have been identified and a restricted diet has been followed for some time, gradual desensitization may be achieved by adding small quantities of one allergen at a time to the diet and then adding a little more of the same food until the person has built up a resistance to that particular food.

Recent studies of children with learning problems and hyperkinesis have indicated a possible allergic sensitivity to salicylates and food colors and flavors used in a wide variety of foods. Some of these children have shown a rapid dramatic improvement in scholastic achievement when treated with a salicylate-free diet.

Table 22-1. Elimination diets

Diet 1	Diet 2	Diet 3	Diet 4
Rice	Corn	Tapioca	Milk, up to 2-3 qt
Tapioca	Rye	White and sweet potato	daily
Rice biscuit	Corn pone	Lima beans	Tapioca cooked with
Rice bread	Corn-rye muffin	Potato bread	milk and milk
	Rye bread	Soybean or lima bean	sugar also may be
	Ry-Krisp	bread	taken
Lettuce	Tomato	Beets	
Spinach	Squash	Carrots	
Carrot	Asparagus	Lima beans	
Beet	Peas	String beans	
Artichoke	String beans	Tomato	
Lamb	Chicken	Beef	
	Bacon	Bacon	
Lemon	Pineapple	Lemon	
Grapefruit	Peaches	Grapefruit	
Pear	Apricots	Peaches	
	Prunes	Apricots	
Cane sugar	Cane sugar	Cane sugar	
Wesson oil*	Mazola oil	Olive oil	
Olive oil	Wesson oil*	Wesson oil*	
Salt	Salt	Gelatin	
Gelatin	Karo corn syrup	Salt	
Syrup made of maple	Gelatin	Olives	
sugar or cane sugar		Syrup made of maple	
flavored with		sugar or cane sugar	
maple†		flavored with	
Olives		maple†	
Pear butter			

From Rowe, A.H.: Elimination diets and the patient's allergies, ed. 2, Philadelphia, 1944, Lea & Febiger.
*If patient has shown by skin test to be allergic to cottonseed, omit Wesson oil.
†If allergy to cane sugar is suspected, use beet sugar or corn glucose.

Questions on allergy

1. What is an allergen?
2. In what ways do allergens enter the body?
3. What are the foods that most often cause allergic symptoms?
4. How does heredity affect the appearance of allergy?
5. In what ways does an allergen usually manifest itself in children?
6. To what foods are children most likely to be allergic?
7. If a child is allergic to cow's milk, what other types of milk can usually be given?

8. If a person is allergic to raw tomatoes, would it be possible to eat cooked tomatoes?
9. Plan a diet based on Rowe's elimination diets 1 and 2.
10. Plan a diet based on Rowe's diet 3.

Suggestions for additional study

1. Make a report on the various ways in which food allergies can affect a person.
2. Read the labels on various cereals and determine which ones can be used on a wheat-free diet and which ones can be used on a corn-free diet.
3. A patient is on an egg-free, wheat-free diet. May he have the following foods: orange juice, broiled lamp chop, oatmeal, rye bread, mashed potatoes, apple dumpling, baked apple, noodles, buttermilk, shredded wheat, gelatin with fruit?

Suggested readings

Clark, M., Shapiro, D., and Lindsay, J.: Allergy: new insights, Newsweek, pp. 40-45, Aug. 23, 1982.

Fiengold, B.F.: Why your child is hyperactive, New York, 1975, Random House, Inc.

Rowe, A.H.: Elimination diets and the patient's allergies, ed. 2, Philadelphia, 1944, Lea & Febiger.

Speer, F.: Food allergy, Littleton, Mass., 1979, PSG Publishing Co., Inc.

Williams, S.R.: Nutrition and diet therapy, ed. 4, St. Louis, 1981, The C.V. Mosby Co.

Williams, S.R.: Essentials of nutrition and diet therapy, ed. 3, St. Louis, 1982, The C.V. Mosby Co.

23

Surgery

A patient undergoing surgery faces great physiological and psychological stress on the body. During this period nutritional demands are greatly increased. Deficiencies can easily develop. If these deficiencies are not met, serious clinical problems can develop. It is imperative, therefore, that careful attention be given to preparation of the patient for surgery and to the nutritional therapy needs that follow. If these needs are met, there will be less risk of complications, and resources will be provided for better wound healing and a more rapid recovery.

PREOPERATIVE NUTRITIONAL CARE
Nutrient reserves

When the surgery is elective, not an emergency, reserves of nutrients can be built up in the body to serve the patient's needs during the surgical procedure and immediately after, when no food intake will be possible. Particular needs center on protein, calories, vitamins, and minerals.

PROTEIN. Protein deficiencies among surgical patients are far more commonly encountered than one would assume. Surveys among surgical wards in large city hospitals have revealed frank protein-calorie malnutrition and multiple postsurgical complications. It is imperative that the patient facing surgery be fortified with adequate protein in tissue and plasma reserves to counteract blood losses during surgery and to prevent tissue breakdown in the immediate postoperative period.

CALORIES. Any time that increased protein for tissue building is necessary, attention must also be given to increasing calories to provide for energy demands and to spare the protein for its tissue-building work. For example, increased carbohydrate would be necessary to provide optimum glycogen stores in the liver as a necessary resource for energy demands to spare protein for tissue synthesis. Also, if the patient is underweight to any degree, extra calories would need to be provided to build the weight up to a maintenance level before surgery. If the patient is overweight, some weight reduction may be indicated to help reduce surgical risks.

237

VITAMINS AND MINERALS. When additional protein and calories are required for any purpose, additional vitamins and minerals involved in protein and energy metabolism must also be supplied. Any deficiency state, such as anemia, should be corrected. Water balance should be ensured, since both electrolytes and fluids are necessary to prevent dehydration.

Immediate preoperative period

The usual preparation for surgery calls for nothing to be taken orally for at least 8 hours before the surgery. This is necessary to ensure that the stomach has no retained food in it at the time of the operation. Food in the stomach may cause complications resulting from vomiting or aspiration of food particles during anesthesia or during recovery from the anesthesia. In addition, any food present in the stomach may increase the possibility of postoperative gastric retention or expansion or interfere with the surgical procedure itself.

If the surgery is an emergency, there is no time available for building up nutritional reserves. This is all the more reason for persons to maintain a well-balanced diet as a regular habit. In this way optimum nutrient reserves will be available to supply needs at any time of stress.

POSTOPERATIVE NUTRITIONAL CARE
Nutrient needs for healing

Nutritional support is necessary to aid recovery from surgery. In surgical disease, as well as related surgical procedures, nutrient losses are greatly increased. At the same time food intake is greatly diminished or even absent for a period of time. Therefore to provide this additional nutritional support, several nutrients require particular attention.

PROTEIN. Optimum protein intake in the postoperative recovery period is of primary concern for all patients. Protein is needed to replace losses occurring during surgery and to supply the increased demands of the healing process. During the period immediately after surgery the body usually undergoes considerable *catabolism*. This means that the process of tissue breakdown and loss exceeds the process of tissue buildup. During this period a negative nitrogen balance of as much as 20 g/day may occur. This negative balance represents an actual loss of tissue protein of over a pound a day. In addition to these protein losses from tissue breakdown caused by metabolic imbalance, there are added losses of protein from the body. These losses include plasma protein loss through hemorrhage, wound bleeding, or various body fluid losses. In addition, there may be increased loss from extensive tissue destruction, inflammation, infection, and trauma. It is evident that if any degree of prior malnutrition or chronic infection existed, the patient's protein deficiency could easily become severe and cause serious complications. There are a number of reasons for this increased protein demand:

Building tissue. The process of wound healing requires the building of a great deal of new body tissue. This can only be done when a sufficient amount of the essential amino acids from protein intake or body stores can be brought to the tissue by the circulating blood. The eight essential amino acids cannot be made by the body and must be present for tissue to be made. After surgery, when food intake is usually not possible, attention must be given to supplying these essential amino acids through intravenous injection. This is particularly true if the period of inability to eat normally is extended for any period of time. These tissue protein deficiencies are best met by oral feedings. Thus it is important that a patient be helped to eat as early as possible after surgery. Sometimes protein must be increased to 100 to 200 g/day to restore lost protein tissues and synthesize new tissues at the wound site.

Controlling shock. A sufficient supply of plasma protein, usually albumin, is necessary to protect the blood volume (p. 93). If the plasma protein level drops, there is insufficient pressure to keep tissue fluid circulating between the capillaries and the cells. If this situation occurs, the water leaves the blood capillaries and cannot be drawn back into circulation. Shock symptoms result from a shrinking blood volume and the body's effort to restore it.

Controlling edema. When the serum protein level is low, as previously described, *edema* develops as a result of this loss of the osmotic pressure required to maintain the normal movement of fluid between the capillaries and surrounding interstitial tissues. The condition of edema is characterized by puffiness or swelling in the tissue resulting from excess fluid being held there rather than being returned to circulation. Generalized edema may affect heart and lung action. Local edema at the site of the surgical wound also interferes with closure of the wound and hinders the normal healing process.

Healing bone. Any bone surgery, such as in orthopedic problems, involves extensive bone healing. Protein, as well as mineral matter, is essential in the bone tissue for proper bone formation. Protein provides a matrix for the laying down of calcium and phosphorus to form the bone. Protein anchors the mineral matter to build strong bone tissue.

Resisting infection. The major components of the body's immune system, which provide its defense against infection, are protein tissues. These defense agents include special white cells called lymphocytes, as well as antibodies and various other blood cells, hormones, and enzymes. The strength of the tissue is a major defense barrier against infection at all times.

Transporting lipids. Fat is also an important component of tissue structure. It forms the center of cell walls and participates in many other necessary activities of metabolism. Protein is required for carrying fat in the bloodstream to all tissues for maintaining these structures and activities. Also, protein is necessary to carry fat to the liver for necessary work in fat metabolism. Protein present in the liver combines with fat and helps to remove it from the liver, thus avoiding the danger of fatty infiltration, which would lead to liver disease.

• • •

From the previous discussion it is evident that protein deficiency can lead to many clinical problems in surgery, such as poor wound healing, rupture of the suture lines, delayed healing of fractures, depressed heart and lung function, anemia, reduced resistance to infection, liver damage, extensive weight loss, and increased mortality risks.

WATER. Water balance after surgery is a constant concern. Sufficient fluid intake is necessary to prevent dehydration. In patients who have complications or who are seriously ill and have extensive drainage, as much as 7 L of fluid daily may be required. In addition, during the postoperative period large water losses may occur from vomiting, hemorrhage, fever, or excessive urination. A comparison of daily water volume requirements of surgical patients is given in Table 23-1. The usual intravenous fluids after surgery will supply some initial needs. However, oral intake should begin as soon as possible and be maintained in sufficient quantity.

CALORIES. Again, as is always the case when increased protein is demanded for tissue building, a sufficient amount of nonprotein calories must be supplied for energy to spare protein for its vital tissue-building function. The fuel nutrients, carbohydrate and fat, must therefore be in sufficient supply in the total diet. Since excess fat intake presents problems in digestion and general tissue health, carbohydrate becomes the major source of needed fuel. The total calories in the diet after surgery should be increased to 2500 to 3000 calories per day before protein can be used for tissue repair and not be converted in part to provide energy itself. In situations of acute stress, as in extensive surgery or burns, calorie needs may increase to as much as 4000 to 6000 calories. Carbohydrate not only spares protein for tissue building but also helps to avoid liver damage by maintaining an adequate amount of glycogen reserves in the liver tissue. Excessive body fat should be avoided, since fatty tissue heals poorly and is more susceptible to infection.

VITAMINS. Several vitamins require particular attention in wound healing. Vitamin C is a necessary material for the building of strong tissue. It deposits a cementlike substance between the cells and thus forms strong tissue. It also helps to build connective tissue, new capillary walls, and general tissue ground substance. If extensive tissue building is required, 1 g or more daily of vitamin C may be needed. Also, as calories and protein are increased, the B vitamins, especially thiamin, riboflavin, and niacin, must be increased. These vitamins provide essential coenzyme factors needed to metabolize carbohydrate and protein. Other B-complex vitamins, folic acid, B_{12}, pyridoxine, and pantothenic acid, also play important roles in building hemoglobin, thus meeting the de-

Table 23-1. Daily water requirements of the surgical patient

Type of case and fluid needs	Average fluid required (ml)
Uncomplicated cases	
For vaporizations	1000-1500
For urine	1000-1500
	2000-3000 TOTAL
Complicated cases (sepsis, elevation of temperature, humid weather, renal damage)	
For vaporization	2000-2500
For urine	1000-1500
	3000-4000 TOTAL
Seriously ill patients with drainage	
For vaporization	2000
For urine	1000
For replacement of body fluid losses	
1000 ml bile drainage	1000
3000 ml Wangensteen drainage	3000
	7000 TOTAL

Modified from Zintel, H.A.: Nutrition in the care of the surgical patient. In Wohl, M., and Goodhart, R., editors: Modern nutrition in health and disease, ed. 3, Philadephia, 1964, Lea & Febiger, p. 1055.

mands of an increased blood supply, and in meeting general stress needs in the body. Vitamin K, essential for blood clotting, is usually present through the action of intestinal bacteria.

MINERALS. Attention to any mineral deficiencies, that is, continued adequate amounts in the diet, is essential. When tissue is broken down, as is the case after surgery, cell potassium and phosphorus are lost. Also, electrolyte imbalances of sodium and chloride result from water losses. Iron deficiency anemia may develop from blood loss or from faulty iron absorption. Another important mineral in wound healing is zinc (pp. 77-78). An adequate amount of protein usually meets this need, since most dietary zinc is found in protein foods of animal origin. Sometimes in extensive surgery zinc supplements may be used.

Diet management

After surgery, patients may be fed by two basic methods: liquid feedings through the veins or oral feedings.

PERIPHERAL VEIN FEEDINGS. Usually, in the immediate postoperative period the patient receives intravenous feedings to supply necessary water and electrolytes. In some cases there may be additions to the feedings of amino acids, dextrose, and vitamins and minerals. When these feedings have to be used more than a few hours, a fat solution is available for added calories. However, this fat emulsion cannot be added to the regular intravenous feeding but must be given separately between feedings.

SPECIAL CENTRAL VEIN FEEDINGS. In cases of extended illness or malnutrition, especially when the gastrointestinal tract is involved and regular eating is impossible, a special procedure is used to sustain nutritional support. A catheter is placed into a larger central vein, and special concentrated formulas are used to ensure adequate nutrient intake. This procedure is called *hyperalimentation*, or *total parenteral nutrition* (TPN). In such a larger central vein concentrated solutions may be used that contain a high percentage of glucose (20% to 50%), crystalline amino acids, electrolytes, minerals, and vitamins. Intermittent use of a lipid solution can supply additional needed calories and essential fatty acids. Since this method of feeding requires a special surgical procedure for insertion of the feeding tube, as well as careful monitoring throughout, successful use of this feeding method depends on a well-trained team of specialists. This team includes the physician, nurse, nutritionist, and pharmacist. Much support for the patient needs to be provided throughout this feeding process.

ORAL FEEDINGS. The majority of surgical patients can and should progress to oral feedings as soon as possible. Oral feedings allow for greater additions of needed nutrients and help to stimulate normal action of the gastrointestinal tract. Food can usually be taken orally as soon as regular bowel sounds return. It must be remembered that a plain fluid-electrolyte intravenous solution cannot meet the postoperative nutritional demands. It can only compete with starvation. Thus it is important that such limited intravenous feeding not be maintained any longer than is absolutely necessary. A rapid return to regular eating should be encouraged and maintained. When oral feedings do begin, the patient usually progresses from clear to full liquids and then to a soft or regular diet. Examples of this progressive routine used in hospitals is given in Table 13-1 (p. 145). Individual tolerances and needs will always be a guide, but encouragement and help should be supplied in patient care to enable the patient to eat as soon as possible.

NUTRITIONAL CARE AFTER GASTROINTESTINAL SURGERY

Since the gastrointestinal system is uniquely designed to handle food, a surgical procedure on any part of this system requires special dietary attention or modification.

Mouth, throat, or neck surgery

Surgery involving the mouth, throat, or neck requires modification in the manner of feeding. The patient usually cannot chew or swallow normally, and accommodations must be made in each case according to individual limitations.

ORAL LIQUID FEEDINGS. Concentrated feedings in liquid form should be planned to ensure adequate nutrition in less volume of food. A formula can be made up using enriching materials to secure the needed protein, calories, vitamins, and minerals. Supplements of protein and carbohydrate can be added to general milk-based beverages and soups; lactose or other sugars can be added to fruit juices. Eggnogs with nutrient supplements can supply frequent reinforced nourishment. An example of a concentrated milk shake formula is given in Table 15-1 (p. 164). Such a formula may be supplemented with powdered skimmed milk or a protein concentrate such as Casec. This type of concentrated milk shake could supply as much as 20 g of protein and 400 calories.

TUBE FEEDINGS. In cases of radical neck or facial surgery, or when the patient is comatose or severely debilitated, tube feedings may be indicated. In such cases the patient cannot chew or swallow normally at all. Usually a nasogastric tube is inserted. However, if there is obstruction in the esophagus, the tube is inserted into an opening in the abdominal wall, made by the surgeon at the time of surgery. This procedure is called a *gastrostomy*. In any form of tube feeding it is important that the amount of the formula and the rate at which it is given are carefully watched. Usually 2 L are sufficient for a 24-hour period. Feedings should not exceed 8 to 12 ounces in each 3- to 4-hour interval. Formulas are prescribed by the nutritionist or the physician according to need of and tolerance by the individual patient. Two general types of forumula are used: prepared commercial formulas or blended food mixtures.

Commercial formulas. A wide variety of commercial formulas are available. They are designed in their composition to meet particular needs. For example, Lonalac is a low-sodium formula. Sustagen and similar products are general protein-calorie formulas. Some of these formulas are also useful for oral feedings when they are sufficiently palatable. The so-called elemental formula is usually less palatable and frequently used for tube feeding. Commercial formulas have the advantage of being standard in composition and immediately available for use. They are also sterile and may be stored.

Blended food mixtures. In cases in which a patient requires an individual ratio of nutrients a special tube feeding may be calculated, using regular foods mixed in a blender. The use of regular foods often provides the patient with needed psychological support, although the foods themselves are not tasted. An example of such a planned formula, made with blended food mixtures and a protein supplement, is given in Tables 24-1 and 24-2 (pp. 257 and 258). Such a planned formula would give a 3000-calorie tube feeding with a balanced ratio of nutrient ingredients. Ingredients in a blended food formula may include baby food or any regular food that liquifies in a blender. Usually patients not only tolerate such food mixtures better but also feel they are getting regular food. The usual ingredients include a milk base with additions of egg, strained meat, vegetable, fruit, fruit juice, nonfat dry milk, cream, brewer's yeast, and ascorbic acid.

Stomach surgery

Since the stomach is the first major food reservoir in the gastrointestinal tract, stomach surgery poses special problems in maintaining adequate nutrition. A number of these nutritional problems may develop immediately after the surgery, depending on the type of surgical procedure used and the individual patient's response. Other complications may occur later when the patient begins to eat in a more regular fashion.

IMMEDIATE POSTOPERATIVE PERIOD. Immediately after surgery, especially when a total gastrectomy has been performed, serious nutritional deficits may occur. If the gastric resection also involved a *vagotomy* (cutting of the vagus nerve, which supplies a major stimulus for gastric secretions), increased gastric fullness and distention may result. Lacking the normal nerve stimulus, the stomach becomes atonic and empties poorly. Food fermentation occurs, producing flatus or gas, as well as diarrhea. After extensive gastric surgery, weight loss is common. At least half of these patients fail to regain weight to optimum levels.

In most cases, after gastric surgery oral feedings are *slowly* resumed according to the individual patient's tolerances and the extent of the surgery. A typical pattern of this gradual addition of foods is given on p. 245. Usually a diet pattern of this gradual type will cover about a 2-week period after the surgery. The basic principles of diet therapy for this postgastrectomy period follow: (1) keep meals small and frequent and (2) eat only simple, easily digested, mild, low-bulk foods. An outline for planning the immediate postoperative diet following gastrectomy is given on p. 245.

LATER "DUMPING SYNDROME." The so-called dumping syndrome is a frequently encountered complication following extensive gastric resection. After the initial recovery from surgery, when the patient begins to feel better and eats a regular diet in greater volume and variety, discomfort may be experienced about 15 minutes after meals. The patient has a cramping, full feeling. The pulse becomes rapid. A wave of weakness, cold sweating, and dizziness may follow. Frequently the patient may become nauseated and vomit. These distressing reactions to food intake only increase the patient's anxiety. As a result, less and less food is eaten. Increasing loss of weight and general malnutrition result.

The symptoms described here are those of a shock syndrome that results when a meal containing a large proportion of readily soluble carbohydrate rapidly enters the small intestine. When the stomach has been removed, the food passes directly from the esophagus into the small intestine. This rapidly entering food mass is a concentrated solution in relation to the surrounding circulating blood. Therefore to achieve an osmotic balance, or a state of *isotonicity* (p. 96), water is drawn from the blood circulation into the intestine. This water shift causes a rapid shrinking of the vascular fluid volume. As a result, the blood pressure drops, and signs of heart action to rebuild the blood volume appear—rapid pulse, sweating, weakness, and tremors. Later, in about 2 hours, a second sequence of events may follow. The initial concentrated solution of carbohydrate has been rapidly digested and absorbed. The blood glucose rises rapidly and stimulates an overproduction of insulin. In turn there is an eventual drop in the blood sugar below normal fasting levels, and symptoms of mild hypoglycemia (lowered blood sugar) occur. Dramatic relief from all of these distressing symptoms, as well as gradual regaining of lost weight follows careful control of the diet. Principals of this postgastrectomy diet for treatment of the dumping syndrome are given on p. 246.

GASTRECTOMY DIETS

No. 1	No. 2	No. 3	No. 4
Breakfast	*Breakfast*	*Breakfast*	*Breakfast*
Soft-cooked egg	Soft-cooked egg	Same as No. 2	Egg, not fried
Salt	or poached egg		Cereal
Sugar	Butter		Toast
	White toast		Butter
	Strained cereal		Canned fruit
	Cream		Cream
10:00 AM	*10:00 AM*	*10:00 AM*	*10:00 AM*
Jell-O with cream	Same as No. 1	Same as No. 1	Same as No. 1
Luncheon	*Luncheon*	*Luncheon*	*Luncheon*
Mashed potato	Sliced turkey or	Roast beef	Tender meat
with butter	plain tender	Mashed potatoes	Potato or substitute
Salt	meat	Pureed vegetable	Whole vegetables
Sugar	Baked potato	White bread	Bread, butter
	with butter	Butter	Dessert (no fresh fruit)
	Salt, sugar	Plain pudding	
2:00 PM	*2:00 PM*	*2:00 PM*	*2:00 PM*
Baked custard	Same as No. 1	Same as No. 1	Same as No. 1
Dinner	*Dinner*	*Dinner*	*Dinner*
Baked potato	Small tender	Small tender	Tender meat
	steak	steak	Potato or substitute
	Baked potato	Baked potato	Whole vegetables
	with butter	Pureed vegetable	Bread, butter
	White toast	White bread	Dessert (no fresh fruit)
	Butter	Butter	
		Vanilla ice cream	
8:00 PM	*8:00 PM*	*8:00 PM*	*8:00 PM*
Plain pudding	Same as No. 1	Plain pudding	Same as No. 3
		with cookie	

NOTE: All meals are small in portions. Fluids, such as soup, milk, fruit juices, and other beverages, should be taken in moderation.

Gallbladder surgery

Treatment of acute gallbladder disease or gallstones usually involves surgical removal of the gallbladder. Since the function of the gallbladder is to concentrate and store bile, which aids in the digestion of fat, the main dietary modification is a reduction in the dietary fat. Depending on individual toleration and response, a relatively low-fat diet may need to be followed, not only immediately after the surgery but also for use at home. Such a low-fat diet is outlined on p. 167 and may serve as a general guide.

DIET FOR POSTOPERATIVE GASTRIC DUMPING SYNDROME

General description
1. Five or six small meals daily.
2. Relatively high fat content to retard passage of food and help maintain weight.
3. High protein content (meat, egg, cheese) to rebuild tissue and maintain weight.
4. Relatively low carbohydrate content to prevent rapid passage of quickly used foods.
5. No milk; no sugar, sweets, or desserts; no alcohol or sweet carbonated beverages.
6. Liquids between meals only; avoid fluids for at least 1 hour before and after meals.
7. Relatively low roughage foods; raw foods as tolerated.

Meal pattern

Breakfast	2 scrambled eggs with 1 or 2 tbs butter or margarine
	½-1 slice bread or small serving cereal with butter or margarine
	2 crisp bacon
	1 serving solid fruit*
Midmorning	1 slice bread
sandwich of:	butter or margarine
	2 oz (56 g) lean meat
Lunch	4 oz (112 g) lean meat with 1 or 2 tbs butter or margarine
	green or colored vegetable† with butter or margarine
	½-1 slice bread with butter or margarine
	½ banana or other solid fruit*
Midafternoon	Same snack as midmorning
Dinner	4 oz (112 g) lean meat with 1 or 2 tbs butter or margarine
	green or colored vegetable† with butter or margarine
	½-1 slice bread with butter or margarine (or small serving starchy vegetable substitute)
	1 serving solid fruit*
Bedtime	2 oz (56 g) meat or 2 eggs or 2 oz (56 g) cheese or cottage cheese
	1 slice bread or 5 crackers
	butter or margarine

---

*Fruit choice: applesauce, baked apple, canned fruit (drained), banana, orange or grapefruit sections.
†Vegetable choice: asparagus, spinach, green beans, squash, beets, carrots, green peas.

Intestinal surgery

In cases of intestinal disease involving lesions or obstructions resection of the intestine may be done. Sometimes an opening to the outside from the intestine is needed for the elimination of fecal waste materials. If the opening is in the area of the ileum (first section of the large intestine)—an ileostomy—the food mass is more liquid, and more problems may be encountered in management. If the opening is farther along the colon in the last part of the large intestine—a colostomy—the feces are more formed, and management is easier. In any of these cases general attention is given postoperatively to reducing the fiber or residue content of the diet to diminish muscle stimulation of the gastrointestinal tract and rapid food transit. A general low-residue diet pattern is given on p. 153. Very soon, however, for both physiological and psychological reasons, progression to a regular diet provides optimum nutrition, as well as physical and emotional rehabilitation. Regular food provides much psychological support to the patient, and adjustments to individual tolerances for specific foods can easily be made.

Rectal surgery

For a brief period after rectal surgery (hemorrhoidectomy), a clear fluid or nonresidue diet (below and p. 248) may be indicated. A residue-free elemental

---

NONRESIDUE DIET

General description
1. This diet includes only those foods free from fiber, seeds, and skins and with the minimum amount of residue.
2. Fruits and vegetables are omitted except for strained fruit juices.
3. Milk is omitted.
4. The diet is adequate in protein and calories, containing approximately 75 g protein, 110 g fat, 250 g carbohydrate, and 2260 calories. It is likely to be inadequate in vitamin A, calcium, and riboflavin.
5. If patients are to remain for a long length of time on this diet, supplementary vitamins and minerals should be given.

	Allowed	Not allowed
Beverages	Carbonated beverages, coffee, tea	Milk, milk drinks
Bread	Crackers, melba or rusks	Whole-grain bread
Cereals	Refined as Cream of Wheat, Farina, fine cornmeal, Malt-o-Meal, pablum, rice, strained oatmeal, cornflakes, puffed rice, Rice Krispies	Whole-grain and other cereals

Continued.

NONRESIDUE DIET—cont'd

	Allowed	Not allowed
Cheese		None allowed
Desserts	Plain cakes and cookies, gelatin desserts, water ices, angel food cake, arrowroot cookies, tapioca puddings made with fruit juice only	Pastries, all others
Eggs	As desired, preferably hard cooked	Fried eggs
Fats	Butter or substitute, small amount cream	None
Fruits	Strained fruit juices	All others
Meat, fish, poultry	Tender beef, chicken, fish, lamb, liver, veal; crisp bacon	Fried or tough meat, pork
Potatoes or substitute	Only macaroni, noodles, spaghetti, refined rice	Potatoes, corn, hominy, unrefined rice
Soup	Bouillon and broth only	All others
Sweets	Hard candy, fondant, gumdrops, jelly, marshmallows, sugar, syrup, honey	Other candy, jam, marmalade
Vegetables	Tomato juice	All others
Miscellaneous	Salt	Pepper

NOTE: Fruit juice and hard candies may be taken between meals to increase caloric intake.

POSTSURGICAL NONRESIDUE DIET
General description
1. This diet is slightly higher in residue but has greater variety, including potatoes, white bread products, processed cheese, sauces, desserts made with milk, and cream for coffee and cereal.
2. The average daily menu will contain 85 g protein, 2300 calories, and is slightly higher in vitamins and minerals.

Selection of foods
To the above add
Cheese: Processed cheese, mild cream cheeses
Potatoes: Prepared any way, no skin
Bread: Any kind without bran, white bread, rolls, pancakes, waffles
Fats: 2 oz cream or half-and-half per meal, cream sauce, cream gravy
Desserts: All desserts except those containing fruit and nuts
Condiments: As desired

diet formula, such as Vivonex, may be used. However, healing is usually rapid, and return to a regular diet follows.

Questions on surgery

1. Name the essential nutrients required by a patient who has had surgery to support the healing process and recovery. Give reasons for each need and ways of meeting the needs.
2. What is catabolism? Why does it occur after surgery? How is it met in planning the diet?
3. What basic methods are used in managing the diet of a patient who has had surgery?
4. What special needs might the patient with mouth, throat, or neck surgery have? How would they be met?
5. What basic problem would a patient who has had a gastrectomy have after full eating is resumed? How would this problem be solved?
6. What nutrient is of special concern after gallbladder surgery? Why?
7. What feeding routine would be observed for a patient with a colostomy? Why?
8. Outline a diet for a patient who has had a hemorrhoidectomy.

Suggestions for additional study

1. Make a survey to discover as many different commercial products as are available for use in tube feedings or oral supplement feeding. Visit a local pharmacy and discuss these items with the pharmacist.
2. Interview one of the hospital clinical dietitians concerning the types of these products that are used by the hospital.
3. Make arrangements with the hospital pharmacist to observe the mixing of the formula solutions for use in TPN feedings.
4. Compare the cost of commercial and food-blended tube feedings. What are advantages of each type?

The patient with a gastrectomy

After a long experience with peptic ulcer disease and little relief gained by conservative medical management, Charles Thompson and his physician decided that surgery would be the best treatment to follow. Charles then entered the hospital for a total gastrectomy.

The following day the surgeon performed the operation and established an anastomosis between the jejunum and the remaining portion of the esophagus. Charles withstood the surgery well. Gradually, over the next 2-week period immediately after surgery, a refeeding program was initiated. In the first 24 to 48 hours immediately after surgery Charles received nothing orally but was fed by intravenous therapy, with close attention given to maintaining fluid and electrolyte balances. When he received his initial liquid in the form of ice chips or sips of water adjusted in temperature for the best tolerance, the nurse observed carefully to see what his responses were.

Since Charles tolerated the initial water by mouth well, the next few days he received 1 or 2 ounces of milk between the small amounts of water. Gradually the amount of milk was increased a bit and a single soft food item added at one or two of the feedings during the day. Soft foods such as eggs, soft-cooked cereal, baked custard, baked potatoes, or plain puddings were used. By the end of the second week, Charles was tolerating a full soft diet in small feedings about six times during the day. The nurse cautioned him to use fluids, such as milk, soup, fruit juice, and other beverages, in moderation.

After Charles recovered from the surgery and was improved enough to go home, he gradually felt his strength returning. The physician had emphasized that he should observe his tolerances, eat smaller amounts at a time, and stress the use of protein foods. When Charles had recovered from the surgery itself and began to resume more and more of his usual activities, his food intake increased. Because he felt so much better, he began to eat a greater volume of food and in greater variety. Friends invited the family out for meals, and they began to do more entertaining themselves. Also, he began to become involved more in his old business activities, in which many luncheon business conferences with rich foods and alcohol were included.

As time went by, Charles began experiencing increasing discomfort after his meals. About 10 to 15 minutes after he had eaten, he would have a cramping, full feeling. He felt his heart begin to beat more rapidly, and a wave of weakness would suddenly come over him. He would break out in a cold sweat and feel dizzy. Often he would become nauseated and vomit. As these episodes increased, his anxiety about himself increased accordingly, and as a result he started to eat less and less. His weight began to drop. He was already fairly thin, and this increased weight loss made him look more emaciated and debilitated. Soon he was in a general state of malnutrition.

When Charles returned to seek medical help, the physician initiated a change in his eating habits. The clinic nurse described in general what the diet changes would be and made arrangements for both Charles and his wife to see the nutritionist, who then explained the diet in detail and worked out a food plan that would be acceptable in his situation. The diet seemed strange to Charles, but be began to follow it carefully. Because he felt so ill, he was glad to make any changes that might be helpful. To his pleased surprise he found that the symptoms he had experienced before disappeared almost completely. Because he felt so much better on the new diet plan, he formed his new eating habits around it. His weight gradually increased, and his general state of nutrition improved markedly. He found that he always fared better if he would "nibble," rather than consume a large, heavy meal at one time.

QUESTIONS TO GUIDE YOUR INQUIRY

1. What were Charles' nutritional needs immediately after surgery and in the next 2 weeks? Why was it necessary for his feedings to be resumed cautiously?

2. Why was an emphasis placed on protein intake after Charles' surgery as he began to tolerate food? Why is a negative nitrogen balance a usual follow-up to surgical

procedures? Why does the body need protein after surgery? What are its functions during this period?

3. Why do sufficient calories have to be consumed as soon as food is tolerated?

4. Why is fluid therapy of paramount importance after surgery?

5. What minerals and vitamins should be increased after surgery?

6. When Charles began to feel better and resumed heavier eating habits, why did he experience the symptoms he did after consuming a meal? What is this response called? Why?

7. What principles of diet therapy would have been observed in the corrective diet suggestions given to Charles by the physician, nurse, and nutritionist? Give the reasons for each of these principles.

8. Outline a day's meal pattern for Charles on his newly adjusted diet pattern.

Suggested readings

Williams, S.R.: Nutrition and diet therapy, ed. 4, St. Louis, 1981, The C.V. Mosby Co.

Williams, S.R.: Essentials of nutrition and diet therapy, ed. 3, St. Louis, 1982, The C.V. Mosby Co.

24

Cancer

Over the past few years, with accumulating environmental problems and changing life-styles, cancer has become an increasing health problem. It now ranks second, after heart disease, as a leading cause of death in the United States, accounting for about 20% of the total number of deaths each year. Since cancer is generally associated with the aging process, the increasing life expectancy has contributed in some measure to this increasing incidence.

One of the problems in the study and treatment of cancer is that it is not a single problem. It has a highly varying nature and expresses itself in multiple forms. The general term *cancer* is used to designate a malignant tumor or *neoplasm* ("new growth"). However, there are many forms of cancer, varying worldwide and changing with population migrations to different environments. It would be more correct, therefore, to use the plural term *cancers* in discussing this great variety of neoplasms.

For these reasons there is no one specific treatment or a "special diet" for cancer, despite various fad diets and claims. Rather, relationships of nutrition and cancer care center on two fundamental areas: (1) *prevention* in relation to the environment and to the body's natural defense system and (2) *therapy* in relation to nutritional support for medical treatment and rehabilitation.

THE BODY'S DEFENSE SYSTEM

The defense system of the human body is complex but remarkably efficient. It is composed of special types of cells and tissues that not only protect against external invaders, such as bacteria and viruses, but also fend off internal "aliens," such as malignant tumor cells. Both the immune system and the tissue-healing process are part of this overall defense complex.

The immune system

Special white blood cells called *lymphocytes* provide the immune system's primary line of defense for detecting and destroying malignant cells arising daily in the body. The two types of lymphocytes are called *T cells* and *B cells* according to the tissue from which they arise. The T cells come from the thymus gland, and the B cells come from special bursal lymphoid tissue in the gut. Together these cells destroy harmful agents, make antibodies that counteract the harmful substances (antigens), and initiate an inflammatory response, which supports healing. All of these materials and the tissues from which they arise are basically composed of protein. Hence nutritional support is essential to maintain the strength and integrity of this efficient immune system. Studies of severely malnourished populations have shown loss of immune powers with deterioration of basic tissues involved: liver, bowel wall, bone marrow, spleen, and lymphoid tissue.

The healing process

The strength of any body tissue is maintained through constant synthesis of tissue protein, building and rebuilding. Such strong tissue is a front line of the body's defense. This process of tissue building and healing requires optimum nutritional intake. Specific nutrients, protein and key vitamins and minerals, as well as nonprotein energy sources, must constantly be supplied in the diet.

NUTRITIONAL SUPPORT FOR CANCER TREATMENT

Three major forms of therapy are used today as medical treatment for cancer: (1) surgery, (2) radiation, and (3) chemotherapy. Each one requires nutritional support.

Surgery

Any surgery, as discussed in Chapter 23, requires nutritional support for the healing process. This is particularly true for patients with cancer because their general condition is often weakened by the disease process and its drain on the body's resources. With early diagnosis and sound nutritional support before and after surgery, many tumors can successfully be removed, and recovery is often ensured. Nutritional therapy will also include any needed modifications in food texture or in specific nutrients, depending on the site of the surgery or the function of the organ involved. Various methods of feeding patients after surgery are discussed in Chapter 23 and may be reviewed there.

Radiation

Depending on the site and intensity of the radiation treatment, the patient may experience numerous nutritional problems. For example, radiation to the area of the head, neck, or esophagus affects the oral mucosa and salivary secretions. This will influence taste sensations and sensitivity to food texture and temperature. In a similar manner radiation to the abdominal area affects the intestinal mucosa. This causes loss of villi and absorbing surface; hence malabsorption problems may follow. Also, ulcers or inflammation and obstruction or fistulas may develop from the tissue breakdown. Fistulas, from the Latin word for "pipe," are abnormal openings or passageways within the body or to the outside. As such, they interfere with normal functioning of the involved tissue. The general malabsorption problem may be further compounded by lack of food intake resulting from loss of appetite and nausea.

Chemotherapy

A number of drugs have been developed in the past few years to combat cancer. They are often used in combinations to achieve a desired effect of killing the cancer cells. However, because these drugs are toxic, they have similar effects on normal cells and have to be regulated very carefully. This accounts for the particular toxic side effects experienced by patients and creates the attendant problems in nutritional management:

1. *Gastrointestinal tract effects*. Numerous problems may develop that interfere with food tolerance: nausea and vomiting, loss of appetite, diarrhea, ulcers, malabsorption, or stomatitis (inflammation of the tissues in the mouth).
2. *Bone marrow effects*. Interference with the production of specific blood factors causes related problems: reduced red blood cells causing anemia, reduced white blood cells causing lowered resistance to infections, and reduced blood platelets causing bleeding.
3. *Hair follicle effects*. Interference with normal hair growth results in general hair loss or baldness.

NUTRITIONAL THERAPY
Objectives

In general, in care of the patient with cancer, problems in nutritional care stem from the disease process itself and from its treatment. Thus there are two basic objectives in a strong nutrition program in cancer care:

PREVENTION OF CATABOLISM. Every effort is made to meet the increased metabolic demands of the disease and thus prevent extensive catabolic, or tissue breakdown, effects. It is far easier to maintain a state of good nutrition than it is to rebuild the body from a state of extensive malnutrition. This catabolic effect may be increased by the medical treatment.

RELIEF OF SYMPTOMS. The symptoms of the disease or side effects of the treatment can be devastating for the patient. Relief for the patient requires much individual counseling with the patient and family to devise ways of meeting needs and helping the patient to eat. The types of foods used, their texture and temperature, or the process of feeding may have to be changed frequently according to individual situations or responses and needs.

Although the clinical nutritionist and the physician have the primary responsibility for planning and managing the nutritional care program, a tremendous contribution is made by the nursing staff and other health care personnel in the day-to-day support and counsel in helping the patient to eat. It is often just this kind of constant care that makes the difference in combating the course of the disease and in ensuring the comfort and well-being of the patient.

Principles of nutritional care

Two basic principles underlie all sound patient care. These are identifying needs and planning care based on these needs. Only then can it be determined if real needs have been met. Thus nutrition assessment and nutritional care planning are of primary concern:

ASSESSMENT OF NUTRITION. Determining the nutritional status of each patient is the primary responsibility of the clinical nutritionist, but other support staff in nursing often assist. Procedures used include body measurements and calculations of body composition, laboratory tests, physical examination and clinical observations, and dietary analysis.

NUTRITIONAL PLAN OF CARE. Based on the information gathered about each patient, including living situation and social needs, the clinical nutritionist, in consultation with the physician, develops a personal plan of nutritional therapy for each patient. This outline is then incorporated in the nursing care plan, since the nutritionist works with the nursing staff to carry it out. The day-to-day plan is constantly checked with the patient and family and changed as needed to meet the nutritional demands of the patient's condition.

Nutritional needs

Individual needs will, of course, vary. However, guidelines for nutritional therapy must meet specific nutrient needs related to the accelerated metabolism, which demands increased protein tissue synthesis and energy.

ENERGY. The hypermetabolic nature of the disease and its healing requirements place great energy demands on the patient with cancer. Sufficient fuel from carbohydrate, and to a lesser extent from fat, must be available to spare protein for vital tissue building. An adult patient with good nutritional status will need about 2000 kilocalories for maintenance requirements. A malnourished patient will require 3000 to 4000 kilocalories, depending on the degree of malnutrition or extent of tissue injury.

PROTEIN. The necessary tissue building for healing requires essential amino acids and nitrogen. Efficient protein use depends on an optimum protein/calorie ratio to promote tissue building and prevent tissue wastage (catabolism). An adult patient with good nutritional status will need about 80 to 100 g of high-quality protein to meet maintenance requirements. A malnourished patient will need 100 to 200 g to replenish tissue and restore positive nitrogen balance.

VITAMINS AND MINERALS. Key vitamins and minerals control protein and energy metabolism through their roles as coenzyme partners in cell enzyme systems (see Chapters 6 and 7). They also play important roles in building and maintaining strong tissue. Thus an optimum intake of vitamins and minerals, at least to the level of the recommended dietary allowances, but more frequently to higher potency levels, is required. Supplements to the dietary sources are usually indicated.

FLUID. Adequate fluid intake must be ensured for two reasons: (1) to replace gastrointestinal tract losses or losses from fever or infection and (2) to help the kidneys dispose of metabolic breakdown products from destroyed cancer cells and from toxic drugs used in chemotherapy. Some of these drugs, such as cyclophosphamide (Cytoxan), require as much as 2 to 3 L of forced fluids daily to prevent hemorrhagic cystitis.

Nutritional management

Achieving these nutritional objectives and needs, in the face of frequent poor tolerance of food or inability to eat, poses a great challenge to the health care team. The specific method of feeding depends on the patient's condition. However, four basic methods are available to the clinical nutritionist and the physician in managing a particular patient's nutritional care. Two of these are enteral (using the gut); two are parenteral (using a vein).

ENTERAL: ORAL DIET WITH NUTRIENT SUPPLEMENTATION. An oral diet with supplementation is the most desired form of feeding, of course, whenever it is possible. A personal food plan needs to be worked out with the patient and family, based on the nutrition assessment information gathered. It needs to

Table 24-1. Sample tube feeding formula (2500 ml, 3000 calories)

Ingredients	Amount	Protein	Fat	Carbohydrate
Homogenized milk	1 L	32	40	48
Eggs	3	21	16	
Apple juice	400 ml			55
Vegetable oil	30 ml		30	
Strained baby food (4 oz [112 g] jars)				
Beef liver	4 yars	56	12	14
Beets	2 jars	3		20
Peaches	2 jars	1	1	59
Sustagen	1½ cups (225 g)	52	7	150
(Water as needed to total 2500 ml)		___	___	___
TOTALS		165	106	346
TOTAL CALORIES			2998	

Table 24-2. Types of tube feedings

Ingredients	Calories	Protein (g)	Fat (g)	Carbohydrates (g)
Regular tube feeding				
6 eggs	452	36.6	33.0	—
1 L homogenized milk	666	34.2	38.1	47.8
1 cup nonfat milk solids	434	42.7	1.2	121.3
½ cup Karo syrup	469			62.4
1 tablet brewer's yeast				
75 mg ascorbic acid				
¼ tsp salt				
1500 ml				
TOTAL	2021	113.5	72.3	231.5
Sustagen				
3 cups Sustagen	1755	105.0	15.0	300.0
4 cups water				
1200 ml				
600 g Sustagen (4 cups)	2300	140.0	20.0	400.0
1200 ml water				
1400 ml				
Add for banana Sustagen:				
2 tsp banana flakes	88	1.2	—	23.0
or				
1 mashed banana				
Low-calcium tube feeding				
6 cans strained meat	540	80.4	25.2	0
1 L fruit juice	432	0	2.0	108.0
¼ cup Karo syrup	234			61.0
ascorbic acid				
brewer's yeast				
1800 ml				
TOTAL	1206	80.4	27.2	169.0
Low-sodium tube feeding				
1 L low-sodium milk	666	34.2	38.1	47.8
Casec 90 g—3 oz 18 tbs	306	75.0		
¼ cup Karo syrup	234			61.0
1000 ml				
TOTAL	1206	109.2	38.1	108.8

include adjustments in food texture and temperature, food choices, and tolerances. It should provide as much calorie and nutrient density as possible in smaller volumes of food. It must give special attention to eating problems such as loss of appetite, mouth problems, and gastrointestinal tract problems with supportive care procedures. A number of excellent suggestions and resources are available for the patient and family (Fleming, Weaver, and Brown, 1977; Rosenbaum et al., 1980).

ENTERAL: TUBE FEEDING. When the gut can still be used but the patient requires still more assistance, tube feeding may be indicated. Many commercial formulas are available, but they must be selected with care. Many patients prefer a blended mixture of food items, which is often better tolerated and may provide more additional emotional support (see Chapter 23). Also, if needed for a longer period of time, the food-blended formula is far less costly than commercial products. However, commercial products have the advantage of convenience, standard composition, and easy storage.

PARENTERAL: PERIPHERAL VEIN FEEDING. When the gastrointestinal tract cannot be used, intravenous feeding must be initiated (Tables 24-1 and 24-2). When the nutrient demands are not excessive and the need extends for only a brief time, feeding through a peripheral vein instead of a larger central vein carries less risk and can provide satisfactory nutritional support. Commercial solutions containing dextrose, amino acids, vitamins, and minerals are used. A separately administered fat emulsion, Intralipid, is also used to supply calories and essential fatty acid.

PARENTERAL: CENTRAL VEIN FEEDING. When nutritional demands are greater and the vein feeding must continue over an extended period of time, central vein feeding has often provided a lifesaving alternative. A skilled team of professionals, including physician, nutritionist, nurse, and pharmacist, is required to avoid complications. In this TPN feeding method a formula of greater nutrient density can be used, providing increased nutritional support for patients in greater need.

CONCLUSIONS: CANCER THERAPY AND PREVENTION

As indicated in the beginning of this chapter, relationships of nutrition and cancer center on therapy and prevention.

Treatment

There is ample evidence at this point that vigorous nutritional support increases the chances for success of medical treatments in the care of cancer. The fundamental reasons for this possible outcome have been reviewed briefly. It is also evident that much effort on the part of the health care team, the patient, and the family, all working together, is necessary for this vigorous nutritional support to become a reality.

Prevention

On the basis of studies thus far the National Research Council Committee on Diet, Nutrition, and Cancer issued dietary guidelines in a 1982 report. The committee indicated that these were intended to serve as interim guidelines until more information is available but that they are consistent with good nutritional practices and are likely to reduce the risk of cancer. The six dietary guidelines follow:

1. *Fat*. Reduce fat intake from the present American average of 40% of

total calories to 30% to reduce the risk of breast and colon cancer associated with high-fat diets.

2. *Fiber*. Increase the use of fruits, vegetables, and whole-grain cereal products in the diet to ensure sufficient fiber to reduce the risk of colon cancer.

3. *Vitamins A and C*. Emphasize the use of citrus fruits, carotene-rich vegetables, and vegetables of the Cruciferae (cabbage) family.

4. *Processed meats*. Minimize consumption of salt-cured, pickled, or smoked foods, including smoked sausages, hot dogs, ham, and smoked fish. These smoke-cured foods have been associated with cancer in some populations.

5. *Food additives*. Minimize contamination of foods by carcinogens from any source, whether avoidable or unavoidable. Intentional food additives, direct and indirect, should continue to be evaluated for carcinogenic activity before they are approved for use in the food supply.

6. *Alcohol*. Moderate the use of alcoholic beverages, if they are used at all.

Questions on cancer

1. Why is cancer an increasing health problem?
2. In what two main areas does nutrition relate to cancer care?
3. Describe the components of the body's defense system.
4. Describe the nutritional problems associated with each of the major medical treatments of cancer.
5. Describe the three main side effects of chemotherapy used in cancer treatment.
6. What are the basic objectives of nutritional therapy in the care of patients with cancer?
7. Why is nutrition assessment an important first step in planning the nutritional care of a patient with cancer?
8. Discuss the nutritional needs of a patient with cancer. Give the reasons for each need.
9. What are the four basic methods of feeding a patient with cancer to ensure that the nutritional demands are met? Describe each method.
10. What are the dietary guidelines of the National Research Council for diet recommended to prevent cancer?

Suggestions for additional study

1. Visit the local chapter of the American Cancer Society. Interview a staff member about the chapter's work. Obtain any patient education materials and evaluate them with your classmates.
2. Write a list of suggestions for helping a patient suffering the side effects of chemotherapy to eat.

The patient requiring tube feeding

Mr. and Mrs. Wilson, both age 70, lived on their small farm in a rural area of the county. They had no family, since their two sons had been killed in World War II. Mr.

Wilson had tended his small farm as long as he was able to do so, but now he was unable to work. They had gradually sold off parcels of their land until they had only the farmhouse and a small plot of land remaining. Their income was small, and they could scarcely meet the taxes for the land. They were both in poor health and worried about their future care. Their closest relationship was with the small church in the community, where they had been members most of their lives, but they now were unable to attend. The present pastor of the church was a young man with several small children, whose wife was a dietitian. The pastor's family had a warm affection for Mr. and Mrs. Wilson and visited frequently in their small home.

Mrs. Wilson began to have some symptoms of difficulty in swallowing and pain in the area of her throat and neck. Cancer eventually developed. Finally radical neck surgery became necessary. After the surgery she was unable to consume food in the normal manner and had to be fed through a tube.

The first formula ordered by the doctor was a water dilution of Sustagen to provide 1700 calories a day. Mrs. Wilson tolerated this feeding fairly well and gradually improved. As her need for protein and calories was increased, the doctor ordered an increase in her diet to 3000 calories. At first this increase in calories was also a Sustagen formula, but Mrs. Wilson began to have gastrointestinal difficulties and diarrhea. To counteract this problem, the formula was changed to a calculated food mixture yielding a better balance of nutrients at the same calorie level. The doctor wanted her to have 2500 ml of the formula each day.

In the days that followed Mrs. Wilson continued to improve and regain her strength. Her pastor and his wife visited frequently and brought Mr. Wilson with them. Soon the day came when the doctor indicated that Mrs. Wilson would be able to go home. He discussed her needs for home care with the nurse and home care coordinator. He felt reasonably sure that after a period of continued use of the tube feeding, Mrs. Wilson would be able to gradually resume small liquid to soft-textured oral feedings. Her need for optimum nutrition was evident.

The day Mrs. Wilson was to go home, the pastor and his wife and Mr. Wilson came to get her. The doctor discussed her needs with all of them, and the pastor and his wife assured him that they would do what was necessary to see that she had the care she needed.

QUESTIONS TO GUIDE YOUR INQUIRY

1. What nutritional needs did Mrs. Wilson have in preparing her for surgery? What solutions to these needs can you propose? How would you involve the physician, the clinic nurse, and the pastor and his wife in your solutions?

2. What are some of the indications for tube feeding?

3. What are the implications of such a method of feeding for Mrs. Wilson? What are her needs? Her husband's needs?

4. What is Sustagen? What measure of Sustagen in Mrs. Wilson's initial tube-feeding formula was necessary to achieve 1500 calories? What are the food values in this amount of Sustagen?

5. Why did gastrointestinal tract difficulties result when the tube feeding using Sustagen alone was increased to 3000 calories?

6. What solution was found for meeting this problem? Why was the calculated mixed tube feeding better tolerated? Outline such a tube feeding: 3000 calories, 165 g protein, and not more than 350 g carbohydrate.

7. In planning for Mrs. Wilson's home care, what problems do you see? What solutions can you propose? What persons would you involve?

Suggested readings

Chernoff, R., and Bloch, A.S.: Liquid feedings: considerations and alternatives, J. Am. Diet. Assoc. **70**:389, 1977.

Fleming, S.M., Weaver, A.W., and Brown, J.M.: The patient with cancer affecting the head and neck: problems in nutrition, J. Am. Diet. Assoc. **70**:391, 1977.

Rosenbaum, E.H., et al.: Nutrition for the cancer patient, Palo Alto, Calif., 1980, Bull Publishing Co.

Williams, S.R.: Nutrition and diet therapy, ed. 4, St. Louis, 1981, The C.V. Mosby Co.

Williams, S.R.: Essentials of nutrition and diet therapy, ed. 3, St. Louis, 1982, The C.V. Mosby Co.

APPENDIX

Table A. Food values

	Approximate measure	Calories	Protein (g)	Fat (g)	Carbo-hydrate (g)
Beverages					
Coca-Cola	1 bottle (6 oz)	78	0	0	20.4
Ginger ale	1 glass (6 oz)	60	0	0	15.3
Chocolate milk shake	1 regular (8 oz milk)	421	11.2	17.8	58.0
Chocolate malted milk shake	1 regular (8 oz milk)	502	13.1	19.5	72.1
Cider, sweet	1 glass (6 oz)	94	0.2	0	25.8
Cocoa, all milk	1 cup (6 oz milk)	174	6.9	8.5	20.3
Eggnog	1 glass (6 oz milk)	233	12.5	12.6	17.7
Lemonade	1 large glass, 1 oz lemon juice	104	0.2	0	27.2
Milk, buttermilk	½ pt	86	8.5	0.2	12.4
Milk, chocolate	½ pt	185	8.0	5.5	26.5
Milk, skimmed	½ pt	87	8.6	0.2	12.5
Milk, whole	½ pt	166	8.5	9.5	12.0
Soda, ice cream, vanilla	1 regular	261	2.3	7.1	48.7
Soda, ice cream, chocolate	1 regular	255	2.7	8.3	46.0
Breads					
Bread, corn	1 piece (2 in square)	139	3.2	4.3	21.6
Bread, rye	1 slice	57	2.1	0.3	12.1
Bread, white, enriched	1 slice	63	2.0	0.7	11.9
Bread, whole-wheat	1 slice	55	2.1	0.6	11.3
Biscuit, baking powder	1 average (2 in diameter)	109	2.4	4.1	14.9
Bun, cinnamon, plain	1 average	158	3.1	4.8	25.6
Doughnut, cake type, plain	1 average	135	2.2	6.5	17.5
Doughnut, sugared or iced	1 average	151	2.2	6.5	21.7
Muffin, white flour	1 average, 12 from 2 cups flour	120	3.2	4.3	17.1
Muffin, whole-wheat	1 average, 12 from 2 cups flour	120	3.4	4.3	17.1
Pancake, various flours	1 average (4 in diameter)	62	2.3	1.2	10.7
Roll, white, soft	1 Parker House	81	2.1	1.6	13.6

From Church, C.F., and Church, H.N.: Food values of portions commonly used, ed. 11, Philadelphia,
Abbreviations: g, gram; IU, international unit; lb, pound; µg, microgram; mg, milligram; oz, ounce; tbs,
figure; 0, none; tr, trace.
Equivalents: 1000 micrograms (µg) = 1 milligram (mg); 1000 milligrams (mg) = 1 gram (g); 28.34 g = 1

Calcium (mg)	Iron (mg)	Vitamin A (IU)	Thiamin (µg)	Ribo-flavin (µg)	Niacin (mg)	Ascorbic acid (mg)
0	0	0	0	0	0	0
0	0	0	0	0	0	0
363	0.9	687	120	547	0.5	4
420	1.3	891	186	655	0.5	4
11	0.9	75	37	56	tr	2
224	0.9	295	80	334	0.3	2
242	1.5	843	123	451	0.2	2
4	tr	0	20	tr	tr	15
288	0.2	10	90	430	0.3	3
272	0.2	230	80	400	0.2	2
303	0.2	10	90	440	0.3	3
288	0.2	390	90	420	0.3	3
69	0.1	295	24	106	0.1	1
75	0.7	297	30	127	0.2	1
29	0.7	229	90	102	0.7	(0)
17	0.4	0	40	20	0.4	(0)
18	0.4	0	60	40	0.5	0
22	0.5	0	70	30	0.7	0
19	0.5	20	86	70	0.6	0
27	0.9	205	85	87	0.8	0
12	0.6	41	72	63	0.5	tr
12	0.6	41	72	63	0.5	tr
30	0.7	193	78	95	0.6	0
33	0.7	193	88	85	0.5	0
96	0.3	44	30	53	0.2	0
19	0.5	73	72	64	0.5	0

1970, J.B. Lippincott Co.
tablespoonful, level; tsp, teaspoonful, level; ( ), tentative data; —, data inadequate to give a specific oz.

Continued.

Table A. Food values—cont'd

	Approximate measure	Calories	Protein (g)	Fat (g)	Carbo-hydrate (g)
Breads—cont'd					
Roll, white, sweet	1 average commercial	178	4.7	4.3	29.6
Waffle, plain, average	1 waffle (5½ in diameter)	232	5.1	14.0	21.4
Cereals and cereal products					
Cheerios	1 oz (1⅛ cups)	104	4.1	2.0	19.7
Cornflakes	1 oz (1⅓ cups)	105	2.1	0.1	24.4
Cream of Wheat, cooked	¾ cup	102	3.5	0.3	21.7
Grapenuts	1 oz (¼ cup)	110	2.8	0.2	24.0
Macaroni, cooked	½ cup (1 in pieces)	105	3.6	0.4	21.2
Macaroni and cheese, baked	1 cup	366	15.3	19.9	31.4
Noodles, egg, enriched, cooked	¾ cup	81	2.7	0.75	15.3
Oatmeal, cooked	¾ cup	111	4.0	2.1	19.5
Popcorn	1 cup	54	1.8	0.7	10.7
Post Toasties	1¼ cups (1 oz)	100	2.1	0.1	24.0
Rice, white, cooked	¾ cup	150	3.2	0.15	33.0
Rice Krispies	1 cup	107	1.6	0.1	25.1
Rice, puffed	1 cup	107	1.8	0.1	24.7
Spaghetti, cooked	¾ cup	162	5.5	0.6	33.0
Spaghetti, Italian style	1 average serving with meat sauce	396	12.7	20.7	39.4
Sugar Crisp	1 oz (individual package)	110	1.9	0.3	25.0
Wheat, shredded	1 large biscuit (4 in × 2¼ in)	106	3.2	0.5	22.1
Cracker, graham	1 (2½ in square)	28	0.5	0.7	5.0
Cracker, Ritz	1 cracker	16	0.2	0.8	2.0
Cracker, saltine	1 cracker	14	0.3	0.3	2.3
Matzoth	1 piece (6 in diameter)	78	2.1	0.2	17.3
Pretzel sticks	7 average thin sticks	37	0.9	0.3	7.5
Ry-Krisp	1 double square wafer	20	0.7	0.1	4.1
Zwieback	1 piece (61 to 1 lb)	31	0.9	0.7	5.3
Dairy products					
Butter	1 tsp	36	0	4.1	0
Butter	1 tbs	100	0.1	11.3	0.1
Cheese, cheddar, American	1 oz (1 slice ¼ in thick)	113	7.1	9.1	0.6
Cheese, cottage	½ cup	107	22.0	0.55	2.2

*Vitamin A and D values for butter and cream are average year-round figures; vitamin A and D content

Calcium (mg)	Iron (mg)	Vitamin A (IU)	Thiamin (μg)	Ribo-flavin (μg)	Niacin (mg)	Ascorbic acid (mg)
35	0.3	0	30	70	0.6	0
59	0.9	178	122	159	0.8	tr
47	2.1	(0)	325	56	0.6	0
2	0.5	(0)	120	20	0.6	0
10	1.1	0	17	17	0.2	0
—	1.0	(0)	130	—	1.5	0
7	0.75	(0)	120	75	1.0	0
355	1.2	818	96	355	0.9	tr
4	0.6	45	165	75	1.35	0
15	1.2	(0)	165	38	0.3	0
(2)	(0.4)	(0)	(50)	(20)	(0.3)	0
—	0.4	(0)	110	—	0.5	0
9	0.4	(0)	15	7	0.5	0
7	0.5	(0)	110	10	2.0	0
4	0.5	(0)	125	11	1.5	0
10	1.2	(0)	186	113	0.5	0
27	2.1	901	120	117	3.0	(24)
3	0.5	(0)	14	—	0.7	0
13	1.0	(0)	60	30	1.3	0
1	0.1	(0)	20	10	0.1	0
1	0.1	(0)	—	—	—	0
1	0.1	(0)	tr	tr	tr	0
—	—	0	—	—	—	0
1	0.1	0	1	4	0.1	0
3	0.2	0	20	10	0.1	0
8	0.1	0	—	—	—	0
1	0	165*	tr	tr	tr	0
3	—	460*	tr	tr	tr	0
206	0.3	400	10	120	tr	(0)
108	0.35	25	20	345	0.1	(0)

varies with the seasons.

Continued.

Table A. Food values—cont'd

	Approximate measure	Calories	Protein (g)	Fat (g)	Carbo- hydrate (g)
Dairy products—cont'd					
Cheese, cream	2 tbs	106	2.6	10.5	0.6
Cream, light	1 tbs	30	0.4	3.0	0.6
Cream, heavy, sweet or sour	1 tbs	50	0.3	5.2	0.5
Cream, heavy, whipped	1 heaping tbs, sweetened	52	0.3	5.2	1.3
Milk, buttermilk	½ pt	86	8.5	0.2	12.4
Milk, chocolate	½ pt	185	8.0	5.5	26.5
Milk, skimmed	½ pt	87	8.6	0.2	12.5
Milk, whole	½ pt	166	8.5	9.5	12.0
Desserts					
Blancmange, vanilla	½ cup	152	4.2	4.7	23.8
Brownies	1 (2 in × 2 in × ¾ in)	141	1.8	8.4	16.6
Cake, angel	1 piece (⅒ of average cake)	145	3.4	0.1	33.0
Cake, chocolate, 2 layer	1 piece (1/12 of cake with white icing)	356	3.1	7.7	45.0
Cake, sponge cake	1 piece (⅒ of average cake)	145	3.2	2.3	28.1
Cake, white, 2 layer, chocolate icing	3 in section of layer cake	314	4.0	10.4	52.6
Cookies, oatmeal	1 large (3½ in diameter)	114	1.6	4.4	17.5
Cookies, sugar	1 cookie (3½ in diameter)	64	1.0	2.6	9.1
Custard baked	1 custard (4 from 1 pt milk)	205	8.8	9.1	22.8
Fig bars, commercial	1 small, average	56	0.7	0.8	12.1
Gingerbread, using hot water and 1 egg	1 small piece (2 in cube)	206	2.2	9.9	26.9
Ice cream, vanilla	¼ of 1 pt	147	2.8	8.9	14.6
Jell-O, plain	1 serving (5 to 1 package)	65	1.6	0	15.1
Jell-O with whipped cream	1 serving, 1 tbs cream	117	1.8	5.4	16.4
Pie, apple	⅙ of medium pie	377	3.8	14.3	60.2
Pie, blueberry	⅙ of medium pie	372	3.9	15.4	56.9
Pie, cherry	⅙ of medium pie	360	4.3	12.4	59.6
Pie, chocolate	⅙ of medium pie	294	6.9	13.7	37.7
Pie, custard	⅙ of medium pie	266	7.6	12.1	32.7

*Vitamin A and D values for butter and cream are average year-round figures; vitamin A and D content

Calcium (mg)	Iron (mg)	Vitamin A (IU)	Thiamin (µg)	Ribo-flavin (µg)	Niacin (mg)	Ascorbic acid (mg)
19	0.1	(410)	tr	60	tr	(0)
15	0	120*	4	20	tr	tr
12	0	220*	tr	20	tr	tr
12	0	220*	tr	20	tr	tr
288	0.2	(390)	90	420	0.3	3
272	0.2	230	80	400	0.2	2
303	0.2	(10)	90	440	0.3	3
(288)	0.2	10	90	430	0.3	1
144	0.1	195	45	210	0.1	1
11	0.5	226	38	41	0.2	(0)
3	0.1	(0)	3	66	0.1	0
24	0.5	265	17	70	0.1	(0)
88	0.4	390	20	70	0.2	(0)
12	0.6	220	24	59	0.1	(0)
12	0.5	27	59	36	0.2	(0)
5	0.2	25	32	27	0.2	(0)
163	1.1	607	82	315	0.1	(0)
11	0.2	0	3	10	0.1	(0)
45	1.4	69	66	54	0.5	0
87	0.1	369	29	135	0.1	1
(0)	(0)	(0)	(0)	(0)	(0)	(0)
12	(0)	212	4	16	tr	tr
11	0.5	156	46	26	0.4	1
14	0.7	166	25	29	0.4	5
16	0.6	601	41	26	0.4	2
118	0.8	325	30	128	0.2	(0)
111	0.8	305	63	215	0.2	(0)

varies with the seasons.

Continued.

Table A. Food values—cont'd

	Approximate measure	Calories	Protein (g)	Fat (g)	Carbo-hydrate (g)
Desserts—cont'd					
Pie, lemon meringue	⅙ of medium pie	281	3.8	9.8	45.3
Pie, mince	⅙ of medium pie	398	3.9	10.9	71.8
Pie, pumpkin	⅙ of medium pie	330	6.7	10.7	53.5
Pie, raisin	⅙ of medium pie	437	4.6	12.4	81.2
Sherbet, average	½ cup commercial	118	1.4	0	28.8
Shortcake, biscuit, strawberries	1 cup berries, 1 medium biscuit	399	4.8	8.9	61.2
Pudding, cornstarch, chocolate	½ cup	219	4.5	6.6	37.1
Pudding, cornstarch, vanilla	½ cup	152	4.2	4.7	23.8
Pudding, tapioca, cream	½ cup	133	4.9	5.0	17.3
Eggs					
Egg, cooked, boiled	1 medium	77	6.1	5.5	0.3
Egg, fried	1 medium, 1 tsp margarine	110	6.1	9.2	0.3
Egg, omelet, plain	1 medium	120	6.6	9.8	1.0
Egg, omelet, Spanish	2 eggs, 4 tbs sauce	329	14.6	26.9	7.6
Egg, scrambled	1 medium, 1 tbs milk, 1 tsp fat	120	6.6	9.8	1.0
Fats and oils					
Butter	1 tsp	36	tr	4.1	tr
Butter	1 tbs	100	0.1	11.3	0.1
Dressing, commercial French	1 tbs	59	0.1	5.3	3.0
Dressing, commercial mayonnaise	1 tbs	58	0.2	5.5	2.1
Dressing, homemade French	1 tbs	86	0.0	9.2	0.7
Dressing, homemade mayonnaise	1 tbs	92	0.2	10.1	0.4
Dressing, Thousand Island	1 rounded tbs	98	0.3	10.0	2.4
Margarine	1 tsp	36	tr	4.1	tr
Margarine	1 tbs	100	0.1	11.3	0.1
Fish					
Flounder or sole, baked	¼ lb	204	16.9	20.0	0
Haddock, cooked, fried	1 fillet (3 in × 3 in × ½ in)	214	23.5	9.0	8.1
Halibut steak, cooked	1 serving (4 to 1 lb)	205	21.0	12.2	0
Herring, pickled	2 small	223	20.4	15.1	0

Calcium (mg)	Iron (mg)	Vitamin A (IU)	Thiamin (µg)	Ribo-flavin (µg)	Niacin (mg)	Ascorbic acid (mg)
13	0.5	260	29	52	0.1	1
35	3.4	12	106	55	0.5	1
47	2.0	27	98	53	0.5	(0)
48	0	0	20	70	0	(0)
103	2.2	2278	58	163	0.5	(0)
73	2.0	429	167	207	1.3	(89)
147	0.2	196	45	217	0.2	(0)
144	0.1	195	45	210	0.1	(0)
105	0.5	313	46	186	0.1	1
26	1.3	550	40	130	tr	0
27	1.3	702	40	130	tr	0
44	1.3	726	46	153	tr	0
103	3.4	2008	110	260	1.0	13
44	1.3	726	56	165	tr	0
1	0	165	tr	tr	tr	0
3	0	460	tr	tr	tr	0
tr	tr	0	0	0	0	0
1	0.1	20	tr	tr	(0)	(0)
tr	tr	(0)	(0)	(0)	(0)	0
2	0.1	34	3	3	tr	0
3	0.2	109	9	5	0.1	1
1	0	165	(0)	(0)	(0)	(0)
3	0	460	(0)	(0)	(0)	(0)
69	0.9	—	49	54	1.6	0
44	1.4	139	69	134	2.6	—
15	0.8	497	55	61	8.8	—
22	1.1		—	—	—	0

Continued.

Table A. Food values—cont'd

	Approximate measure	Calories	Protein (g)	Fat (g)	Carbo-hydrate (g)
Fish—cont'd					
Oysters, raw	½ cup (6-9 medium)	100	11.8	2.5	6.7
Oysters, escalloped	1 serving 6 oysters	356	15.9	18.0	31.6
Oysters, fried	6 oysters	412	15.1	29.6	18.2
Salmon, pink	⅔ cup	143	20.5	6.2	0
Salmon, red	⅔ cup	173	20.2	9.6	0
Scallops, fried	5-6 medium	426	23.8	28.4	19.3
Scallops, raw	2-3 (12 to 1 lb)	78	14.8	0.1	3.4
Shrimp, canned	4-6 shrimp	64	13.4	0.7	0
Tuna, canned	⅝ cup solids	198	29.0	8.2	0
Fruits					
Apple, baked, un-pared	1 large, 2 tbs sugar	213	0.6	0.8	64.9
Apple, raw	1 small (2¼ in diameter)	50	0.3	0.4	13.0
Apple, raw	1 large (3 in diameter)	117	0.6	0.8	30.1
Applesauce, canned	½ cup, sweetened	92	0.3	0.2	25.0
Applesauce, canned	½ cup	50	0.3	0.3	13.1
Apricots, raw	2-3 medium	51	1.0	0.1	12.9
Apricots, canned in syrup	4 halves, 2 tbs juice	80	0.6	0.1	21.4
Apricots, canned in water	4 halves	32	0.5	0.1	8.1
Avocado	½ small pear	245	1.7	26.4	5.1
Banana, raw	1 small	88	1.2	0.2	23.0
Banana, raw	1 medium	132	1.8	0.3	34.5
Banana, raw	1 large	176	2.4	0.4	46.0
Blueberries, canned in syrup	½ cup	123	0.5	0.5	32.4
Blueberries, canned in water	½ cup	45	0.5	0.5	10.9
Blueberries, frozen, no sugar	⅝ cup	61	0.6	0.6	15.1
Cantaloupe, diced	½ cup	24	0.7	0.2	5.5
Cherries, canned, sweet, in syrup	½ cup red	105	0.6	0.1	28.5
Cherries, canned in water	½ cup red	51	0.8	0.4	12.6
Cherries, maraschino	1 cherry	19	tr	tr	5.2
Cranberry jelly	1 rounded tbs	47	tr	tr	13.0
Cranberry sauce	1 rounded tbs	40	tr	0.1	10.3
Dates, dried and fresh	3-4 pitted	85	0.6	0.2	22.6
Figs, canned in syrup	3 figs, 2 tbs juice	113	0.8	0.3	30.0
Figs, dried	2 small	81	1.2	0.4	20.5
Fruit cocktail, canned	6 tbs fruit and juice	70	0.4	0.2	18.6

Calcium (mg)	Iron (mg)	Vitamin A (IU)	Thiamin (μg)	Ribo-lavin (μg)	Niacin (mg)	Ascorbic acid (mg)
113	6.7	385	175	240	1.4	—
158	7.0	894	143	277	1.5	0
134	6.4	1539	134	274	1.2	0
187	0.8	70	30	180	8.0	(0)
259	1.2	230	40	160	7.3	(0)
41	3.1	0	91	173	2.3	(0)
26	1.8	0	(40)	100	1.4	—
58	1.6	30	5	15	1.1	(0)
(8)	1.4	80	50	120	12.8	(0)
12	0.6	(180)	40	45	0.3	(2)
5	0.3	80	33	27	0.1	4
12	0.6	180	80	60	0.4	9
5	0.5	40	25	15	0.1	1-2
5	0.5	35	25	10	0.1	1-2
16	0.5	2790	30	50	0.8	7
10	0.3	1350	20	20	0.3	4
10	0.3	1350	20	20	0.3	4
10	0.6	290	60	130	1.1	16
8	0.6	430	40	50	0.7	10
12	0.9	645	60	75	1.0	15
16	1.2	860	80	100	1.4	20
14	0.6	50	15	15	0.3	17
14	0.6	50	15	15	0.3	16
16	0.8	240	20	20	0.3	14
20	0.5	4104	60	48	0.6	40
11	0.3	430	30	20	0.1	3
11	0.3	120	30	20	0.1	3
1	tr	35	(3)	(2)	tr	tr
tr	tr					
(2)	(0.1)	(6)	(4)	(4)	tr	tr
22	0.6	18	27	30	0.7	(0)
35	0.4	50	30	30	0.4	tr
56	0.9	24	48	36	0.5	(0)
9	0.4	160	10	10	0.4	2

Continued.

Table A. Food values—cont'd

	Approximate measure	Calories	Protein (g)	Fat (g)	Carbo-hydrate (g)
Fruits—cont'd					
Grapefruit, raw	½ small	40	0.5	0.2	10.1
Grapefruit, raw	½ large (5 in diameter)	100	1.3	0.5	25.3
Grapes, green seedless	60	66	0.8	0.4	16.7
Grapes, Tokay	22	66	0.8	0.4	16.7
Honeydew melon	¼ of 5 in diameter melon	32	0.5	0	8.5
Lemons, raw	1 medium	32	0.9	0.6	8.7
Limes, raw	1 large	37	0.8	0.1	12.3
Olives, green	1 large	7	0.1	0.7	0.2
Olives, ripe	1 large or 2 small	7	0.1	0.7	0.2
Orange, whole	1 small (2½ in diameter)	45	0.9	0.2	11.2
Orange, whole	1 large (3⅜ in diameter)	106	2.1	0.5	26.3
Orange sections	½ cup	44	0.9	0.2	10.8
Peaches, raw	1 medium large	46	0.5	0.1	12.0
Peaches, raw	1 cup, sliced	77	0.8	0.2	20.2
Peaches, canned in syrup	2 halves, 1 tbs juice	68	0.4	0.1	18.2
Peaches, canned water-pack	2 halves, 2 tbs juice	27	0.5	0.1	6.8
Peaches, frozen	½ cup, scant	78	0.4	0.1	20.2
Pears, raw	1 medium pear	63	0.7	0.4	15.8
Pears, canned in syrup	2 halves, 1 tbs juice	68	0.2	0.1	18.4
Pears, canned in water	2 halves, 1 tbs juice	31	0.3	0.1	8.2
Pineapple, canned in syrup	½ cup, crushed	102	0.5	0.2	27.5
Pineapple, canned in syrup	1 large or 2 small slices, 1 tbs juice	78	0.4	0.1	21.1
Pineapple, canned in juice	1 large or 2 small slices, 2 tbs juice	55	0.5	0.1	14.5
Plums, raw	2 medium	50	0.7	0.2	12.9
Plums, canned in syrup	2 medium, 2 tbs juice	76	0.4	0.1	20.4
Prunes, dried, raw	3 medium or 4 small	67	0.6	0.2	17.8
Prunes, cooked, no sugar	4 medium, 2 tbs juice	86	0.7	0.2	22.7
Prunes, cooked, with sugar	4 medium, 2 tbs juice	119	0.7	0.2	31.2
Raisins, dried	1 tbs	27	0.2	0.1	7.2
Raisins, dried	1 cup	429	3.7	0.8	113.9

Calcium (mg)	Iron (mg)	Vitamin A (IU)	Thiamin (µg)	Ribo-flavin (µg)	Niacin (mg)	Ascorbic acid (mg)
22	0.2	tr	40	20	0.2	40
55	0.5	tr	100	50	0.5	100
17	0.6	80	60	40	0.2	4
17	0.6	80	60	40	0.2	4
(17)	(0.4)	40	50	30	0.2	23
40	0.6	0	40	tr	0.1	50
(40)	0.6	0	(40)	tr	(0.1)	27
5	0.1	16	tr	—	—	—
5	0.1	3	tr	tr	—	—
33	0.4	(190)	80	30	0.2	49
78	0.9	(447)	188	71	0.5	115
32	0.4	(180)	75	25	0.3	48
8	0.6	880	20	50	0.9	8
13	1.0	1478	34	84	1.5	13
5	0.4	450	10	20	0.7	4
5	0.4	450	10	20	0.7	4
6	0.4	520	10	30	0.5	4
13	0.3	20	20	40	0.1	4
8	0.2	tr	10	20	0.1	2
8	0.2	tr	10	20	0.1	2
38	0.8	105	100	20	0.2	12
29	0.6	80	70	20	0.2	9
29	0.6	80	70	20	0.2	9
17	0.5	350	60	40	0.5	5
8	1.1	230	30	30	0.4	1
14	1.0	473	25	40	0.2	tr
17	1.3	545	22	45	0.4	tr
17	1.3	545	22	45	0.4	tr
8	0.3	5	15	8	0.1	—'
125	5.3	80	240	130	0.8	tr

Continued.

Table A. Food values—cont'd

	Approximate measure	Calories	Protein (g)	Fat (g)	Carbo-hydrate (g)
Fruits—cont'd					
Raspberries, black, raw	⅔ cup	74	1.5	1.6	15.7
Raspberries, red, raw	¾ cup	57	1.2	0.4	13.8
Rhubarb, cooked, sweetened	½ cup fruit and syrup	137	0.3	0.1	35.1
Strawberries, raw	10 large	37	0.8	0.5	8.3
Strawberries, frozen, sweetened	½ cup, scant	106	0.6	0.4	26.6
Watermelon	½ cup cubes	28	0.5	0.2	6.9
Watermelon	1 slice (6 in diameter, 1½ in thick)	168	3.0	1.2	41.4
Fruit juices					
Apple juice, canned	2 tbs	16	0.03	0	4.3
Apple juice, canned	3 fl oz	48	0.1	0	13.8
Apricot juice	3 fl oz	44	0.5	0.4	10.2
Grape juice, commercial	3 fl oz	67	0.4	0	18.2
Grapefruit juice, fresh	3¼ fl oz	36	0.5	0.1	9.2
Grapefruit juice, canned	3¼ fl oz sweetened	52	0.5	0.1	13.7
Grapefruit juice, canned	3¼ fl oz	38	0.5	0.1	9.8
Lemon juice, fresh	1 tbs	4	0.1	tr	1.2
Orange juice, fresh	3¼ fl oz	44	0.8	0.2	11.0
Orange juice, canned	3¼ fl oz sweetened	54	0.6	0.2	13.9
Orange juice, canned	3⅛ fl oz	44	0.8	0.2	11.1
Pineapple juice, canned	3¼ fl oz	49	0.3	0.1	13.0
Prune juice, canned	3 fl oz	63	0.3	0	17.4
Tomato juice, canned	3 fl oz	21	0.9	0.2	4.3
Meats					
Bacon	1 strip, drained (6 in)	48	1.8	4.4	0.2
Bacon, Canadian, cooked	1 slice (2¼ in diameter, ³⁄₁₆ in thick)	57	6.6	3.1	0.1
Beef brisket, cooked	3 pieces (2 in × 1 in × 1 in)	338	15.8	30.0	0
Beef, chuck, pot roast	1 slice (2 in × 1½ in × ½ in)	93	7.8	6.6	0
Beef, hamburger, average cooked	1 small patty (2 oz)	118	12.9	7.1	0
Beef, hamburger, average cooked	1 medium patty (5 to 1 lb)	246	14.6	20.4	0

*Calcium may not be available because of high oxalic acid content.

Calcium (mg)	Iron (mg)	Vitamin A (IU)	Thiamin (μg)	Ribo-flavin (μg)	Niacin (mg)	Ascorbic acid (mg)
40	0.9	0	20	(70)	(0.3)	(24)
40	0.9	130	20	(70)	(0.3)	24
26*	0.2	16	2	—	tr	2
28	0.8	60	30	70	0.3	60
22	0.6	40	20	50	0.2	41
7	0.2	590	50	50	0.2	6
42	1.2	3540	300	300	1.2	36
2	0.2	12	6	9	tr	tr
6	0.5	40	20	30	tr	1
10	0.3	—	40	50	0.2	tr
8	0.3	tr	40	20	0.2	40
8	0.3	tr	30	20	0.2	35
8	0.3	tr	30	20	0.2	35
2	tr	0	6	tr	tr	8
19	0.2	(190)	80	30	0.2	49
10	0.3	(100)	70	20	0.2	42
10	0.3	(100)	70	20	0.2	42
15	0.5	80	50	20	0.2	9
(24)	(1.5)	—	27	72	0.3	tr
(6)	(0.3)	978	48	27	0.6	15
3	0.2	(0)	40	22	0.3	0
4	1.0	(0)	164	67	1.4	0
0	2.4	(0)	100	130	4.4	0
3	0.9	(0)	15	60	1.2	0
7	1.9	(0)	38	102	2.6	0
8	2.2	0	43	115	3.0	0

Continued.

Table A. Food values—cont'd

	Approximate measure	Calories	Protein (g)	Fat (g)	Carbo-hydrate (g)
Meats—cont'd					
Beef, hamburger, average cooked	1 large patty (4 to 1 lb)	300	18.2	24.6	0
Beef, hamburger on bun	1 average, plain	332	17.1	21.9	15.4
Beef, porterhouse, broiled	1 large steak with gravy (5 oz)	513	34.5	40.5	0
Beef, rib, roasted	1 slice (3 in × 2¼ in × ¼ in)	96	7.2	7.2	0
Beef, round, cubed, cooked	1 piece, 3 oz (4 in × 3 in × ⅜ in)	214	24.7	12.0	0
Beef, rump, pot roast	1 slice (5 in × 3½ in × ¼ in)	320	17.8	27.2	0
Beef steak, club broiled	1 large (4 oz)	410	27.6	32.4	0
Beef stew with potatoes, carrots, onions, gravy	3 oz chuck, 2 small potatoes, 1 small carrot, 1 onion	529	28.1	19.6	56.1
Beef tongue, medium cooked	3 slices, 2 oz (3 in × 2 in × ⅛ in)	160	11.6	12.2	0.2
Chili con carne (no beans)	½ cup, scant, 60% meat	200	10.3	14.8	5.8
Frankfurter, cooked	1 average (5½ in long × ¾ in diameter)	124	7.0	10.0	1.0
Ham, smoked, cooked	1 slice, 1 oz (4 in × 2½ in × ⅛ in)	119	6.9	9.9	(0.1)
Lamb chop, rib, cooked	1 chop	128	7.9	(10.5)	0
Lamb, ground, cooked	1 patty, 2 oz (2 in diameter, ½ in thick)	130	8.2	10.5	0
Lamb, leg, roasted	1 slice, 1 oz (3 in × 2¾ in × ⅛ in)	82	7.2	5.7	0
Liver, beef, fried	1 slice, 1½ oz (3 in × 2¼ in × ⅜ in)	86	8.8	2.9	5.6
Liver, calf, cooked	1 slice, 1⅓ oz (3 in × 2¼ in × ⅜ in)	74	8.8	3.6	1.0
Liver, chicken, cooked	1 medium large liver	74	8.8	3.6	1.0
Meat loaf, beef and pork	1 slice, 2⅓ oz (4 in × 3 in × ⅜ in)	264	10.4	19.2	11.5
Meat gravy	1 tbs	41	0.3	3.5	2.0
Pork chop, loin, fried	1 medium (2⅓ oz)	233	16.1	18.2	0
Pork, loin, roasted	1 slice, 1 oz (3 in × 2½ in × ¼ in)	100	6.9	7.8	0
Pork, spareribs, roasted	Meat from 6 average ribs (3 oz)	246	15.4	(20.0)	0
Veal chop, loin, fried	1 medium (3 oz)	186	21.8	9.4	0

Calcium (mg)	Iron (mg)	Vitamin A (IU)	Thiamin (μg)	Ribo-flavin (μg)	Niacin (mg)	Ascorbic acid (mg)
11	2.7	0	54	144	3.7	0
23	2.4	0	63	145	3.3	0
17	4.5	(0)	90	270	7.1	0
3	0.9	(0)	18	54	1.9	0
10	3.1	(0)	74	202	5.1	0
7	2.1	(0)	34	128	2.6	0
13	3.6	(0)	72	216	5.6	0
86	5.0	5590	255	280	5.5	(20)
4	(1.5)	(0)	(30)	(130)	(1.5)	0
38	1.4	150	20	120	2.2	0
3	0.6	(0)	80	90	1.2	0
3	0.9	(0)	162	63	1.3	0
4	1.1	(0)	45	80	1.9	0
4	1.0	(0)	85	150	2.7	0
3	0.9	(0)	42	75	1.5	0
4	2.9	18658	90	1283	5.1	(10)
3	4.5	9565	63	1193	5.9	(8)
6	3.0	12880	56	886	4.7	(4)
26	1.7	50	118	111	2.0	(0)
tr	(0.1)	0	(10)	(7)	tr	—
8	2.1	(0)	580	168	3.5	(0)
3	0.9	(0)	249	72	1.5	0
8	2.2	(0)	400	150	2.8	0
10	3.0	(0)	110	265	6.7	0

Continued.

Table A. Food values—cont'd

	Approximate measure	Calories	Protein (g)	Fat (g)	Carbo-hydrate (g)
Meats—cont'd					
Veal cutlet, breaded, baked	1 average serving, 3 oz	217	23.8	9.4	8.0
Veal, leg, roasted	1 slice, 1 oz (3 in × 2 in × ⅛ in)	70	8.4	3.8	0
Veal, stew, carrots, onions	½ cup	121	8.8	7.8	3.6
Sausages					
Bologna	1 slice, 1 oz (4½-in diameter, ⅛ in thick)	66	4.4	4.8	1.1
Liver sausage	1 slice, 1 oz (3 in diameter, ¼ in thick)	79	5.0	6.2	0.5
Luncheon meat	1 slice (1 oz)	81	4.6	6.8	0.5
Salami	1 slice, 1 oz (3¾ in diameter, ¼ in thick)	130	7.2	11.0	0
Nuts					
Almonds, chocolate	5 medium	84	2.0	6.9	5.1
Cashew nuts, roasted	6 to 8 nuts	88	2.8	7.2	4.1
Coconut, shredded, dried	2 tbs	83	0.5	5.9	8.0
Peanut butter	1 tbs, scant	86	4.0	7.2	3.2
Peanuts, roasted	15 to 17 nuts	84	4.0	6.6	3.5
Pecans, shelled	12 halves or 2 tbs, chopped	104	1.4	11.0	2.0
Poultry					
Chicken, broiler, fried	¼ chicken, no bone	232	22.4	13.6	3.1
Chicken, canned	⅓ cup boned meat	169	25.	6.8	0
Chicken, creamed	½ cup, scant	208	17.6	12.1	6.6
Chicken, fryer, fried	½ breast (4 oz raw)	232	26.8	11.9	3.1
Chicken, fryer, leg, fried	1 small leg	64	10.5	5.3	1.5
Chicken, hen, stewed	1 medium thigh or ½ breast	207	26.5	10.4	0
Chicken pie with peas, potatoes	2 in square serving 4 oz)	230	9.6	12.1	20.2
Chicken, roasted	3 slices (3½ in × 2½ in × ¼ in)	198	28.3	(8.6)	0
Duck, roasted	3 slices (3½ in × 3 in × ¼ in)	310	22.8	23.6	0
Goose	3 slices (3½ in × 3 in × ¼ in)	322	28.1	22.4	0
Turkey	3 slices (3½ in × 2½ in × ¼ in)	200	30.9	(7.6)	0

Calcium (mg)	Iron (mg)	Vitamin A (IU)	Thiamin (μg)	Ribo-flavin (μg)	Niacin (mg)	Ascorbic acid (mg)
22	3.0	(0)	102	256	6.5	0
4	1.1	(0)	40	95	2.4	0
16	1.5	1627	34	83	1.5	(0)
(3)	1.6	(0)	54	57	0.8	0
3	1.6	1725	51	36	1.4	(0)
6	0.4	(0)	110	54	1.1	(0)
4	1.1	(0)	75	63	0.9	0
28	0.5	0	(27)	(75)	(0.5)	tr
7	0.8	—	95	29	0.3	0
6	0.5	0	tr	tr	tr	(0)
11	0.3	0	18	20	2.4	(0)
11	0.3	0	45	20	2.4	(0)
11	0.4	8	108	17	0.1	tr
18	1.8	230	74	168	9.7	(0)
12	1.5	(0)	32	136	5.4	0
83	1.1	328	(40)	180	3.8	tr
19	1.3	460	67	101	10.2	0
9	1.0	161	43	113	2.4	0
16	1.6	(0)	52	150	6.0	(0)
19	1.2	143	87	68	2.3	(6)
20	2.1	(0)	80	180	9.0	(0)
19	5.8	(0)				
10	4.6	(0)				
30	5.1	0-20	81	173	9.8	0

Continued.

Table A. Food values—cont'd

	Approximate measure	Calories	Protein (g)	Fat (g)	Carbo-hydrate (g)
Salads					
Cabbage slaw	⅔ cup	68	2.3	3.5	7.9
Carrot and raisin	3 heaping tbs, lettuce leaf	153	1.9	5.8	27.9
Chicken with celery	½ cup, lettuce leaf	185	16.1	10.9	5.7
Gelatin with chopped vegetables	1 square, ¼ head lettuce	115	2.2	5.7	15.1
Gelatin with fruit	1 square, ¼ head lettuce	139	2.1	5.7	21.6
Lettuce with French dressing	1 wedge	133	1.4	10.8	6.9
Potato with onion, parsley	½ cup potato with French dressing	184	1.9	10.8	21.2
Prunes, stuffed with peanut butter	4 prunes	414	13.4	28.5	32.9
Sandwiches					
Bacon, lettuce, and tomato	1 sandwich	282	6.3	15.6	28.8
Chicken, hot with gravy	1 sandwich, 3 tbs gravy	356	21.9	15.3	29.8
Chicken salad	1 sandwich	245	14.3	8.6	26.6
Chicken, sliced, lettuce	1 sandwich	303	15.8	14.4	26.6
Club (bacon, chicken, and tomato)	1 average, 3 slices toast, lettuce	590	35.6	20.8	41.7
Cream cheese and jelly	1 sandwich	368	6.6	16.0	50.4
Egg salad on white bread	1 average	279	10.5	12.5	30.6
Peanut butter	1 average	328	11.8	19.5	30.0
Roast beef, hot with gravy	1 average, 3 tbs gravy	429	19.3	24.5	29.8
Tuna fish salad	1 average, white bread	278	11.0	14.2	25.8
Soups					
Asparagus, cream (Campbell's)	⅞ cup (3 to 1 can)	131	5.9	6.4	12.8
Bean, homemade	¾ cup	195	6.1	11	18.6
Beef, noodle (Campbell's)	⅞ cup	52	3.3	2.4	4.5
Celery, cream (Campbell's)	⅞ cup	146	4.9	8.6	12.2
Chicken, cream (Campbell's)	⅞ cup	145	6.5	9.9	7.7
Chicken, gumbo (Campbell's)	⅞ cup	51	1.9	0.9	8.8

Calcium (mg)	Iron (mg)	Vitamin A (IU)	Thiamin (μg)	Ribo-flavin (μg)	Niacin (mg)	Ascorbic acid (mg)
53	0.5	200	50	85	0.2	(12)
48	1.5	4708	83	81	0.5	(6)
32	1.3	290	53	130	3.4	(5)
24	0.5	1977	37	58	0.3	(8)
23	0.5	391	42	50	0.3	16
22	0.5	540	40	80	0.2	8
21	0.8	243	70	38	0.8	(16)
63	2.3	800	110	140	7.9	5
53	1.5	870	160	142	1.6	13
49	2.4	(0)	178	209	6.5	0
50	1.5	10	142	140	3.2	1
52	1.8	320	162	172	4.6	2
103	4.3	1705	384	410	10.2	27
60	1.1	575	120	140	1.0	2
68	2.4	580	160	210	1.0	2
61	1.0	165	96	80	5.4	(0)
43	2.9	(0)	166	209	4.9	(0)
48	1.2	231	142	113	4.1	1
(126)	(0.1)	(171)	(40)	(182)	(0.1)	(1)
52	1.9	1364	120	70	0.5	(0)
(126)	(0.1)	(171)	(40)	(182)	(0.1)	(1)
(126)	(0.1)	(171)	(43)	(182)	(0.1)	(1)

Continued.

Table A. Food values—cont'd

	Approximate measure	Calories	Protein (g)	Fat (g)	Carbo-hydrate (g)
Soups—cont'd					
Chicken, noodle (Campbell's)	⅞ cup	56	3.1	19.0	6.6
Chicken, rice (Campbell's)	⅞ cup	36	2.7	1.3	3.5
Clam chowder (Campbell's)	⅞ cup	64	2.2	2.4	8.3
Green pea (Campbell's)	⅞ cup	110	5.4	1.9	17.9
Oyster stew, home-made	1 serving, 8 oz milk, 4 oysters	321	15.0	22.2	15.7
Scotch broth (Campbell's)	⅞ cup	96	5.8	2.8	11.8
Split pea, homemade	1 serving, ¾ cup	201	7.1	11.1	19.4
Tomato (Campbell's)	⅞ cup	141	5.6	6.1	15.9
Vegetable (Campbell's)	⅞ cup	68	2.9	1.5	10.9
Vegetable, beef (Campbell's)	⅞ cup	77	5.9	2.1	7.9
Syrups and sugars					
Honey, strained	1 tbs	62	0.1	0	16.7
Molasses	1 tbs	50	—	0	13.0
Sorghum syrup	1 tbs	52	—	0	13.4
Sugar, brown	1 tbs	52	(0)	0	13.4
Sugar, powdered	1 tbs	42	(0)	0	10.9
Sugar, white, granulated	1 tbs	48	(0)	0	12.4
Sweets					
Caramels, plain	1 medium	42	0.3	1.2	7.8
Chocolate creams	1 average (35 to 1 lb)	51	0.5	1.8	9.4
Chocolate fudge, milk	1 piece 1¼ in square (15 to 1 lb)	118	0.5	3.1	23.7
Chocolate mints	1 medium (20 to 1 lb)	87	0.9	3.1	15.8
Gumdrops	1 large or 8 small	33	0	0	8.6
Hershey's milk chocolate	1 bar, plain, small (1 oz)	154	2.4	9.5	15.8
Hershey's Mr. Good-bar	1 bar	158	4.2	10.4	12.9
Jelly beans	10 jelly beans	66	0	0	16.7
Mars, Candy Bar	1 bar, 1⅜ oz	177	2.4	8.3	24.2
Mars, Forever Yours	1 bar	122	1.1	1.6	26.7
Mars, Milky Way	1 bar	121	1.2	2.0	24.8
Mars, Snickers	1 bar	122	1.9	3.0	22.8

Calcium (mg)	Iron (mg)	Vitamin A (IU)	Thiamin (μg)	Ribo-flavin (μg)	Niacin (mg)	Ascorbic acid (mg)
352	3.8	1058	188	550	1.1	(3)
44	1.6	1446	139	81	1.0	(2)
(126)	(0.1)	(171)	(43)	(182)	(0.1)	(1)
1	0.2	(0)	tr	10	tr	1
33	0.9	—	14	12	tr	—
30	2.4	—	—	—	—	—
11	0.4	(0)	(0)	(0)	(0)	(0)
—	—	(0)	(0)	(0)	(0)	(0)
—	—	(0)	(0)	(0)	(0)	(0)
13	0.2	17	2	14	tr	tr
—	—	—	—	—	—	—
14	0.2	64	3	19	tr	tr
—	—	—	—	—	—	—
(0)	(0)	0	0	0	0	0
57	0.7	43	27	145	0.1	tr
34	0.5	36	47	72	2.0	tr
52	0.4	0	17	121	0.27	tr
22	0.2	0	15	53	0.14	tr
29	0.2	0	15	107	0.13	tr
27	0.1	0	10	102	0.08	tr

Continued.

Table A. Food values—cont'd

	Approximate measure	Calories	Protein (g)	Fat (g)	Carbo-hydrate (g)
Sweets—cont'd					
Mars, Three Muske-teers	1 bar	147	0.8	0.9	35.1
Marshmallow, plain	1 average (60 to 1 lb)	25	0.2	0	6.2
Mints, cream	10 mints (½ in cubes)	53	0	0	13.7
Peanut brittle	1 piece (2½ in × 2½ in × ⅜ in)	110	2.1	3.9	18.2
Preserves and jellies					
Assorted jams, commercial	1 tbs	55	0.1	0.1	14.2
Assorted jellies	1 tbs	50	0	0	13.0
Vegetables					
Asparagus, canned, green	6 medium stalks	21	2.4	0.2	3.9
Beans, dry with pork and tomato sauce	½ cup	147	7.5	2.7	24.0
Beans, green limas, cooked	½ cup	76	4.0	0.3	14.7
Beans, green limas, frozen	½ cup	109	6.4	0.7	19.9
Beans, green, canned	1 cup	27	1.8	0.2	5.9
Beans, green, frozen	½ cup	35	2.4	0.2	7.7
Beans, yellow, canned	1 cup	27	1.8	0.2	5.9
Beets, canned	½ cup	34	0.8	0.1	8.1
Broccoli, cooked	⅔ cup	29	3.3	0.2	5.5
Brussels sprouts, cooked	½ cup (5-6)	33	3.1	0.4	6.2
Cabbage, raw	½ cup	12	0.7	0.1	2.7
Cabbage, cooked	½ cup	20	1.2	0.2	4.5
Carrots, cooked	½ cup	35	0.6	0.5	7.5
Cauliflower, cooked	½ cup	15	1.5	0.1	3.0
Celery, raw	1 large outer stalk (8 in long)	7	0.5	0.1	1.5
Celery, raw	1 cup, diced	18	1.3	0.2	3.7
Celery, cooked	½ cup	12	0.9	0.2	2.4
Corn, canned	½ cup	70	2.3	0.6	16.7
Cucumber, raw	½ medium (6-8 slices)	6	0.4	0	1.4
Garlic bulbs, peeled	5 bulbs	9	0.4	tr	2.0
Kale, cooked	½ cup	20	2.0	0.3	3.6
Lettuce wedge	Small	15	1.0	0.3	2.7
Mushroom, fresh	10 small or 4 large	16	2.4	0.3	4.0
Mushroom, canned	½ cup	14	1.7	0.3	4.5
Parsley, raw	10 small sprigs	5	0.4	0.1	0.9

*Calcium may not be available because of presence of oxalic acid.

Calcium (mg)	Iron (mg)	Vitamin A (IU)	Thiamin (µg)	Ribo-flavin (µg)	Niacin (mg)	Ascorbic acid (mg)
15	0.2	0	6	43	0.04	tr
(0)	(0)	(0)	(0)	(0)	0	0
10	0.5	7	22	12	1.2	0
2	0.1	2	4	4	0.04	1
(2)	(0.1)	(2)	(4)	(4)	(0.04)	1
23	2.1	760	90	120	1.1	18
53	2.3	110	165	45	0.6	3
23	1.4	230	110	70	0.9	12
53	1.9	220	100	70	0.8	17
45	2.1	620	40	70	0.5	7
65	1.1	450	70	100	0.6	11
45	2.1	150	40	70	0.5	7
18	0.6	15	15	35	0.2	5
130	1.3	3400	70	150	0.8	74
24	0.9	280	28	84	0.4	33
23	0.3	40	30	25	0.2	25
39	0.4	75	40	40	0.3	27
27	0.8	14,760	30	25	0.4	3
13	0.7	54	35	50	0.3	17
20	0.2	0	20	20	0.2	3
50	0.5	0	50	40	0.4	7
33	0.3	0	25	20	0.2	3
4	0.5	190	30	50	0.8	5
5	0.2	0	20	20	0.1	4
1	0.2	—	—	—	—	3
113	1.1	4190	35	115	0.9	26
22	0.5	540	40	80	0.2	8
9	1.0	0	100	440	4.9	5
(9)	(1.0)	0	20	300	2.4	(0)
19*	0.4	823	11	28	0.1	19

Continued.

Table A. Food values—cont'd

	Approximate measure	Calories	Protein (g)	Fat (g)	Carbo-hydrate (g)
Vegetables—cont'd					
Parsnips, cooked	½ cup	47	0.8	0.4	10.7
Peas, green, cooked	½ cup	73	3.6	0.5	13.8
Pepper, shell, baked	1 shell, no filling	`17	0.8	0.1	3.9
Peppers, green, raw	1 tbs chopped	3	0.1	tr	0.6
Pickles, sour	1 large (4 in diameter × 1¾ in)	15	0.7	0.3	3.0
Pickles, sweet	1 pickle (2 in × ⅝ in)	11	0.1	tr	2.6
Pimento, canned	1 medium	9	0.3	0.2	2.0
Potatoes, white, baked	1 medium (2½ in diameter)	98	2.4	0.1	22.5
Potatoes, white, boiled	1 medium (2¼ in diameter)	83	2.0	0.1	19.1
Potatoes, white, french fried	10 pieces (2 in × ½ in × ½ in)	197	2.7	9.6	26.0
Potatoes, white, mashed with milk and margarine	½ cup	123	2.1	6.0	15.9
Potato chips	10 pieces (2 in diameter)	108	1.3	7.4	9.8
Radish, red, raw	1 small	2	0.1	tr	0.4
Sauerkraut, canned	⅔ cup	22	1.4	0.3	4.4
Spinach	½ cup	23	2.8	0.6	3.3
Squash, summer, cooked	½ cup, scant	16	0.6	0.1	3.9
Squash, winter, baked	½ cup	47	1.9	0.4	11.0
Sweet potatoes, baked	1 medium, peeled (5 in × 2 in)	183	2.6	1.1	41.3
Sweet potatoes, candied	1 half (3¾ in × 2¼ in)	358	3.0	7.2	72.4
Tomato catsup	1 tbs	17	0.3	0.1	4.2
Tomatoes, canned	½ cup	23	1.2	0.2	4.7
Tomatoes, raw	1 small	20	1.0	0.3	4.0
Miscellaneous					
Cocoa, dry	1 tbs	21	(0.6)	1.7	3.4
Cornstarch	1 tbs	29	0	0	7.0
Gelatin, dry, plain	1 tbs	34	8.6	0	0
Postum	1 tsb	4	0.06	tr	0.8
Tapioca	1 tbs	36	0.06	tr	8.6
Alcoholic beverages†				Alcoholic grams	
Beer, average	8 oz	112	1.4	8.9	10.6

*Calcium may not be available because of presence of oxalic acid.
†Calories in the alcoholic beverages are derived from the alcohol content.

Calcium (mg)	Iron (mg)	Vitamin A (IU)	Thiamin (μg)	Ribo-flavin (μg)	Niacin (mg)	Ascorbic acid (mg)
44	0.6	0	45	80	0.1	10
20	1.7	535	95	50	0.8	8
7	0.3	481	26	46	0.3	64
1	tr	63	4	7	tr	12
34	1.6	420	tr	90	tr	8
2	0.1	11	(0)	2	tr	1
2	0.5	805	7	21	0.1	33
13	0.8	20	110	50	1.4	17
11	0.7	20	90	30	1.0	14
15	1.0	25	90	55	1.7	14
37	0.6	260	80	50	0.8	7
(6)	(0.4)	(10)	(40)	(20)	(0.6)	2
4	0.1	3	3	2	tr	8
36	(0.5)	40	30	60	0.1	16
111*	1.8	10600	70	180	0.6	27
15	0.4	260	40	70	0.6	11
24	0.8	6190	50	150	0.6	7
44	1.1	11410	120	80	0.9	28
72	1.8	12500	80	80	1.0	18
2	0.1	(320)	15	12	0.4	2
(13)	0.7	1260	72	36	0.8	19
11	0.6	1100	60	40	0.5	23
9*	0.8	2	8	27	0.2	(0)
(0)	(0)	(0)	(0)	(0)	(0)	(0)
(0)	(0)	(0)	(0)	(0)	(0)	(0)
1	tr	—	—	—	—	—
1	0.1	(0)	(0)	(0)	(0)	(0)
10	0.0	(0)	tr	72	0.5	0

Continued.

Table A. Food values—cont'd

	Approximate measure	Calories	Protein (g)	Fat (g)	Carbo-hydrate (g)
Alcoholic beverages —cont'd					
Eggnog, Christmas type	1 punch cup	335	3.9	15.0	18.0
Gin, dry	1 jigger (1½ oz)	105	—	15.1	
Highball	1 glass	166	—	24.0	
Manhattan	1 cocktail	164	tr	19.2	7.9
Martini	1 cocktail	140	0.1	18.5	0.3
Old-fashioned	1 glass	179	—	24.0	3.5
Rum	1 jigger (1½ oz)	105	—	15.1	0
Tom Collins	1 cocktail	180	—	21.5	9.0
Whiskey, bourbon	1 jigger (1½ oz)	119	—	17.2	0
Whiskey, Scotch	1 jigger (1½ oz)	105	—	15.1	0
Wine, California, red	1 wine glass (3⅓ oz)	72	0.2	10.0	0.5
Wine, port	1 wine glass (3⅓ oz)	158	0.2	15.0	14.0

Table B. Estimated safe and adequate daily dietary intakes of additional selected

	Age (yr)	Vitamins			Trace elements†	
		Vitamin K (μg)	Biotin (μg)	Pantothenic acid (mg)	Copper (mg)	Manganese (mg)
Infants	0-0.5	12	35	2	0.5-0.7	0.5-0.7
	0.5-1	10-20	50	3	0.7-1.0	0.7-1.0
Children and	1-3	15-30	65	3	1.0-1.5	1.0-1.5
	4-6	20-40	85	3-4	1.5-2.0	1.5-2.0
Adolescents	7-10	30-60	120	4-5	2.0-2.5	2.0-3.0
	11+	50-100	100-200	4-7	2.0-3.0	2.5-5.0
Adults		70-140	100-200	4-7	2.0-3.0	2.5-5.0

*Because there is less information on which to base allowances, these figures are not given in the main Nutrition Board, National Academy of Sciences–National Research Council; Recommended dietary al-
†Since the toxic levels for many trace elements may be only several times usual intakes, the upper levels

Calcium (mg)	Iron (mg)	Vitamin A (IU)	Thiamin (µg)	Ribo-flavin (µg)	Niacin (mg)	Ascorbic acid (mg)
44	0.7	01	35	113	tr	tr
—	—	—	—	—	—	—
—	—	—	—	—	—	—
1	tr	35	3	2	tr	(0)
5	0.1	4	tr	tr	tr	(0)
—	—	—	—	—	—	—
—	—	—	—	—	—	—
—	—	—	—	—	—	—
—	—	—	—	—	—	—
—	—	—	—	—	—	—

vitamins and minerals*

	Trace elements†			Electrolytes		
Fluoride (mg)	Chromium (mg)	Selenium (mg)	Molybdenum (mg)	Sodium (mg)	Potassium (mg)	Chloride (mg)
0.1-0.5	0.01-0.04	0.01-0.04	0.03-0.06	115-350	350-925	275-700
0.2-1.0	0.02-0.06	0.02-0.06	0.04-0.08	250-750	425-1275	400-1200
0.5-1.5	0.02-0.08	0.02-0.08	0.05-0.1	325-975	550-1650	500-1500
1.0-2.5	0.03-0.12	0.03-0.12	0.06-0.15	450-1350	775-2325	700-2100
1.5-2.5	0.05-0.2	0.05-0.2	0.1-0.3	600-1800	1000-3000	925-2775
1.5-2.5	0.05-0.2	0.05-0.2	0.15-0.5	900-2700	1525-4575	1400-4200
1.5-4.0	0.05-0.2	0.05-0.2	0.15-0.5.	1100-3300	1875-5625	1700-5100

table of the RDA and are provided here in the form of ranges of recommended intakes. From Food and lowances, Washington, D.C., rev. 1980, The Academy.
for the trace elements given in this table should not be habitually exceeded.

Glossary

Nutrition

absorption process by which food is transferred from the digestive system to the blood.

accelerate to increase the speed.

accessory something joined to or added to another product but not essentially a part of it.

acid-base balance a balance between the acid and basic elements caused partly by the balance between the intake of foods that leave an acid ash and those that leave an alkaline ash in the body.

acidosis an abnormal state in which the blood and body tissues become excessively acid.

additives elements that are added to a natural food.

adolescence the period between childhood and maturity.

alkaline medium a medium that is alkaline, as opposed to an acid medium.

amenities acceptable social behavior.

atherosclerosis fat deposits in the walls of the arteries, usually in older persons.

bacteria one-cell vegetable microorganisms concerned with fermentation and putrefaction.

basal metabolism the minimal amount or number of calories needed to support the basic metabolic processes of a person at rest and 12 hours after taking food.

biological value how useful a nutrient is to the body for maintenance or growth.

calorie, large the amount of heat required to raise 1 kg of water 1° C; the calorie of this unit value is used in all the discussions and calculations in this text.

capillary minute blood vessel carrying blood and forming a part of the capillary system.

caries decay of bone or tooth tissue.

cartilage a translucent elastic tissue commonly called a gristle.

cell a small mass of protoplasm bounded externally by a semipermeable membrane.

cellular debris waste matter resulting from the breakdown of cells.

choline a decomposition product of lecithin essential for functioning of the liver.

colon the large intestine from the cecum to the rectum.

compound a substance composed of definite proportions of two or more elements.

The following were used as references: Webster's New International Dictionary of the English Language (unabridged), ed. 2, Springfield, Mass., 1950, G & C Merriam Co.; Webster's New Collegiate Dictionary, Springfield, Mass., 1959, G & C Merriam Co.; Dorland's Illustrated Medical Dictionary, ed. 26, Philadelphia, 1981, W.B. Saunders Co.

concentrate condensed amount of certain nutrients.

condiment an ingredient added to food to enhance the flavor of the food.

conjunctivitis inflammation of the mucous membrane that lines the eyelids and covers the exposed surface of the eyeball.

contamination the process of rendering food or water unfit for use.

cortisone a hormone from the adrenal cortex.

creatine a colorless, crystalline substance that can be isolated from various animal organs and body fluids.

culture a medium prepared in the laboratory in which to grow microorganisms.

deficiency disease a disease caused by the lack of essential constitutents in the diet or by defective metabolism.

duodenum the first part of the small intestine.

emulsified the combination of two liquids not mutually soluble.

endocrine pertaining to a gland that produces an internal secretion.

enzyme a chemical substance that acts on other substances and accelerates the specific chemical reaction but does not itself become a part of the final product.

facilitate to make less difficult.

fetal pertaining to the product of conception during the last 6 months of pregnancy.

fortified foods foods with additions made to give increased nutritional value.

geriatrics study and treatment of the diseases of old age.

glycogen the form in which carbohydrate is stored in the animal body for future conversion into sugar and for subsequent use in performing muscular work or for liberating heat.

grams (g) 28.3 grams equal 1 ounce; for practical purposes in calculating diets, 30 grams are considered equal to 1 ounce.

granule a small grainlike body.

homogenize a process that breaks up the fat globules in milk.

hormone a chemical substance that originates in a specific organ or gland in the body and is conveyed through the blood to another part of the body, stimulating it to activity.

hypoglycemia deficiency of sugar in the blood.

insecticide an agent or preparation for killing insects.

lacteal an intestinal lymphatic that conveys the chyle to the lymph circulation.

lubricant an agent that produces smoothness.

malformation abnormal shape or structure.

mammary pertaining to the breast.

metabolism the changes that foods undergo after absorption from the digestive tract.

milligram (mg) $\frac{1}{1000}$ of a gram.

molecule the smallest quantity into which a substance may be divided without the loss of its characteristics.

mucus a viscid fluid secreted by mucous membranes and glands.

nonconductor a substance that does not transmit heat or electricity.
nutrients foods that supply the body with necessary elements.

optimum amounts amounts producing the best results.
organic pertaining to the internal organs of the body.
oxidation process by which a substance is combined with oxygen.
oxytocin a postpituitary hormone that stimulates uterine contraction after delivery of the placenta, avoiding postpartum hemorrhage.

pasteurized the partial sterilization of a fluid by heating it at 144° to 149° F, which destroys certain organisms and undesirable bacteria that could produce disease, without destroying the chemical composition of the fluid.
pathological caused by a disease.
pellagra a deficiency disease caused by improper diet and characterized by skin lesions, gastrointestinal tract disturbances, and nervousness.
peristalsis rhythmic contractions of the alimentary canal.
physiologist one versed in the study of the functions of the organs of the body.
plasma the liquid part of the lymph and blood.

quacks those who pretend a knowledge they do not possess.

radiation the discharge of rays in all directions from a common center.

seborrheic afflicted with abnormal discharge of sebum from the glands of the skin.
senile physiological deterioration accompanying the aging process, especially loss of mental faculties in old age.
specific anything especially adapted to a certain purpose.
structural pertaining to structure rather than another aspect.
subclinical pertaining to the period of time before appearance of typical symptoms of a disease.
supplement a nutrient that is added to supply that which is lacking in a product or to reinforce it.
synthesize the process of building a product from separated elements.

tissue a collection of similar cells and fibers that form structural material in the body.
toxemia distribution through the body of poisonous products of bacteria that grow in a focal site.
toxic poisonous.

urea constituent of urine and the final product of protein metabolism in the body.

viscera internal organs, especially the abdominal.

Diet therapy

adequate sufficient for specific requirements.
allergen any substance causing allergic symptoms.
amino acids the "building blocks" of protein.
anorexia loss of appetite.

bland diet meal plan in which all food that causes chemical, mechanical, or thermal irritation is avoided.
bulk large volume.

cardiovascular pertaining to the heart and blood vessels.
cirrhosis a chronic, progressive disease of the liver, essentially inflammatory.
constituents component parts.
corpuscle a blood cell
cystic duct the duct of the gallbladder that unites with the hepatic duct from the liver to form the common bile duct.

defecation evacuation of the bowels.
desensitize to lessen or eradicate sensitivity to a product.
diverticulitis inflammation of one or more diverticula in the colon, causing stagnation of feces in the small distended sacs.

edema a condition in which excess fluids form within the body.
elimination excretion of waste products from the body by the skin, kidneys, and intestines.
erythrocytes red blood cells.
extracellular outside of and surrounding the cell.

fibrinogen a soluble protein in the blood plasma that is essential in the clotting of blood.

gastrointestinal pertaining to the stomach and intestines.
glomerulus a tuft of capillary loops projecting into the inside of the renal capsule.

hemicellulose a substance that increases bulk in the stool and promotes regular evacuation from the bowels.
hepatic pertaining to the liver.
hepatic duct the canal that receives bile from the liver and unites with the cystic duct to form the common bile duct.
hypersensitivity excessively sensitive.
hyperthyroidism a condition caused by excessive secretion of the thyroid glands.
hypoglycemia pertaining to deficiency of sugar in the blood.

inflammation a response to an injury to the tissues.
inhibit to hold in check or restrain.
inorganic composed of inanimate matter.
insulin a protein hormone of the internal secretion of the islands of Langerhans in the pancreas that controls the level of blood sugar.
intracellular within or into a vein.

jaundice yellowness of the skin caused by bile pigments in the blood.

kilogram (kg) 1000 grams.

lesion an injury or wound.
leukocytes white blood corpuscles.
liter (L) 1.056 quarts.

macrocytes red blood corpuscles larger than normal.
microorganism a minute living organism not perceptible to the naked eye.
milliliter (ml) $\frac{1}{1000}$ of a liter.
millimeter $\frac{1}{1000}$ of a meter.
misnomer an incorrect designation.
monosaccharide a sugar that cannot be separated into smaller units.
mucous membrane the membrane lining passages and cavities that secrete mucus.

nephrosis a condition in which there are degenerative changes in the kidneys without the occurrence of inflammation.
neurological pertaining to the study of nervous diseases.
neurotic an emotionally unstable individual.

obesity an abnormal condition caused by excessive deposits of fat in the body.
occlusion the closing of a passage.
osmotic pressure pressure causing the passage of solutions of different concentrations through a membrane.

parenterally either within or into a vein or subcutaneously (beneath the skin).
pericarditis inflammation of the membranous sac enclosing the heart.
peritoneal cavity the region containing all the abdominal organs except the kidneys.
plasma the liquid part of the blood in which the corpuscles and platelets float.
platelet a small circular or oval disk that is found in the blood and takes part in the coagulation of the blood.
polyuria excessive secretion and discharge of urine.
prothrombin substance present in the blood plasma and essential for the clotting of blood.
psychotherapy any mental method of treating disease, especially nervous disorders.

regeneration repair, regrowth, or restoration of a part.
residue that which remains after roughage is removed.
retina the sensitive membrane of the eye that receives the image formed by the lens and that is connected with the brain by the optic nerve.
roughage the indigestible fibers of fruits and vegetables.

satiety satisfaction.
spleen an organ that disintegrates the red blood cell when its usefulness is ended and sets free the iron contained in the cell.

therapeutic nutrition that branch of nutrition concerned with the treatment of disease.
thermal pertaining to heat.

uremia the retention in the blood or urinary constituents caused by failure of the kidneys to excrete them.
ureter one of the two tubes carrying urine from the kidneys to the bladder.

varices enlarged, twisted veins.
vascular pertaining to or composed of blood vessels.

Index